PSYCHOSOCIAL RESEARCH ON PEDIATRIC HOSPITALIZATION AND HEALTH CARE

PSYCHOSOCIAL RESEARCH ON PEDIATRIC HOSPITALIZATION AND HEALTH CARE

A REVIEW OF THE LITERATURE

By

RICHARD H. THOMPSON, Ph.D.

Director of the Child Life and Family Education Department
Wyler Children's Hospital, University of Chicago
Chicago, Illinois

CHARLES C THOMAS • PUBLISHER
Springfield • Illinois • U.S.A.

Published and Distributed Throughout the World by

CHARLES C THOMAS • PUBLISHER
2600 South First Street
Springfield, Illinois 62717

ISBN 0-398-05070-8

Library of Congress Catalog Card Number: 84-16464

With THOMAS BOOKS *careful attention is given to all details of manufacturing and design. It is the Publisher's desire to present books that are satisfactory as to their physical qualities and artistic possibilities and appropriate for their particular use.* THOMAS BOOKS *will be true to those laws of quality that assure a good name and good will.*

Printed in the United States of America
SC-R-3

Library of Congress Cataloging in Publication Data

Thompson, Richard H.
Psychosocial research on pediatric hospitalization and health care.

Bibliography: p.
Includes index.
1. Children—Hospital care—Psychological aspects.
I. Title. [DNLM: 1. Child, Hospitalized—psychology.
WS 105.5.H7 T475p]
RJ242.T49 1985 362.1'1'088054 84-16464
ISBN 0-398-05070-8

To Lynn

ACKNOWLEDGEMENT

Completion of this review was made possible, in part, by a grant from the Association for the Care of Children's Health, 3615 Wisconsin Avenue, N.W., Washington, D.C. 20016.

CONTENTS

PSYCHOSOCIAL RESEARCH ON PEDIATRIC HOSPITALIZATION AND HEALTH CARE

Chapter 1

FOCUS OF THE LITERATURE REVIEW

The past two decades have witnessed a tremendous increase in the literature concerning the psychosocial aspects of childhood hospitalization and health care, the magnitude of which may be illustrated by comparing the volume of recent publications to that existing prior to 1965. In their classic review of the literature on the hospitalization and illness of children, Vernon, Foley, Sipowicz, and Schulman (1965) cite some 208 articles including theoretical and descriptive pieces, case studies, and reports of more formally structured research projects. A relatively small percentage of these articles fall into the latter category, providing data collected through formal research procedures. However, since 1965 alone more than 300 reports of formal research pertaining to childhood hospitalization and health care have been published. It is this body of research literature, published in 1965 or later, that will be the subject of the present review.

SELECTION OF THE RESEARCH TO BE REVIEWED

An effort has been made to conduct a comprehensive search of the psychosocial research literature on the hospitalization of children and adolescents. The research literature concerning children in other health care settings (i.e., outpatient medical or dental clinics) has also been examined to identify studies relevant to a given topic, such as children's reactions to specific medical procedures or psychological preparation for health care encounters. However, the nonhospital-based research is less exhaustively reviewed in the present volume than is that concerning childhood or adolescent hospitalization.

The studies to be discussed in the following chapters (all of which have been published in journals or books, or are dissertations available through University Microfilms International) were located by several methods. Computerized searches of the Psychological Abstracts, Dissertation Abstracts, Educational Resources Information Center (ERIC), and Medline data bases were conducted. On the basis of a preliminary review of the literature, topic areas considered to be of greatest importance were selected to focus the computerized search process. These topics included: 1) children's concepts of hospitalization, illness, and health care, 2) children's psychological responses to hospitalization and health care, 3) responses of other family members to a child's hospitalization, 4) non-medical aspects of children's hospital experience, such as their everyday activities and their interactions with parents and staff, and 5) interventions designed to minimize children's psychological upset, including parental presence, preparation, and play experiences.

In addition to the computerized literature searches, other published bibliographic references were examined, including *The Hospitalized Child* by Akins, Mace, and Akins (1981). Citations of potential relevance were located and their content assessed. Finally, as research articles were identified, the reference list of each was examined for further related studies.

Research has been selected for inclusion in the present review if, in addition to relevant subject matter, it is characterized by systematic attempts to define a question of interest, to collect data pertinent to the question in a methodical manner, to analyze the data (not necessarily using statistical methods), and to discuss their implications. Case studies have been typically excluded from consideration. However, an exception has been made if a particular study includes a minimum of four subjects and provides information on a topic of considerable interest to health care professionals for which little other research exists. Examples of such topic areas include children's reactions to isolation or intensive care units.

Studies otherwise appropriate for inclusion in the review, yet providing information specific to a single illness or condition, are also typically omitted. A wealth of literature exists, for example, on children's reactions to various forms of chronic illness or the accompanying treatment, but consideration of this literature would extend the present review beyond the manageable. Research pertaining to children with specific illnesses is, however, included when its focus is not solely on the illness, but rather provides information on conditions applicable to other categories of patients as well. Thus included are studies on topics such as the preparation of cardiac patients for surgery or the effects of rooming-in by parents of cancer patients.

THE RESEARCH IDENTIFIED

Using the criteria described above, a total of 306 research reports have been identified. For purposes of this and other summary figures provided in the text, results of research reported in more than one source (e.g., a dissertation that is subsequently published in article form) are counted as a single study. Nevertheless, all citations are given in the text to provide the reader with greater flexibility in locating the material. Separate articles reporting on different aspects of a research project, though drawn from the same sample, are counted individually.

The 306 identified reports have been categorized on the basis of their research design. Seventy-seven of the studies are *experimental*, incorporating deliberate assignment of subjects to varying treatment conditions. Forty-three use *nonexperimental* designs, wherein differences among preexisting groups of subjects are compared. The groups compared typically consist of subjects who have or have not, of their own accord, participated in intervention programs such as preadmission visits to the hospital or parent rooming-in. Another 72 studies are *correlational* in nature, examining relationships among varying levels of child and/or parent characteristics. Among the relationships commonly investigated is that between parent and child anxiety or the association between child variables (e.g., age, measures of personality characteristics, length of hospitalization, etc.) and indices of children's psychological upset. Seventy studies are *descriptive*, documenting the frequency and distribution of subjects' activities, behaviors, and contacts with others, without using the data gathered to formally test hypotheses. Also in this group are studies exploring children's conceptions of health care and illness. A final group of 44 studies are *surveys*, which either assess patient, parent, or staff attitudes and knowledge about designated topics, or determine the types of services offered by health care institutions.

The identified studies were further categorized according to the major topic investigated by each. Although this process was somewhat subjective (since many projects address more than a single topic) and was undertaken primarily to organize the presentation of material, the results are indicative of the distribution of researchers' efforts in recent years. For example, the most frequently addressed subject is the preparation of children and parents for hospitalization and health care procedures. Sixty-five studies, or more than 20 percent of all research identified, are devoted to this topic. Research investigating children's emotional reactions to health care (either documenting the nature or occurrence of children's responses, or examining the relationship between these responses and other variables) is also common, with 53 studies addressing this topic. Another 28 studies focus on subjects' responses to specific medical procedures or environments. Twenty-five studies examine either the effects of children's separation from parents during hospitalization or the value of rooming-in programs designed to minimize the amount of separation experienced.

A surprisingly small amount of research on adolescent hospitalization was discovered. Only 27 studies specifically consider this age group. Of these studies, more than two-thirds (N = 19) are surveys concerning adolescent health care. Direct observation of adolescents is rare; experimental research is nonexistent.

The effects of hospitalization on nonhospitalized family members is also addressed in the research literature. The reactions and activities of parents during hospitalization are examined in 27 studies, with most of these limiting their investigation to *mothers'* responses. Another seven articles consider the impact of a child's hospitalization on nonhospitalized siblings.

Twenty-seven studies concern play in the hospital or other medical settings, though eight of these are surveys of the prevalence and characteristics of hospital-based play programs, rather than direct investigations of children's play behavior. Twenty-seven articles examine children's concepts of health care and illness. The remaining twenty studies document children's activities when in the hospital or their interactions with health care personnel.

FORMAT OF THE LITERATURE REVIEW

Within the body of the review that follows, a description of all major studies is provided, which includes sample characteristics (sample size, ages, and conditions of subjects), a brief presentation of methodology and assessment procedures, and a summary of principal findings. This information is intended to assist the reader in making a critical evaluation of the research design, the merits of the study, and the applicability of the findings to children and families in other settings. Though this primary description is given only in the chapter most closely related to the content of the study, research pertaining to more than one topic is cited in all appropriate chapters. In such cases, reference to the primary description will be made, if necessary for fuller understanding of the secondary citation. An overview of the content of the remaining chapters of the book is given below.

Chapter 2: Children's Responses to Hospitalization and Health Care

A construct central to much of the literature to be reviewed in this text is the *psychological upset* of children subjected to medical care. Methods used to assess this construct in the *immediate* or *post-hospital* periods and the frequency of their application in the research literature are discussed in Chapter 2. Also considered are data on the occurrence and incidence of psychological upset among children, both while undergoing health care and in the period following discharge from the hospital. This chapter concludes with a review of the research findings on a range of factors potentially associated with the upset experienced by children in health care settings.

Chapter 3: Children's Conceptions of Hospitalization, Illness, and Health Care

Studies documenting children's explanations and beliefs about the causes of hospitalization and illness are presented. Four areas in particular are examined. First, it has been suggested that children, especially young children, view illness and injury as being a product of their own actions. Therefore, hospitalization and medical care may be interpreted as punishment for their misdeeds. Research assessing the prevalence of this belief is considered. Second, studies investigating possible age-related changes in children's causal explanations of illness and health are reviewed. Relationships between the development of health care explanations and other domains of cognitive development are also examined. Next, the potential impact of hospitalization or illness on the development and sophistication of children's health care concepts is considered. The chapter concludes with an examination of research on children's conceptions of hospital-related phenomena such as medical instruments, procedures, and personnel.

Chapter 4: Research on Specific Procedures and Environments

In addition to investigating the effects of hospitalization as a whole on children's responses, researchers have also isolated more limited aspects of the medical experience for consideration. Typically, these isolated components consist of medical procedures or hospital settings that represent a particularly intense emotional threat to the children receiving care. In Chapter 4 research is reviewed concerning children's responses to specific procedures and medical techniques, such as injections, the use of restraints, rectal temperatures, binocular bandaging, cardiac catheterization, and anesthesia induction. Also reviewed is research concerning reactions to medical environments, including isolation and intensive care units, recovery rooms, and emergency rooms.

Chapter 5: Separation and Rooming-in

Despite the liberalization of visiting policies of hospitals in recent years, separation from parents and other family members remains a common part of many children's hospital experience. Studies examining the effects of separation from parents on children's immediate and posthospital reactions are examined in Chapter 5. Data are also presented on the effectiveness of interventions designed to reduce children's upset associated with separation, such as parental visitation, rooming-in, and presence during procedures, and the use of parent voice recordings.

Chapter 6: Parent and Sibling Responses to Hospitalization

The nature of parents' responses to the hospitalization of a child, and the factors influencing those reactions are discussed in Chapter 6. Evidence suggesting a relationship between the anxiety level of parents and their children during health care episodes is presented. Also examined are the results of interventions designed to reduce parents' anxiety during hospitalization.

Until recently, the response of children to a sibling's hospitalization was virtually unexamined. Though literature pertaining to sibling responses (also presented in Chapter 6) is still limited, it appears to be increasing. Data currently exist on the adjustments children make when a sibling is hospitalized, on their participation in the child's hospitalization, and on the possible effects of visiting a newborn sibling in the hospital.

Chapter 7: Adolescent Hospitalization, Health Care, and Illness

As noted earlier, the literature on adolescent hospitalization and illness is limited and primarily consists of surveys either of hospital services for adolescents or of the attitudes of patients, parents, and staff members toward adolescent care. Gaps in this area of the literature are readily apparent. For example, despite the frequency with which psychological preparation has been examined, no study has been solely devoted to the preparation of adolescents for health care experiences. Similarly, only a single study considers adolescent health care concepts. The data presented in Chapter 7 include documentation of the conditions for which adolescents are hospitalized, adolescent preferences for care and information providers during hospitalization, parent responses to adolescent hospitalization, and information on the necessity for and functioning of separate adolescent hospital units. Finally, surveys of staff members' knowledge and attitudes about adolescents are reviewed.

Chapter 8: The Hospital Milieu

Though considerable research effort has been devoted to children's psychological reactions to hospitalization, less documentation of children's typical activities during the course of a hospital stay exists. In Chapter 8, research detailing this area of children's behavior is presented. Included is information on children's television viewing habits, the amount and type of contact they have with others in the hospital setting, the nature of their communications with adults, and their sleep patterns.

Chapter 9: Play and the Hospitalized Child

The paradoxical relationship between children's play behavior and their stress responses in health care settings is examined in Chapter 9. A portion of the research findings considered in this chapter suggest that play behavior is disrupted when children are confronted by the stressful circumstances of hospitalization. However, another group of studies indicate that spontaneous or structured play may be useful in reducing children's psychological upset and in modifying specific behaviors manifested in medical environments. In addition to presenting data on both of these relationships, the chapter briefly considers the current status of play programs in hospitals.

Chapter 10: Psychological Preparation for Hospitalization and Health Care Procedures

As mentioned earlier, the most frequently examined topic in the literature on childhood hospitalization and health care (accounting for more than one-fifth of all identified research projects) is the psychological preparation of subjects for impending events. Methods used to prepare children and parents for health care experiences vary considerably and include the rudimentary, didactic presentation of information, the elaboration of this technique to include information about sensory experiences, the incorporation of play activities in the preparation process, the use of filmed modeling, instruction in relaxation techniques, and the providing of emotional support, as well as differing combinations of these elements. Experimental research on each of these methods is reviewed in Chapter 10. Also reviewed in this chapter are nonexperimental studies that examine the effectiveness of preadmission programs and compare the characteristics of families who chose to participate in these sessions with those who do not. The chapter concludes with a consideration of survey data on the status of preparation practices in acute care hospitals.

Chapter 11: Summary and Conclusions

The literature review concludes with a reconsideration of the impact of hospitalization and illness on children. In particular, evidence pertaining to the occurrence of psychological upset, including the likely determinants of children's emotional distress, is presented. The focus then shifts to consideration of the quality of the research contained in the review. Specific criticisms of the research literature, originally raised by Vernon, Foley, Sipowicz, and Schulman (1965), are examined, and suggestions are made for broadening the scope of future investigations.

Chapter 2

CHILDREN'S RESPONSES TO HOSPITALIZATION AND HEALTH CARE

A primary function of the research on childhood hospitalization and health care has been the documentation of children's upset during the period of treatment and following discharge from the hospital. Indices of emotional distress, whether behavioral, subjective, or physiological, have been used in experimental and nonexperimental studies to assess the effectiveness of interventions, and in correlational research to examine the relative vulnerabilities of children differing in sociodemographic, psychological, and personal or experiential characteristics. The principal task of the present chapter is to briefly review the research on factors potentially related to children's responses in health care settings. However, before proceeding to this review, consideration must be given to the methods and instruments used by researchers for assessing children's emotional responses to health care.

ASSESSING PSYCHOLOGICAL UPSET

Of the 306 research studies reviewed in this volume, 161 include an assessment of children's emotional responses to health care, be it hospitalization, outpatient medical care, or dental treatment. The *immediate responses* of children (defined as those detectable during the period of health care treatment) have been examined in 143 studies. Deferred or continuing reactions, measurable in the period following discharge from the hospital, have been documented in 66 studies. The timing of assessment of the *posthospital responses* has varied from two days postdischarge to more than a decade later, with the latter, long-term data coming from a limited number of retrospective studies. Most posthospital assessments have been completed within a month of the child's discharge. Forty-eight of the studies assessing children's responses to hospitalization have considered both immediate and posthospital reactions.

Responses manifested by children during or subsequent to health care treatment, and which purport to indicate disturbance or deterioration in their emotional status, will be referred to by the general label of *psychological upset,* a term used by Vernon, et al. (1965). Psychological upset (or the other constructs subsumed by this term, such as emotional distress, anxiety, fear, etc.) has been described as a multidimensional phenomenon, which includes behavioral, subjective, and physiological components. Assessment strategies used in the research reviewed in this volume reflect this multidimensionality. Behavioral indices of psychological upset have been most frequently used in both the immediate and posthospital periods, followed in each case by subjective reports and physiological indicators of upset.

Assessment of Immediate Responses

Of the 143 studies examining children's immediate responses to health care, 113 (79.0%) have included a behavioral assessment. In most cases, direct observations of children have been made by trained observers, though indirect measures of behavior have also been used, including summary parent reports (used in 19 studies) or a recording of the amount of time required to perform procedures (an index of children's cooperative behavior; see Sawtell, Simon, & Simeonsson, 1974).

Two principal approaches to the direct behavioral observation of children appear in the literature: 1) documentation of the *occurrence* and/or *frequency* of designated behaviors (used in 67 studies), and 2) the *rating* of some dimension of children's behavior under specified circumstances using a Likert-type scale (51 studies). Systems of the first type, used for documenting the presence or frequency of behaviors, have typically been developed for the individual research project, though two instruments developed by Melamed and colleagues have received multiple use. These are the Observer Rating Scale of Anxiety (Melamed & Siegel, 1975), a measure used to assess the occurrence of 29 behaviors believed to be indicative of the presence or absence of children's anxiety in medical settings, and a similar instrument for use in dental settings, the Behavioral Profile Rating Scale (Melamed, Weinstein, Hawes, & Katin-Borland, 1975).

Instruments commonly used to provide a rating of the intensity of children's behavioral responses (the second approach to direct behavioral observation) include the Global Mood Scale (originally developed by Foley, 1962; see Vernon, Foley, & Schulman, 1967), the Manifest Upset and Cooperation Scales (Wolfer & Visintainer, 1975), and a scale developed by Frankl, Shiere, and Fogels (1962) for use in dental settings.

Subjective or *self-report* measures (which record the affected person's perceptions of events and circumstances, and his or her reaction to them) have been used in 49 (34.3%) of the studies assessing children's immediate responses to health care. Common sources of data in this category include projective assessments (12 studies), children's drawings (6 studies), and direct reports of children's fears, obtained through instruments such as the Hospital Fears Rating Scale (Melamed & Siegel, 1975; used in 9 studies) and the Children's Manifest Anxiety Scale (Castaneda, McCandless, & Palermo, 1956; used in 8 studies).

Thirty-nine studies, or slightly more than one-fourth of those assessing children's immediate reactions, have used at least one measure of *physiological response.* This category includes the direct recording of physiological indices such as vital signs, as well as measures of physical recovery that are presumably affected by one's emotional state. The most frequently used physiological measure is children's heart rate, used in 21 studies. Other commonly used indices in this category include the Palmar Sweat Index (Dabbs, Johnson, & Leventhal, 1968; Johnson & Dabbs, 1967; Thomson & Sutarman, 1953; used in 10 studies), temperature (used in 9 studies), time to first voiding following surgery, ease or volume of postoperative fluid intake, and blood pressure (8 studies each), need for postoperative medications, and incidence of postoperative vomiting (6 studies), respiration rate (5 studies), and urinary cortisol levels and length of hospitalization (each used in 3 studies).

Assessment of Posthospital Responses

As noted above, fewer studies have considered children's posthospital responses (N = 66) than children's immediate reactions to medical or dental treatment (N = 143). Nevertheless, the relative frequency with which the types of measures have been used to assess posthospital psychological upset is comparable to that of assessment of immediate responses, with behavioral measures used in 56 studies (84.8% of all studies examining the posthospital period), subjective measures used in 14 studies (21.2%), and physiological indices used in 11 studies (16.7%).

Methods of collecting data in the posthospital period, however, shift from evaluation through *direct* assessment of behavioral or physiological indices of upset to substantial reliance on parent report. For example, only six of the 56 studies assessing children's behavior following hospitalization have used direct observation. In contrast, 52 studies have included parent-report behavioral measures, with twenty-four of these using the Posthospital Behavior Questionnaire (see Vernon, Schulman, and Foley, 1966) or a modification of this instrument.

The majority of the posthospital physiological data presented in the research is also a product of parent report. For example, in five studies parents were asked to estimate the time required for physical recovery of their child following surgery. Other forms of physiological information obtained from parents include the incidence of fever in children following discharge, whether it was necessary to call a physician about the child's condition (each used in 3 studies), and the occurrence of posthospital vomiting (used twice).

Direct posthospital physiological assessment has been made in only four cases. Barnes, et al. (1972) measured the posthospital urinary cortisol levels of children undergoing open-heart surgery. Melamed and Siegel (1975), Melamed, Meyer, Gee, and Soule (1976), and Zabin and Melamed (1980) each obtained Palmar Sweat Prints from surgical patients at a medical check-up approximately one month after discharge from the hospital.

The relative frequency with which individual types of *subjective* measures have been used following discharge from the hospital is similar to that for assessment during the period of treatment. The Children's Manifest Anxiety Scale was used in six studies, and projective techniques in another five. The Hospital Fears Rating Scale and children's drawings have each been used three times.

Interrelationships of Psychological Upset Measures

The availability of multiple measures to assess each of three components of psychological upset (behavioral, subjective, and physiological) in two separate periods (during hospitalization or treatment, and following discharge) suggests the possibility, if not the necessity, of exploring relationships within and among the domains of upset over time. Although a majority of the studies reviewed employed more than a single measure of psychological upset, information on relationships among measures is sparse—a possible indication that interrelationships have been examined, but found to be nonsignificant.

Of the few studies examining relationships among the identified components of upset, only a limited number of significant associations have been reported. Melamed, Yurcheson, Fleece, Hutcherson, and Hawes (1978) note some significant relationships between subjective and behavioral indices of upset in a dental setting. Significant correlations between behavioral and subjective indices of pain in hospitalized surgical patients have also been reported (Abu-Saad and Holzemer, 1981). Thompson (1983) found an association between children's behavioral responses while receiving an injection in an outpatient setting and a physiological measure, subjects' pulse rates following the procedure. The interrelationships among three types of measures—children's self report of their distress during preparation for hospitalization, observers' ratings of children's behavior, and two parent-report measures—were examined Tarnow and Gutstein (1983). The only significant correlations obtained were between the two parent-report assessments.

Other researchers have dismissed consideration of the relationships across domains of psychological upset, noting that the multidimensionality of the construct implies that upset will manifest itself differently in different subjects and that a change in one domain may occur without a corresponding alteration in another.

This does not, however, explain the absence of examination of relationships among instruments within a given domain.

Also ignored has been consideration of the relationship between children's immediate and posthospital responses. Though 48 studies have collected data on children's reactions during both of these periods, no direct investigation of the association between inhospital and posthospital upset was found. Examination of this relationship is necessary to gain a more comprehensive understanding of the effects of hospitalization on children. For example, it has been suggested that certain behavioral responses exhibited by children in the hospital, such as aggression or crying, should be viewed as normal and adaptive, rather than as an indication of more serious disturbance. Such behavior may, in fact, be associated with better long-term adjustment to hospitalization, than are passive or depressive inhospital behaviors. However, in the absence of research examining the relationship between inhospital and posthospital reactions, this matter remains speculative.

THE IMMEDIATE RESPONSES OF CHILDREN TO HEALTH CARE

Having briefly reviewed the types of measures found in the literature to assess children's immediate and longer-term responses to hospitalization and health care, a more basic question concerning the nature of children's reactions may be addressed. In particular, does the available research indicate that hospitalization, outpatient medical care, or dental treatment results in psychological upset among children during the period of treatment. Early studies, such as that of Prugh, Staub, Sands, Kirschbaum, and Lenihan (1953), conclude that inhospital upset is, indeed, prevalent. Prugh, et al. found that "significant difficulties" in adaptation to the hospital setting were apparent in 92 percent of the children in the control group, who had been cared for under the "traditional practices" of the era, and 68 percent of the experimental group, who had received psychological preparation, frequent parental visitation, and play opportunities.

Among the more recent research examining the inhospital

responses of children is that of O'Donnell (1976), who compared pediatric patients' scores on the Missouri Children's Picture Series administered on the day of admission and again two days later while the subjects were still hospitalized. No significant difference in the overall scores of children was detected between the two administrations. However, test profiles of eleven of the thirty subjects considered (5 to 11 years of age, most of whom were hospitalized for surgical procedures) changed in a negative direction over the course of the study. Scores of another fourteen children remained unchanged, with the remaining five showing improvement.

Two other types of research conducted since 1965 are relevant to the question of children's immediate responses to health care: 1) research comparing the responses of hospitalized and nonhospitalized children, and 2) that evaluating the effectiveness of interventions in reducing children's upset. Few studies of the first type exist. Of these, most compare the subjective (rather than behavioral or physiological) responses of hospitalized and nonhospitalized subjects. Only limited evidence of inhospital upset is apparent from this group of studies.

Astin (1977), for example, compared the self-reported fears of 25 hospitalized children (10 to 12 years of age) and an equal number of nonhospitalized subjects. Fears were identified through completion of a checklist of 71 items representing a total of 11 categories. The groups examined did not differ on total numbers of fears reported, though slight differences were evident in the order of most frequently cited fear categories, with hospitalized children more often expressing fears about home than their nonhospitalized counterparts. The fears of hospitalized children were also rated as more intense than those of subjects in the school group.

The impromptu drawings of 16 leukemia patients, 13 hospitalized children, and 15 nonhospitalized elementary school children were compared by Furth (1973). Though characteristics of the drawings of leukemic children frequently differed from those of the other subjects, few differences between the hospitalized and nonhospitalized subjects were found.

Two additional studies, based on the same sample of children, provide data tangentially related to children's immediate responses.

The sample consisted of 114 nonhospitalized school children and 100 hospitalized subjects, nine to twelve years of age, who were asked to describe pain (Savedra, et al., 1981) and to identify their coping strategies for minimizing pain (Tesler, et al., 1981). Savedra, Tesler, Ward, Wegner, and Gibbons (1981) found that the hospitalized group used a greater modal number of words to describe pain and that, "words more frequently selected by hospitalized children relate to tension, fear, and overall pain intensity" (p. 376).

Tesler, Wegner, Savedra, Gibbons, and Ward (1981) report that nonhospitalized children identified more strategies for pain reduction than did hospitalized subjects. When only the first response given by each child was examined, other group differences emerged. The predominant response of hospitalized children was that medicine, pills, or shots were useful as a means of minimizing pain. Moreover, a greater number of hospitalized than nonhospitalized children said that the presence of their mother or other family members made them feel better.

A more substantive comparison of the subjective responses of hospitalized and nonhospitalized children is provided by Irwin and Kovacs (1979). Thirty children, 6 to 12 years of age, admitted to the hospital for orthopedic surgery, were contrasted with another group of thirty subjects who had never been hospitalized. Projective techniques were used to assess hospitalized children's responses prior to, and three to five days after, surgery. Nonhospitalized subjects were assessed twice with a comparable intervening period. Few initial differences were noted between groups. However, in the days following surgery, hospitalized patients were found to have greater castration concerns, lower self-esteem, and higher dependency than the nonhospitalized group. In a similar study, Sides (1977) found hospitalized children to score higher on the somatization scale of the Missouri Children's Picture Series (Sines, Pauker, & Sines, 1974) than nonhospitalized subjects.

The possible effects of short-term hospitalization for tonsillectomy surgery on the cognitive development of children were examined by Rieveschl (1979). Forty subjects (five to nine years of age, half of whom were hospitalized) were assessed for spatial and affective perspective-taking skills at three times, corresponding to the prehospital, inhospital, and posthospital periods for the surgical group. Comparison of scores for the middle (inhospital) period indicated a greater regression and disorganization of spatial perspective-taking skills for the hospitalized children. In the posthospital period, the affective perspective-taking skills of this group were similarly affected.

Only a single study has compared the spontaneous behavior of hospitalized and nonhospitalized preschool children during free play. In this case, Vredevoe, Kim, Dambacher, and Call (1969) found few significant differences in the play behavior exhibited by surgical patients, medical patients, and nonhospitalized nursery school children.

The absence of more consistent, convincing evidence of immediate psychological upset among hospitalized children in studies comparing their responses with nonhospitalized subjects may, in part, be due to the inability or the failure of researchers to examine the groups under comparable circumstances. For example, the most dramatic immediate responses of hospitalized children are observed during stressful procedures such as injections or anesthesia induction—situations for which there are no naturally occurring, analogous events during which the reactions of nonhospitalized children may be observed. Nevertheless, conditions common to both populations exist, such as social interactions with parents and peers and brief separations from parents. Behaviors of hospitalized and nonhospitalized children in these situations could be compared for evidence of upset among the hospitalized group.

Research evaluating the effectiveness of interventions in health care settings may also be examined for indications of immediate upset. In this research, indices of psychological upset are typically reported for children under varying treatment conditions. A finding of significant group differences attributable to experimental intervention suggests that a degree of psychological upset was indeed present among the population receiving health care, yet was conducive to modification. Failure to find group differences may indicate that the intervention was ineffective, the upset of children was intractable, or, perhaps, that the degree of immediate upset experienced by children was negligible.

A total of 79 studies were found to compare the immediate responses of children exposed to differing treatment conditions, using either experimental or nonexperimental designs. In 65 of these cases, significant group differences were found, thus suggesting that psychological upset was frequently experienced by subjects during the period of health care, yet was modifiable through intervention. The forms of intervention resulting in group differences included psychological preparation (49 studies), parental presence (9 studies), and play (6 studies). No group differences were found in the remaining 14 studies, 12 of which involved preparation.

Alteration in Immediate Behavior as a Coping Response

Information presented in the preceding section (especially that derived from intervention studies) suggests that children frequently experience upset when in health care settings, with this upset often manifesting itself in alterations in behavior. However, changes in children's behavior during health care, even increases in emotionally charged behaviors such as crying or resistance to treatment, are not universally interpreted as valid indices of psychological upset. Depending on the theoretical orientation of the individual researcher, specific behaviors exhibited by children have been given markedly different interpretations.

For example, researchers have repeatedly included the behavior of crying in instruments designed to assess the behavioral component of children's psychological upset (Foley, 1962; Melamed & Siegel, 1975; Wolfer & Visintainer, 1975). Yet others, such as Shaw and Routh (1982) indicate that one must look at the context in which crying occurs, before considering it as evidence of emotional distress. The latter researchers found a greater incidence of crying among children given an injection in the presence of their parents than among those separated from parents during the procedure. Nevertheless, the crying was viewed positively, as an indication of greater security felt by children when their parents were present—a security that allowed them to express, rather than suppress, their feelings.

Other researchers such as Rose (1972) avoid interpretation of behavioral alterations exhibited by children as being either positive or negative. Instead, children's immediate responses to health care are considered to be normal, adaptive efforts to cope with a new and potentially threatening environment. Thus, the function of research adopting this perspective has been to document children's behavioral responses, not for purposes of evaluating the success of children's adaptation, but to gain insight to the adaptation process (e.g., see Taylor, 1983, concerning the postoperative responses of toddlers and preschoolers).

Since changes in children's behavior during hospitalization are interpreted as evidence of their attempts to cope with an unfamiliar situation, Rose (1972) contends that these alterations will be temporary, disappearing soon after children return home. To examine this contention, the behavior of fourteen children, between eighteen months and seven years of age, was observed prior to, during, and after hospitalization for a surgical procedure or cardiac catheterization. Of the 32 behaviors observed, fifteen changed significantly during hospitalization. For example, children spent more time looking and tentatively exploring when in the hospital than when at home. Among other inhospital behavioral changes noted were decreases in pleasure, speech, and attempts to control; increases in sadness, crying, emotionality, and affection were also noted during hospitalization. As predicted, these behaviors reverted toward the prehospital levels following discharge from the hospital.

Other studies have documented the coping behaviors displayed by children during hospitalization (Savedra & Tesler, 1981; Youssef, 1981) or an outpatient examination (Hyson, 1983; Bernheimer, 1981). Savedra and Tesler (1981) observed 33 children, six to twelve years of age, hospitalized for elective surgical procedures of differing severity, recording their "level of involvement" in the coping process during designated stress points. Children were categorized as exhibiting *inactive coping* (silence and nonparticipation), *precoping* or *orienting behavior* (familiarization with the environment), or *active coping* (e.g., attempting to control the situation, cooperating, resisting, etc.). Precoping behaviors were predominant during the presurgical period. Following surgery, the active coping behavior of "attempts to control" was most frequently observed.

Youssef (1981) documented the behavior of ten children, seven through eleven years of age, admitted to the hospital for cardiac catheterization. *Self-control behaviors* (orienting, seeking support from self or others, and expressing feelings) and *loss of control behaviors* were recorded at four periods: at admission, during an echocardiogram, during catheterization, and upon discharge. Overall, children were found to orient and seek support more than they used avoidance or expressed themselves. Orienting behaviors were predominant during admission, echocardiogram, and catheterization, being less evident at discharge. Self-supporting behaviors were common during the echocardiogram, while during catheterization children more frequently sought support from those around them. Avoidance and loss of control behaviors appeared with greater frequency during catheterization than other periods; expressions of feelings were rarely noted.

Among the studies examining coping behaviors in the outpatient setting, Hyson (1983) examined behavior in three categories: *information-seeking* (looking, asking questions), *comfort-seeking* (contact with mother, familiar objects or oneself), and *autonomy* (attempts to control, structure, protest or resist). Forty-eight children, ranging in age from six to sixty months, were observed before, during, and after examination by a physician. Information-seeking behaviors were more common among children of all ages in the period prior to examination. However, beginning with the period of the doctor's examination, autonomy behaviors increased, surpassing information-seeking in frequency. Autonomy behaviors were further subdivided into *instrumental behaviors* (those through which children attempt to directly alter the situation using methods that may or may not be socially desirable) or *expressive behaviors* (crying, fussing, etc.). Instrumental behaviors were more common in the pre-examination period, while expressive behaviors were predominant during the examination. Relationships between autonomy behaviors and age were also noted, with instrumental behaviors increasing with age and expressive behaviors declining. Bernheimer (1981), who also observed the coping behaviors of children undergoing outpatient physical examination, described their behavior as being generally "compliant, nonverbal, and passively apprehensive" (p. xii; see Chapter 3).

Unlike the preceding studies, which have examined overall similarities in the coping behaviors exhibited by children when faced with differing health experiences, other investigators have viewed coping styles as a product of the individual child's personality.

That is, when confronted with potentially stressful circumstances, it is believed that the individual will react by invoking characteristic coping or defense mechanisms. Among the commonly identified coping mechanisms are denial, intellectualism, and projection.

In a study conducted by Knight and colleagues (Knight, 1978; Knight, et al., 1977; Knight et al., 1979) the relationship between the type and effectiveness of coping mechanisms and a physiological index of stress, urinary cortisol levels, was examined. Twenty-five children, between seven and eleven years of age, were interviewed two weeks prior to and during hospitalization for minor elective surgery to assess their ego defense style and the effectiveness of their coping mechanisms. In addition, 24-hour urine collections were made at each time. Levels of cortisol, a hormone secreted by the adrenal cortex during periods of stress, were then measured.

Relationships between coping characteristics and children's cortisol production were nonsignificant prior to hospitalization. However, a significant *inverse* relationship between the effectiveness of one's ego defense and cortisol production was noted during the period of hospitalization. Comparisons were also made of the relative effectiveness of individual coping styles. It was found that children using intellectualization, intellectualization with isolation, or a mixed pattern of defenses had significantly lower cortisol production rates than those children using denial, denial with isolation, displacement, or projection.

Summary of Research on the Immediate Responses to Hospitalization

There is considerable evidence in the literature that hospitalization, or other health care experiences, results in at least brief, transitory changes in children's behavior, in their subjective assessments, and possibly in physiological indices frequently associated with upset. For example, data comparing hospitalized and nonhospitalized children, though extremely limited, indicates that hospitalization may alter children's perceptions of fear and pain, produce fluctuations in psychometric indices, and affect specific areas of their cognitive functioning. Intervention studies have further demonstrated that the alterations observed in children's responses during health care are conducive to modification. Changes in children's behavior during hospitalization and health care have been further documented in the coping literature.

Though there may be agreement on the existence of these changes, the significance of alterations in these indices, behavioral indices in particular, is less clear. The primary point of contention is whether increases in specific behaviors, such as aggression or protest, during the period of treatment are merely normal, adaptive responses that will subside following cessation of health care, or rather are indicators of difficulties in adaptation that may presage further difficulties in the posthospital period. The answer may lie in the investigation of relationships between immediate and post-treatment responses. Unfortunately, with the exception of the small sample considered by Rose (1972), no examination of the relationship between immediate and longer term responses has been conducted.

THE POSTHOSPITAL RESPONSES OF CHILDREN

When considering the psychological responses of children following discharge from the hospital, several issues must be addressed, including the period of time such responses may persist and the manner in which the responses are manifested. The most basic of these issues is whether posthospital psychological upset may, in fact, be found in more than a negligible number of children.

Studies conducted prior to 1965 report that an appreciable percentage of children experienced difficulties in adjustment in the posthospital period. For example, in the earlier mentioned study by Prugh, et al. (1953), 58 percent of the control group children and 44 percent of the experimental group were said to exhibit "disturbing reactions of at least a moderate degree" following discharge from the hospital (p. 85). Woodward (1959) reports that 81 percent of the 198 children hospitalized for burns were slightly to severely upset two to five years after hospitalization. This was compared with the incidence of upset observed among children in several nonhospitalized control groups, which ranged from 7 to 13 percent. Jessner, Blom, and Waldfogel (1952) found 20 percent of the tonsillectomy patients studied to be severely upset following hospitalization, with 70 percent mildly upset and 5 percent classified as improved.

Research appearing since 1965 provides differing estimates of the incidence of posthospital upset among children. Vernon, Schulman, and Foley (1966), for example, had parents of 387 children complete the Posthospital Behavior Questionnaire (PHBQ). This 27-item scale asks parents to compare their child's present (posthospital) behavior with their recollections of the child's prehospital demeanor, indicating whether each behavior in question occurred with more, less, or the same frequency as before hospitalization. After comparing children's total scores, as well as their subscores on six factors, with scores indicative of no change in behavior, Vernon, et al. (1966) concluded that "the combination of illness and hospitalization is a psychologically upsetting experience for children in general, resulting in increased separation anxiety, increased sleep anxiety, and increased aggression toward authority" (p. 593). Despite evidence of posthospital upset among the majority of the subjects, Vernon, et al. (1966) found that the behaviors of 25 percent of the children improved in the posthospital period.

Similar results are reported by Sides (1977), who also used the PHBQ to assess the posthospital responses of his sample—190 children, 5 weeks to 16 years of age, hospitalized for various conditions. In this instance, 120 children (63.2%) were found to display behavioral upset lasting for at least two weeks after discharge, 48 children (25.3%) were unchanged, and 22 (11.6%) were improved in the posthospital period.

A retrospective study by Simons, Bradshaw, and Silva (1980) suggests that much of the apparent posthospital upset subsides within the initial months following discharge. Shortly before their children's fifth birthday, 259 mothers were interviewed concerning the children's previous hospital experiences. In particular, parents were asked to rate their children's behavior in areas such as eating, sleeping, toilet training, and independence at six weeks after admission to the hospital. Simons, et al. report that 62 percent of the children exhibited no change, 15 percent showed improvements, 16 percent deteriorations, and 7 percent displayed both improvements and deteriorations in different behavioral domains.

Dearden (1970) interviewed and observed 36 four-year-old children and their mothers before admission to the hospital for tonsillectomy surgery, and again two weeks, two months, and six months after discharge. Four-fifths of the sample showed some increase in disturbance following hospitalization. The availability of longitudinal data enabled Dearden to further classify children's reactions, based upon prehospital adjustment and duration of posthospital responses. Seven children were found to display consistently high levels of upset before and after hospitalization. Ten children were more upset on the final interview than the initial interview. The remaining 19 children showed some transitory disturbance after discharge, but had returned to prehospital levels within six months.

Each of the studies just cited providing data on the incidence of posthospital upset report that a substantial number of children suffer at least temporary disturbance. As was true of the research on immediate reactions to health care, two additional types of studies offer information on children's posthospital responses. First, a limited number of investigations compare the posthospital responses of hospitalized children with analogous measures of nonhospitalized subjects (Sipowicz & Vernon, 1965; Davenport & Werry, 1970; McGillicuddy, 1976; Riffee, 1981). Another 44 intervention studies present data on the modifiability of posthospital upset.

Studies comparing hospitalized children's emotional status after discharge with that of nonhospitalized samples offer conflicting results. Sipowicz and Vernon (1965) examined the behavior of sets of twins, following the hospitalization of one member of each pair. Six days after the hospitalized child's discharge, parents of the 24 sets of twins were sent a modified version of the PHBQ in which they were asked to identify the twin experiencing greater difficulty in each of 28 behavioral categories. A significantly greater number of hospitalized children were rated as the more upset of the pair, despite the observation that home twins were frequently disturbed by their sibling's hospitalization and their own separation from mother (see Chapter 6).

In contrast, Davenport and Werry (1970) found little evidence that hospitalized children are more upset following discharge than nonhospitalized control subjects. Parents of 145 children scheduled for tonsillectomy surgery were interviewed upon the child's admission to the hospital using the PHBQ, modified for use as a pre- and post-test. Two weeks later, the post-test portion was administered to parents via the telephone. Parents of an equal number of nonhospitalized control children, 50 of whom were siblings of the hospitalized subjects, completed the pre- and post-measures, allowing a two-week intervening period. No group differences in upset were found in the posthospital period; slight improvements in the mean behavior scores of subjects were noted regardless of treatment condition.

McGillicuddy (1976), who also used a modified PHBQ, found a significant difference in the overall behavior scores of children whose mothers remained with them during hospitalization and of a control group of nonhospitalized children, with the difference in favor of the hospitalized subjects. However, the slight regression observed in the behavioral ratings of nonhospitalized subjects was attributed to traumatic events experienced by three children in that group over the course of the research period.

The only study using a self-report measure to compare the posthospital responses of hospitalized children with nonhospitalized subjects was conducted by Riffee (1981). A self-esteem inventory, yielding a total score, as well as scores for four subscales (peer/social, home/family, school, and general self), was completed by 26 surgical patients and 25 nonsurgical hospitalized children on admission to the hospital and again thirty days later. Twenty-eight nonhospitalized children completed the measure twice, with a comparable intervening period. Over the course of the study, surgical patients exhibited a greater decline in the total self-esteem score, and in the peer/social and school subscales, than did subjects in the other groups. Nonsurgical patients, however, differed little from nonhospitalized children, recording a greater decline than the latter group only on the school subscale.

Studies contrasting the posthospital responses of subjects exposed to differing treatment conditions may be interpreted as indicating that psychological upset, which may be ameliorated through intervention, is not uncommon in the period following discharge. Of the 45 studies in this category, 24 (or 53.3%) report posthospital group differences, while the remaining 21 do not. Thirty-eight of these intervention studies considered children's posthospital *behavioral* responses (though all but four of these relied exclusively on parent reports). Of these studies, half (N = 19) report significant behavioral differences attributable to the experimental treatment.

Use of *self-report measures* in the posthospital period to assess the effects of experimental interventions has been rare. Coleman (1975) found no significant differences in the Children's Manifest Anxiety Scale scores of subjects, who had been exposed to varying forms of preparation, in a posthospital assessment conducted one week after discharge. Melamed, Meyer, Gee, and Soule (1976) report no posthospital main effect for treatment condition when using the Hospital Fears Rating Scale (HFRS) as the dependent measure. However, Melamed and Siegel (1975) found that children viewing a modeling film on admission to the hospital had lower HFRS scores than control group children at a follow-up visit approximately one month after discharge.

Physiological indices were used in seven of the 44 intervention studies assessing posthospital responses, all but two of which gathered information through parental report. Children exposed to experimental interventions were said to have fewer posthospital medical complications (Brain & Maclay, 1968; Lehman, 1975; Mahaffy, 1965) and to recover more rapidly (Mahaffy, 1965; Skipper & Leonard, 1968) than control group children. Crocker (1980) failed to find group differences in incidence of fever or vomiting, need to call the physician, or recovery time following discharge. Of the two studies making direct posthospital physiological assessments through the collection of Palmar Sweat Prints (Melamed & Siegel, 1975; Melamed, Meyer, Gee, & Soule, 1976), Melamed and Siegel found lower levels of anxiety among experimental group children.

The Duration of Posthospital Responses

Research bearing on the persistence of posthospital upset has typically used parental ratings of children's behavior as the dependent measure. Several researchers using this procedure report that disturbance is common in the period immediately following discharge from the hospital, but subsides soon thereafter. For example, Lende (1971) found that the majority of the tonsillectomy and adenoidectomy patients studied exhibited signs of upset in the period from ten days to two weeks after discharge. However, significant improvement in their behavior was noted six weeks to two months later. Couture (1976) also reports behavioral regression among elective surgical patients following discharge, further noting that the decline was more precipitous for children whose parents did not room-in. Though children in both "rooming-in" and "non-rooming-in" conditions displayed a similar rate of behavioral recovery in the month following discharge, only those in the rooming-in condition had reached their prehospital level of behavior after one month's time.

Information on the differential effects of an intervention on the posthospital behavior of children over time is also provided by Vernon (1973). The behavior of children hospitalized for minor, elective surgery, half of whom had been prepared for anesthesia, was rated by parents using the PHBQ seven days, and again thirty days, after discharge. Although children in both treatment conditions exhibited improvement in behavior in the period between the two assessments, the rate of recovery of the groups differed. At the initial posthospital assessment, no group differences were found. However, thirty days after discharge, children receiving preparation were significantly less upset than those in the unprepared group.

Gabriel and Danilowicz (1978) also describe a pattern of initial disturbance, followed by relatively rapid recovery, among cardiac surgery patients who had been prepared for medical events. Though the majority of subjects displayed some negative behavioral reactions in the period following discharge, most had subsided within two month's time. For example, sleep disturbances, reported in half of the preschool subjects studied, had disappeared in all but one child by two weeks after discharge. Only one long-term reaction, regressive behavior persisting in one child for more than a year, was noted among the prepared subjects.

Despite the consistency with which longitudinal studies have reported limited periods of behavioral upset after discharge, followed by periods of relatively rapid recovery, caution must be taken in generalizing this pattern to all hospitalized children. Each of the limited longitudinal studies reported above has relied almost exclusively on parent report of children's behavior, rather than using either direct behavioral observation or measures tapping other domains of psychological upset, such as subjective reports or direct physiological assessments. Moreover, with the exception of the Gabriel and Danilowicz (1978) study, which considered cardiac patients, research has been confined to children admitted to the hospital for minor, elective surgery. Thus, knowledge of the patterns of posthospital responses of other classes of patients, such as emergency surgical patients or medical admissions, is severely limited.

The studies providing longitudinal data on children's posthospital behavior have typically used limited periods of assessment as well. Couture (1976) and Vernon (1973) made final assessments of posthospital behavior one month after discharge; Lende's (1971) final assessment was two months postdischarge. More extended periods of assessment were used by Dearden (1970; 6 months after discharge) and by Gabriel and Danilowicz (1978), who provide data on a limited number of children more than a year after discharge.

The lack of diversity in conditions of patients selected for posthospital consideration, the restricted range of dependent measures used, and the limited periods of follow-up may impede detection of certain types of deferred responses. Several recent retrospective studies, in fact, suggest that extended or repeated hospitalization prior to age five, or early hospitalization for major medical or surgical conditions, may be associated with long-term disturbances. For example, Beavers (1974) tested a group of 22 males, seven to fourteen years of age, who had survived surgery for esophageal atresia as infants, comparing their scores on academic and psychological assessment tools with published norms. Though no significant deviations from the norms were found for subjects' general intelligence or academic achievement, the former surgical patients were found to be lower in self-concept, more anxious and less dependent than children on whom the tests were standardized.

Shapiro (1977) used similar academic and psychological tests to compare the responses of 38 childhood cancer survivors, 26 children who had undergone heart surgery, and 34 control children with no history of serious illness. All subjects, 4 to 13 years of age at the time of the study, were examined at least two years after recovery. As in the Beavers (1974) study, academic abilities did not differentiate groups, but cancer patients were found to have more emotional disturbance, more negative perceptions of their mothers, and to display more magical thinking than control group children. Recovered cardiac patients generally achieved intermediate scores, but did not differ significantly from either cancer or control subjects.

Two major retrospective studies of the possible effects of early hospitalization on children's later adjustment have been conducted by Douglas (1975) and Quinton and Rutter (1976). Douglas examined the data gathered over 26 years on a group of British children born in March of 1946, which included records of their early hospital experiences, as well as their behavior and academic performance during adolescence. Depending on the measure selected for examination, data were available on some two to four thousand subjects. Parent reports of children's posthospital behavior indicate that 68 percent were unchanged, 10 percent were improved, and 22 percent were worse upon return home. However, among children who were admitted to the hospital more than once, incidence of behavioral deterioration rose to 38 percent. Deterioration was also found to be more common among children hospitalized for surgery and among those treated in hospitals restricting visitation.

More surprising are Douglas' findings relating early hospitalization to children's adjustment during adolescence. Incidence of troublesome behavior in the classroom, poor reading skills, detention for delinquency, and unstable job patterns were found to be higher among children who had experienced one hospitalization lasting more than a week or repeated hospitalizations before the age of five years.

In an attempted replication, Quinton and Rutter (1976) examined the records of a group of children born in 1959, some thirteen years later than the Douglas sample. Using teacher ratings of children's behavior at ten years of age as the dependent measure, groups of subjects considered to be *disturbed* or *not disturbed* were selected for comparison. Contrary to Douglas' results, single admissions of more than a week in duration, whether occurring before or after five years of age, were unrelated to children's disturbance at age ten. However, Douglas' finding that repeated hospitalizations are associated with emotional disturbance was corroborated. The relationship was found to apply in both "advantaged" and "disadvantaged" groups of subjects, though stronger among advantaged children.

The studies of Douglas (1975) and Quinton and Rutter (1976) are subject to criticism due to their retrospective methodology, the small magnitude of the relationships found, and the fact that subjects examined were hospitalized decades ago under presumably different conditions than exist today. Nevertheless, they are of value in alerting researchers and practitioners to the possibility that hospitalization may result in unexpected, adverse long-term reactions, in addition to the transitory behavioral changes that have been repeatedly documented.

CHILDREN'S RECOLLECTIONS OF THEIR HOSPITAL EXPERIENCES

A small group of studies has examined another form of children's post-treatment responses—recollections of hospitalization, or of particular aspects of the hospital experience, following the period of medical care. In each instance, this research was conducted to investigate children's perceptions of the events in question rather than to assess the effectiveness of experimental intervention. The interval between the medical encounter described and the documentation of children's recollection varied from a few days (Barnes, 1975a, 1975b; Hanna & Sherlock, 1983) to some five years (Holt, 1967, 1968).

Barnes (1975a, 1975b), for example, interviewed thirteen children, six to sixteen years of age, three to four days after leaving the intensive care unit (ICU) where they had been treated following heart surgery. While in the ICU, few of the children had expressed complaints about the setting. However, in the subsequent interviews, subjects freely discussed the unusual and disturbing aspects of the environment, demonstrating an acute awareness of the unit and its activities (see Chapter 4).

Hanna and Sherlock (1983) interviewed fifty Jamaican children (5 to 11 years of age) concerning their recollections of anesthesia and surgery some four to eight days after their operation. Events prior to the induction of anesthesia (e.g., receiving premedication; the ride to, and arrival at, the operating room) were recalled with greater frequency than events occurring in the postoperative period (waking in the recovery room; returning to the ward). Recollection of the actual anesthesia procedures varied with the method of induction. Only 35 percent of the children having inhalational induction remembered placement of the mask on their face, while 80 percent of those having intravenous induction were able to recall the insertion of the needle. Few children expressed any fears in association with the events recalled.

Children's recollections of hospitalization in general were considered in two studies. In a follow-up to a preparation study, Peterson and Shigetomi (1982) interviewed mothers of minor surgery patients one year after discharge from the hospital. Among other questions, mothers were asked if their children continued to discuss the hospital experience. Sixty-seven percent reported that their children still mentioned hospitalization. Spontaneous comments about positive aspects (e.g., ice cream, electric hospital beds, color television) were more common than reference to negative elements such as injections and pain.

Holt (1967, 1968) considered the hospital recollections of thirty children after an interval of five years. Each subject (who had been three to five years of age at the time of admission to the hospital) was interviewed using a set of medical toys, and was further asked to draw the hospital as he or she remembered it. The author reports that intrusive therapeutic and diagnostic procedures were recalled most often and with the greatest affect. Forms of restraint were identified as especially disagreeable. Aside from these elements, most other recollections pertained to pleasant or neutral aspects of hospitalization. Though children seldom referred directly loneliness, isolation, or separation from parents in their descriptions of hospitalization, Holt interprets the absence of people in children's medical play or drawings, and the infrequent mention of interactions with others, as evidence of these concerns.

ILLNESS AS A SOURCE OF PSYCHOLOGICAL UPSET

Much of the research reviewed in the present chapter purports to investigate the effects of "hospitalization" on children during the inhospital or posthospital periods. However, "hospitalization" is, in fact, used as an abbreviation for a constellation of conditions existing within the hospital setting, such as the presence of unfamiliar and often painful stimuli, disruption of routines, and separation from supportive persons. The interaction of these conditions with the personal characteristics of the child results in varying degrees of upset. Research relating specific characteristics of the hospital environment or individual children to indices of psychological upset will be reviewed in the sections to follow. However, before doing so, data from two studies examining the effects of *illness,* in the absence of hospitalization, on children's behavioral responses will be considered (Shrand, 1965; Mattsson & Weisberg, 1970). It is the implication of these studies that the illness suffered by children, apart from other elements of their hospitalization, results in much of the observed behavioral disturbance.

Shrand (1965) considered the responses of 105 children (1 to 12 years of age) sick enough to be hospitalized, but cared for at home by their mothers instead. Parent ratings of children's behavior revealed a pattern of responses similar to that reported in other studies for hospitalized subjects. More than one-third of the children cared for at home exhibited behavioral changes, with subjects between one and four years of age showing greatest vulnerability. Changes were said to persist from a few days to several months after the illness, with most disappearing within two weeks. Types of behavioral changes noted were similar to those found among hospitalized children, except that rejection of mother was not observed in the children nursed at home. No direct comparison was made with hospitalized subjects.

Mattsson and Weisberg (1970) conducted a similar study of 35 preschool children treated at home for acute febrile infections. According to parent reports, all children showed some behavioral changes (e.g., diminished activity, increased sleep, loss of appetite) during the acute phase of the illness. Regression in independence and self-care skills was noted in all children under four years of age, although little loss of bowel or bladder control was reported. The behavior of children toward their mothers differed from that reported by Shrand (1965), with two basic types of reactions observed. *Type I,* characterized by increased clinging and dependence on mothers, was primarily noted among younger subjects. *Type II,* more common among children four years of age or older, consisted of a reduction of interest in physical or verbal contact with mother.

Though neither study included a control group of similar inpatients for purpose of direct comparison, both Shrand (1965) and Mattsson and Weisberg (1970) found that behavioral disturbances of the sort typically documented in hospitalized subjects occur as well in ill children nursed at home. The Shrand data suggest that alteration in parent-child interactions following hospitalization may be a unique product of the hospital setting, possibly due to the increased amount of separation frequently required. Mattsson and Weisberg (1970), however, found behavioral alterations to occur, such as increased clinging or rejection of mother, even in the absence of separation.

FACTORS ASSOCIATED WITH CHILDREN'S PSYCHOLOGICAL UPSET

Vernon, Foley, Sipowicz, and Schulman (1965), and others writing subsequently, have identified a number of factors potentially related to children's psychological upset during and after hospitalization and health care. The remainder of this chapter provides an overview of the research pertinent to four categories of such factors. These include *sociodemographic factors* (age, sex, family configuration, socioeconomic status), *interpersonal factors* (separation from parents, and interactions with others), *intrapersonal factors* (children's personality, emotional adjustment, and understanding of events), and *health care experience factors* (previous hospitalization, reactions in other settings, and the nature of the treatment currently experienced).

Sociodemographic Factors

Age. The relationship between children's age and psychological upset in response to health care has been repeatedly examined.

Vernon, et al. (1965) summarize the findings of previous research as indicating that children between six months and three to four years of age are most vulnerable during hospitalization, with older or younger children exhibiting lesser disturbance. Few studies appearing since 1965 have selected a sample of children with a sufficiently wide age range to test the existence of this proposed U-shaped curve. However, the results of two studies providing data on children less than one year and greater than four years of age conform to the suggested pattern. Vernon, Schulman, and Foley (1966) found that children from six months to nearly four years of age exhibited more behavioral disturbance one week after hospitalization than did children either older or younger. Similarly, Simons, et al. (1980) found that a greater percentage of children 13 to 36 months of age displayed deterioration in behavior six weeks after admission than older or younger subjects.

More commonly, researchers have eliminated children less than one year of age from their samples, examining the influence of age on the reactions of subjects in the preschool and schoolage years. Within this range, upset has been consistently reported to decline with age. This is true of assessments made both during the period of health care and following discharge from the hospital.

Considering children's *immediate responses* first, a decline in upset with age has been noted among children receiving outpatient care (Hyson, et al., 1982; Hyson, 1983), treatment in the emergency room (Gratz, 1977), or treatment at home (Mattsson & Weisberg, 1970). Similar age-related reductions in immediate upset have been reported for hospitalized children. Dependent measures used to assess these reactions include *behavioral observation* (Schulman, et al., 1967; Lee & Greene, 1969; Danilowicz & Gabriel, 1971; Milosavljević, et al., 1972; Visintainer & Wolfer, 1975; Wolfer & Visintainer, 1975, 1979; Dowd, et al., 1977; Powazek, et al., 1978), *self-report* (Melamed & Siegel, 1975; Melamed, et al., 1976; Campbell, 1978; Ferguson, 1979), and *heart rate* (Wolfer & Visintainer, 1975; McGrath, 1979; Burling & Collipp, 1969).

An age-related decline in negative *posthospital* behavior has also been frequently recorded (Aisenberg, et al., 1973; Douglas, 1975; Visintainer & Wolfer, 1975; Shade-Zeldow, 1976; Hackett, 1976;

Rieveschl, 1979; Wolfer & Visintainer, 1975). Brain and Maclay (1968) report that the combined incidence of inhospital and posthospital disturbance declined with increasing age of subjects.

Since few of the studies addressing the age question have considered subjects beyond the late schoolage years, one cannot conclude that a linear reduction in upset continues into the period of adolescence. In fact, one study including subjects from preschool years through adolescence (Gabriel and Danilowicz, 1978) found emotional disturbance to increase again during the adolescent years. Fewer negative reactions were reported among schoolage children (8 to 11 years) than among subjects two to seven *or* twelve to nineteen years of age.

Only a limited number of deviations from the general pattern of decline in psychological upset through the preschool and schoolage years have been reported. Herbertt and Innes (1979) observed the dental behaviors of children in grades one through six and found anxiety to be greatest among children at grade four. The lowest level of cooperative behavior was evident among subjects in grade three. Bothe and Galdston (1972) examined the responses of children four to twelve years of age while undergoing anesthesia induction, finding a greater tendency for older subjects to resist anesthesia than younger children. This result is of interest in light of an earlier report by Jessner, Blom, and Waldfogel (1952) that anesthesia represents a threat to the self-control of schoolage children and is, therefore, a primary source of anxiety for hospitalized children of this age.

Not all research addressing relationships between upset and age has reported significant effects. Nonsignificant age relationships have been reported for children's immediate responses in dental settings (Johnson & Baldwin, 1968, 1969; Nocella & Kaplan, 1982) and in medical settings when *behavioral measures* (Torrance, 1968; Johnson, et al., 1975; Cormier, 1979), *self-report measures* (Lockwood, 1970; Burstein & Meichenbaum, 1979; Fassler, 1980), or a *physiological measure* (urinary cortisol; Knight, 1978) have been used to assess upset. Two studies report no significant age-related effects in the posthospital period (Wolfer & Visintainer, 1975; Burstein & Meichenbaum, 1979). However, since only four of these studies included subjects younger than four years of age (Johnson &

Baldwin, 1968, 1969; Torrance, 1968; Wolfer & Visintainer, 1975), failure of the remaining cases to detect age-related differences may, in part, be attributed to lack of inclusion of subjects in the vulnerable early preschool years.

To summarize, the data are quite consistent in identifying the preschool years as the period of greatest vulnerability to upset associated with hospitalization and health care. There is additional, though more limited, information suggesting a reduced level of vulnerability among children less than one year of age. Susceptibility to upset appears to decline during the schoolage years, possibly increasing again during adolescence (Gabriel & Danilowicz, 1978).

Despite the general agreement of the research concerning age-related patterns of upset, some caution should be exercised in interpreting these results. Whenever an investigation spans a considerable age range (e.g., the period from infancy or toddlerhood through schoolage years) the danger exists that the appropriateness of the instruments used for assessing constructs such as "psychological upset" will vary across age levels, possibly introducing systematic biases.

This problem is especially acute when behavioral measures are used, since the types of behavior considered to be normative change so rapidly in early childhood. Rather than reflecting developmental changes in children's *vulnerability* to upset, some instruments may merely document normative changes in the frequency of occurrence of isolated behaviors typically associated with emotional distress (e.g., crying, protest, or aggression). Though such behaviors may indeed decline with age, they may be supplanted by other, more subtle manifestations of upset that are less readily detected by measures commonly in use. Careful consideration must, therefore, be given to outcome measures used in this area of developmental research, if it is to be determined whether the reportedly lower levels of upset among infants and schoolage subjects are truly a product of their greater invulnerability or are instead an artifact of biased assessment.

Sex. Sex differences in children's responses to hospitalization and health care have seldom been detected. Nonsignificant findings have been reported for reactions to dental care (Johnson &

Baldwin, 1968, 1969; Herbertt & Innes, 1979; Klorman, et al., 1979; Siegel & Peterson, 1980; Nocella & Kaplan, 1982), to hospitalization and medical procedures (Sipowicz & Vernon, 1965; Vernon, et al., 1966; Schulman, et al., 1967; Lee & Greene, 1969; Johnson & Stockdale, 1975; Johnson, Kirchhoff, & Endress, 1975; O'Donnell, 1976; Shade-Zeldow, 1976; Knight, 1978; Burstein & Meichenbaum, 1979; Cormier, 1975, 1979; Fassler, 1980; Eland, 1981; Schulz, et al., 1981; Youssef, 1981; Schwartz, et al., 1983), and to illness treated at home (Shrand, 1965; Mattsson & Weisberg, 1970).

The few studies reporting significant sex differences in response to health care are inconsistent in direction of the effects observed. For example, Torrance (1968) found females to be more upset than males when receiving an injection, though this difference may, in part, be due to the lower mean age of females in the sample selected. Campbell (1978) found that hospitalized male children viewed themselves as less emotional during periods of illness than did females. Melamed, Bennett, et al. (1983) recorded higher levels of self-reported fear among girls receiving dental treatment. Dearden (1970), on the other hand, found a higher percentage of males than females to be in the group of children she identified as being "disturbed" by hospitalization.

Two studies have reported sex-related differences in the mode, rather than absolute level, of children's responses to hospitalization. Aisenberg, et al. (1973) noted differences in the types of aggression demonstrated by males and females following cardiac catheterization. Boys were found to exhibit more physical aggression than girls, who in turn were more verbally aggressive than the males. Savedra and Tesler (1981) noted differences in coping styles used by male and female surgical patients. Females used "precoping" behaviors (orienting or familiarizing themselves with the environment) to a greater extent than males, while boys more often demonstrated attempts to control the situation.

Family Configuration. It has been proposed that first-born and only children may be more vulnerable to psychological upset in response to hospitalization and health care procedures than are later-born children. Schachter (1959), for example, suggested that fear responses of early-born children may be exacerbated by the overprotectiveness of first-time parents. Some support for the birth-order hypothesis is evident. Vernon (1974) found early-born children to be more upset before, but not during, an injection than later-born subjects. Douglas (1975) reports that only children were more likely to experience disturbance in the period immediately following hospitalization and later in adolescence than other children. Dearden (1970) also notes a tendency in her data toward greater upset among only children.

However, a majority of research examining the question of birth order has found no relationship between children's ordinal position and their emotional responses. This includes data on children undergoing hospitalization and medical procedures (Vernon, et al., 1966; Vernon, et al., 1967; Vernon, 1973; Johnson, et al., 1975; Savedra & Tesler, 1981) and on those treated for illness at home (Mattsson & Weisberg, 1970). Brown (1979) reports a tendency toward *less* upset among the only children in her sample of hospitalized patients.

Two studies have provided data on the relationship between *family size* and children's upset (Shade-Zeldow, 1976; Brown, 1979). In neither case was the relationship significant.

Socioeconomic Status. Few significant relationships between family socioeconomic status (SES) and children's responses to hospitalization have been found. Nonsignificant findings are reported in studies conducted by Schulman, et al. (1967), Knight (1978), and Savedra and Tesler (1981). Cormier (1975, 1979) performed a factor analysis on a 45-item checklist of children's behavior during hospitalization. Of the three factors identified through this procedure, one (children's protest behavior) was related to SES. However, the nature of this relationship (which was said to be small in magnitude) was not discussed.

Two studies report significant relationships between parent educational factors and children's responses to hospitalization. Campbell (1978) found mothers' educational level to be inversely related to their children's self-reported emotionality during illness. Clough (1979) found parent educational status to be directly associated with children's observed compliant behavior during hospitalization.

According to Vernon, et al. (1966), parents of lower SES families reported less posthospital upset among their children than did parents at other economic levels. The authors suggest that this difference may be due to the improved environment children experienced while in the hospital, or it may reflect parents' wishes to provide positive responses.

A significant association between family SES and *mothers'* distress in response to hospitalization of their preschool children is reported by Kessler (1969). Middle class mothers were found to be more upset by the experience than either upper or lower class parents.

Interpersonal Factors

Separation. Evidence of the effects of separation from parents on children's emotional status comes from studies of parent rooming-in, visitation, and presence during procedures. The research on parent rooming-in has considered children's inhospital and posthospital responses, with the positive effects of parental contact most unambiguously demonstrated for the posthospital period.

Among those studies addressing inhospital responses, Brain and Maclay (1968) report better adjustment in children whose parents remained with them at night. Lehman (1975) found increased inhospital aggression among children with rooming-in parents. This behavior was interpreted as evidence of the greater comfort and security experienced by rooming-in children, which allowed them to readily express their feelings about hospitalization—an interpretation that is supported by the more favorable posthospital adjustment observed among children in this group. Lee and Greene (1969) report a somewhat greater incidence of crying during anesthesia induction among children whose parents had roomed-in the night before. However, the effects of age may have contributed to this result, since the mean age of rooming-in children was less than that of children whose parents chose not to remain at the hospital overnight. An additional study examining children's immediate responses, Couture (1976), found no difference in the inhospital behavior of children in rooming-in and non-rooming-in treatment conditions.

Each of the five studies examining the *posthospital* effects of rooming-in found positive results to be associated with parental presence (Fagin, 1966, 1969; Brain & Maclay, 1968; Lehman, 1975; McGillicuddy, 1976; Couture, 1976). Despite the unanimity of these findings, care should be taken in their interpretation since the results of each are dependent upon parent report. The favorable results obtained, therefore, may partially be a product of parents' satisfaction with their own experience.

Little information exists on the relationship between the amount of time parents spend visiting their children (exclusive of rooming-in) and children's psychological responses. Lehman (1975) was able to detect the treatment effects reported above, despite the lack of difference in waking time spent with children by rooming-in and non-rooming-in parents. This suggests that rooming-in makes a unique contribution to the modification of children's responses, evident beyond that due to extensive visitation alone. Cormier (1975, 1979) found that children displaying behaviors indicative of depression received almost no parental visitation. O'Donnell (1976) reports that the level of inhospital cooperative behavior was lowest among children who had a *moderate* amount of parental contact, rather than minimal or extensive visitation. The author attributes these results to the moderate group's uncertainty about parental visitation patterns. Savedra and Tesler (1981) found no association between time children spent with parents and the types of coping behaviors exhibited during hospitalization.

The effects of parents' presence during admission procedures (Vernon, et al., 1967), anesthesia induction (Kay, 1966; Schulman, et al., 1967), and injections (Shaw & Routh, 1982) have also been studied. Vernon, et al. (1967) report no differences in the behavior of children during routine admission procedures, whether accompanied by their mothers or not. However, both of the studies reporting on anesthesia induction (Kay, 1966; Schulman, et al., 1967) found parental presence to be associated with reduced child upset during at least part of the procedure.

Shaw and Routh (1982) found increased incidence of crying, and longer periods of fussing, in response to an injection when the mothers of patients were present. However, in an interpretation similar to that given by Lehman (1975) concerning children of rooming-in mothers, Shaw and Routh view the behavior of subjects accompanied by mothers as evidence of their comfort in the presence of a parent, which permits expression of underlying feelings, rather than as an indication of greater upset.

Several studies have examined the impact of children's previous experience with separation on their responses during a subsequent illness or hospitalization. Mattsson and Weisberg (1970) found children's behavior during an illness treated at home to be unrelated to previous separations. Dearden (1970) reports that children having limited experience with normal separation (e.g., being left with a sitter, or visiting away from home overnight) tended to be more upset by hospitalization than those with greater separation experience. Douglas (1975) found children to experience less upset following discharge from the hospital if their mother had begun work outside of the home more than six months prior to the hospitalization. However, children whose mothers started work within six months of admission to the hospital were among the most upset in the sample studied. (For a detailed discussion of the literature on separation, see Chapter 5).

Emotional Responses of Parents. The relationship between parents' anxiety and children's emotional responses has been investigated during dental care, outpatient medical examination, and hospitalization. Johnson and Baldwin (1968, 1969) and Wright and Alpern (1971) report a significant, positive relationship between parent anxiety and children's upset responses during dental treatment. However, other dental studies find this relationship diminished when an intervention is instituted (Johnson & Machen, 1973; Wright, et al., 1973), or when the subjects have had previous experience with dental care (Klorman, et al., 1979). Two studies of outpatient medical care report a significant relationship between parent anxiety and children's reactions (Heffernan & Azarnoff, 1971; Thompson, 1983). Vardaro (1978) reports that child and mother anxiety levels were significantly associated in the period prior to hospitalization.

The relationship between parents' emotional responses and children's upset during hospitalization has been less frequently studied, though indirect evidence of the relationship comes from experimental research examining the value of information provided to parents about their children's hospitalization (Mahaffy, 1965; Skipper & Leonard, 1968). Skipper and Leonard found that an intervention consisting of information given to parents was associated with a reduction in parent anxiety and also with reductions in the inhospital and posthospital upset of their children, who had received no direct intervention. Mahaffy (1965) similarly found that information given to parents resulted in reduced child upset.

Other evidence concerning this relationship during the period of hospitalization is limited and somewhat contradictory. Schulman, et al. (1967) found no relationship between mothers' anxiety and children's responses during anesthesia induction. However, Goslin (1979) found that mothers' state anxiety levels were significantly related to physiological measures of their children, who had been admitted to the hospital for gastroenteritis. Brown (1979) reports that mothers who are anxious about hospitalization tend to have children who are withdrawn when in the hospital. Finally, data provided by Dearden (1970) suggests that the relationship between parent anxiety and child responses may be U-shaped, with either high or low levels of parent anxiety associated with increased child upset.

Parent-Child Relationships. Several studies have documented a relationship between parents' style of discipline or interaction with their children and children's responses to treatment in medical or dental settings. In general, the results of this research indicate that either the avoidance of restriction or the use of harsher forms of discipline (e.g., punishment or force) is associated with increases in children's emotional distress. Dearden (1970) reports that boys (but not girls) with "permissive" parents were more likely to be disturbed by hospitalization than those with so-called "authoritarian" parents. In the same study, ratings of the "emotional atmosphere" of children's homes (the degree to which the child's needs are understood and accepted) were found to be unrelated to children's responses to hospitalization. Shade-Zeldow (1976) reports that mothers' tendency to foster dependency in their children was associated with increases in children's inhospital regression.

Zabin and Melamed (1980) also examined the relationship between parents' disciplinary style and their children's anxiety when in the hospital. Questionnaires, which assessed preferred disciplinary responses to a variety of situations, were sent to the parents of sixty children who had, within the previous year, participated in a research study during hospitalization for minor surgery (Melamed & Siegel, 1975). Sixty percent of the mothers and 54 percent of the fathers completed the questionnaire. Parent responses were then correlated with data on children's anxiety collected in conjunction with the earlier hospital-based research. The pattern of significant relationships indicates that parents' use of positive reinforcement and modeling was associated with lower levels of anxiety, while the use of punishment or force, or the reinforcement of children's dependency behavior, was associated with increased anxiety.

Similar results are reported in dental settings. Fleece (1979) had parents of dental patients complete the same questionnaire as used by Zabin and Melamed to assess disciplinary styles. Parents' use of modeling and reassurance was inversely associated with children's self-reported fear during treatment, while reinforcement of dependency behaviors was directly correlated with children's fear levels. Venham, Murray, and Gaulin-Kremer (1979a) used a different set of instruments to assess parent-child interactions, though the relationships identified were much the same. Higher ratings of behavioral anxiety and increased heart rate during dental treatment were associated with greater parental permissiveness, avoidance of restrictions, and limited use of rewards.

Brown (1979) adopted a different approach to the investigation of the relationships between children's interactions with parents in the home and their behavior in the hospital. A principal components analysis of children's inhospital behavior was conducted, yielding three dimensions: *withdrawal* (the child stays away from, and converses little with, others), *immobility* (the child tends to stay in his or her room), and *distress* (the child shows frank upset and physiological disturbance). The relationship between these inhospital behaviors and three categories of child-family interaction in the home (identified through interviews with mothers) were examined. The three so-called "home experience" factors were *initiation* (the child demonstrates control over his or her own activities), *subordination* (the family extends control over the child's activities), and *proximity* (the child is involved in or integrated into family activities). It was found that children who rated high on any of the three inhospital behavioral factors (distress, immobility, or withdrawal) were low on initiation at home. Moreover, those high in proximity, as well as low in initiation at home, were more likely to be distressed during hospitalization. Children who manifested immobility in the hospital, on the other hand, were *low* in proximity at home, in addition to being low in initiation.

Parent and Child Relationships with the Staff. Research has documented the frequency, duration, and nature of the interactions between parents and staff (Korsch, et al., 1968; Francis, et al., 1969; Gozzi, et al., 1969; Freemon, et al., 1971; Robinson, 1968, 1972) and between children and staff (Pantell, et al., 1982; Cleary, 1977, 1979; Schulman, et al., 1970; Smith, 1976; Grant, 1983). However, in none of these studies were possible relationships between characteristics of those interactions and children's responses to health care examined.

Nevertheless, evidence from correlational studies indicates that variations in staff members' approach to, and interaction with, children can affect patient responses to health care events. Vernon, et al. (1967; also reported in Schulman, et al., 1967) found that children's responses to anesthesia induction differed with the anesthetist conducting the procedure, with this variation possibly related to the extent to which anesthetists attempted to establish rapport with children prior to surgery. In a comparable finding, Hyson, Snyder, and Andujar (1982) report that children exhibited more positive behaviors in an outpatient setting when approached by physicians in a warm, child-oriented manner.

Significant effects have also resulted from experimental research in which the amount or type of interaction occurring between children and health care personnel has been systematically varied. For example, preparation studies, such as those of Fassler (1980) and Minde and Maler (1968), suggest that emotional support provided by staff members can be effective in reducing children's upset, even when substantive information is not provided. Fernald and Corry (1981) contrasted two interactional styles used by medical technicians prior to a blood test and found that an empathic, informative approach to preparing children for the procedure was more effective in reducing children's upset than was a brusque, directive manner.

Melamed, Bennett, et al. (1983) experimentally examined variations in the responses made by dentists to patients' behavior during treatment. It was found that *punishment* responses (i.e., criticism of noncompliant behavior), when used alone, had a detrimental effect on the level of children's cooperation during dental restoration, and increased their self-reported fear. However, criticism was found to be effective in reducing fears and noncompliant behavior, if accompanied by reinforcement of desirable behaviors. Fleece (1979), who also examined variations in reinforcement styles used by dentists, failed to document significant group differences in children's disruptive behavior.

Results similar to those of Melamed, Bennett, et al. (1983) are presented by Weinstein, Getz, Ratener, and Domoto (1982). The authors of this nonexperimental study report that the incidence of children's fear-related behavior was lowest following dentists' use of directive commands or reinforcement of behaviors (see Chapter 8).

Intrapersonal Factors

Unfamiliarity. Vernon, et al. (1965) identified children's unfamiliarity with hospital setting and procedures as one of several factors associated with children's psychological upset. Data from six preparation studies conducted prior to 1965 were cited as evidence that providing children with information about the hospital and their condition is an effective means of reducing emotional distress. In the intervening years, more than 60 preparation studies have been conducted, the results of which, in general, confirm the effectiveness of preparation in reducing children's immediate and posthospital upset (see Chapter 10).

It is unclear, however, whether *information* about unfamiliar elements of the hospital is the operative factor in reducing children's upset since, with few exceptions, researchers have failed to test for knowledge or understanding gained through preparation. Evidence from the few studies making such an assessment indicates that increased information, whether from preparation or other sources, does contribute to reduced upset. Lende (1971) found that, although the type of preparation children received was unrelated to their subsequent upset, a significant relationship existed between children's knowledge of the surgery and their upset behavior. Melamed, Dearborn, and Hermecz (1983) report higher scores on a test of hospital knowledge among subjects who had seen a filmed presentation about hospitalization than among children who had viewed a control film. Test scores of subjects with previous hospital experience were also higher than those of children hospitalized for the first time. Increased information about the hospital was further found to be associated with lower levels of inhospital anxiety. In an outpatient study, Thompson (1983) found a significant relationship between children's ability to identify and ascribe a function to medical instruments and their behavior during a physical examination in which those instruments were used.

Evidence of the role of unfamiliarity in contributing to children's upset could also be obtained through studies manipulating the environment in an effort to eliminate foreign elements, thereby reducing the discrepancy between hospital and home. No research directly adopting this approach was found, though studies indicate that introduction of play experiences to an outpatient waiting area (Williams & Powell, 1980) or an intensive care unit (Cataldo, et al., 1979; Pearson, et al., 1980) positively affected children's behaviors.

Descriptive studies of children's behavior in exceptionally stressful areas such as the emergency room (Roskies, et al., 1975; Resnick & Hergenroeder, 1975; Gratz, 1977), isolation units (Kueffner, 1973, 1975; Hollenbeck, et al., 1980; Powazek, et al., 1978), and intensive care units (Cataldo, et al., 1979; Carty, 1977; Barnes, 1975a, 1975b) have been conducted. However, these studies make no formal assessment of the relationship between children's upset and the unfamiliar elements of these environments (see Chapter 4).

Concepts and Perceptions of Hospitalization and Illness. The development of children's concepts of health care, illness, and hospitalization has been repeatedly examined (see Chapter 3). Yet, despite the frequently expressed belief that children's reactions to medical events are influenced by their understanding and interpretation of their condition (e.g., see A. Freud, 1952), there has been virtually no attempt to systematically relate children's medical concepts to their responses during treatment. Thompson (1983) investigated this issue in an outpatient setting, finding no relationship between the sophistication of five-year-old children's health care concepts and their responses while receiving a physical examination and injection.

The relationship between children's *perceptions*, or subjective evaluations, of medical events and their manifested responses to that experience has been examined in a limited number of studies. Tsigounis (1977) reports generally low and nonsignificant correlations between children's prehospital perceptions of their impending surgery (e.g., ratings of the severity of their surgery, satisfaction with information, and their general expectations concerning hospitalization) and their adjustment following discharge. Clough (1979) notes several significant relationships between children's perceptions and their inhospital behavior. Children who tended to define themselves as being ill were more compliant during hospitalization. Those who found medical treatment to be stressful, or who unfavorably compared hospital life with home life, exhibited more anxiety behavior.

Personality. The relationship between selected personality factors and children's responses to hospitalization has been assessed, though no single area has received exhaustive consideration. For example, two studies have investigated the role of children's temperament. Rose (1972) found that flexibility and rhythmicity were unrelated to the coping behaviors exhibited by children while in the hospital. Bernheimer (1981) found only a limited number of significant relationships between a set of temperament variables and children's coping behavior during an outpatient physical examination.

Knight (1978, Knight, et al., 1977, 1979) examined the style and effectiveness of *defense mechanisms* used by hospitalized children, finding that subjects using intellectualization, intellectualization with isolation, or a mixed pattern of defenses had lower levels of stress than children using denial, denial with isolation, displacement, or projection. Children's stress levels during hospitalization were also inversely related to the *effectiveness* of their defense mechanisms.

Ratings of children's prehospital *anxiety* levels have been significantly related to children's inhospital reactions (Mahon, 1980) and to their rate of posthospital recovery (Tsigounis, 1977). Burstein and Meichenbaum (1979), however, found no relationship between children's prehospital anxiety levels and subsequent inhospital and posthospital assessments of anxiety.

Bolig (1980) assessed children's *field dependence/independence* and *locus of control* (LOC) upon admission to the hospital. Increased levels of field independence on admission were associated with lower anxiety on discharge. Children's LOC, however, was unrelated to discharge anxiety levels. Rothbaum, Wolfer, and Visintainer (1979) also examined the LOC ratings of hospitalized children, relating LOC scores to parents' ratings of children's behavior when upset. Subjects with external locus of control (i.e., who felt that events are controlled by forces other than themselves) were found to exhibit a higher proportion of internal behaviors (withdrawal, worrying, obsessive or compulsive behaviors, etc.) than children with an internal LOC, a finding that was replicated with a second sample.

The effects of personality factors on children's dental behavior was examined by Venham, Murray, and Gaulin-Kremer (1979b). Children rated as having a lower self-concept were found to exhibit significantly higher pulse rates and more anxious behavior during treatment. Increased anxiety was also observed among children who were high in achievement needs, failure avoidance, and motivation.

Prehospital Emotional Adjustment. The adequacy of children's prehospital emotional adjustment has been significantly associated with their responses to hospitalization in several studies. For example, Brain and Maclay (1968) report a significant relationship between children's emotional state prior to admission and incidence of inhospital and posthospital disturbance. Shade-Zeldow (1976) and Sides (1977) each included an index of prehospital adjustment among variables in a regression equation used to predict children's response to hospitalization. In both instances, the prehospital measure contributed significantly to the prediction of *posthospital* upset. However, Shade-Zeldow (1976) found no relationship between children's prehospital adjustment and their *inhospital* response.

The research of Dearden (1970), discussed above, may offer insight to the relationship between prehospital adjustment and subsequent psychological upset. In that study, a portion of the children sampled (nearly 20%) exhibited symptoms of emotional disturbance prior to hospitalization, and maintained a similarly high level of upset throughout the inhospital and posthospital periods. This pattern of disturbance suggests two possibilities. First, children with high levels of prehospital upset may be predisposed, or more vulnerable to upset due to hospitalization. Second, and perhaps more likely, inhospital and posthospital upset noted among children with inadequate prehospital adjustment may merely be a continuation of the prior disturbance. Thus, a portion of the inhospital and posthospital upset observed, and typically attributed to elements of the hospital experience, may exist relatively independent of hospitalization.

This second explanation has received some support in the literature. Stocking et al. (1970, 1972) suggest that, not only is much of the inhospital disturbance noted among children unrelated to the events of hospitalization, but also that the percentage of hospitalized children displaying psychopathology is greater than that in the population as a whole. Parents of a random sample of eighty children admitted to a pediatric hospital were interviewed within 48 hours of the child's admission to identify those children experiencing difficulties in personality development or emotional adjustment deemed severe enough to warrant consultation. Of the eighty children considered, 51 (63.7%) were found to manifest such difficulties. This rate was compared with incidence of psychopathology ranging from six to twelve percent in various studies of nonhospitalized schoolaged children. Only ten percent of the sample was judged to be in need of consultation for problems arising from their treatment or illness. O'Donnell (1976) also reports an unexpectedly high level of disturbance among pediatric inpatients, with 23 of 30 children recording "deviant profiles" on the Missouri Children's Picture Series administered upon admission to the hospital.

If a high incidence of emotional disturbance does, indeed, exist among the population of hospitalized children, what might be the underlying cause of this situation? According to Stocking, et al. (1972), it is perhaps *not* that children requiring medical treatment are more disturbed than others, but rather that disturbed children are frequently hospitalized for inappropriate reasons. They suggest that parents who perceive signs of emotional upset may avoid this awareness, focusing instead on real or imagined physical conditions. Stocking, et al. estimate that thirty percent of the children studied were hospitalized unnecessarily; 24 of the 27 in this group were judged to exhibit emotional disturbance.

The literature on *life events* may provide an alternative explanation for a high percentage of emotional disturbance among hospitalized children, should the figures cited by Stocking, et al. be replicable. Instead of examining the prehospital adjustment of hospitalized subjects, this group of studies determines the total number of "life events," which represent potential psychological stressors (e.g., moving to a new school district, parents divorcing, adding a third adult to the household) experienced by children. Kashani, et al. (1981) found that "normal," nonhospitalized subjects experienced significantly fewer life events than either hospitalized pediatric patients or child psychiatric patients. Similarly, Heisel, et al. (1973) found that groups of children with juvenile rheumatoid arthritis, general pediatric patients, pediatric surgical patients, and psychiatric patients had each experienced more frequent and more severe life events prior to onset of their condition than did their healthy peers.

If previously experienced events of emotional significance are, as the life events literature suggests, associated with the onset of illness and the necessity for hospitalization, it should not be surprising to find a substantial portion of hospitalized children either displaying upset in response to the earlier events, or being vulnerable to further upset associated with hospitalization. However, a direct study of the relationship between life events and children's inhospital or posthospital responses has not been conducted.

Health Care Experience Factors

Prior Health Experiences. The influence of prior hospitalization on children's responses to current health care has been examined. In particular, researchers have sought to determine whether the responses of children previously hospitalized differ from those of children with no hospital experience. The majority of studies examining this question have found that prior hospitalization does not affect children's responses during subsequent health care, be it emergency room treatment (Gratz, 1977), treatment of illness at home (Shrand, 1965), or hospitalization (Vernon, et al., 1966;

Sipowicz & Vernon, 1965; Lockwood, 1970; Knight, 1978; Savedra & Tesler, 1981).

Of those studies finding a significant association between prior hospitalization and later reactions to health care, four have found children's responses to be negatively affected. Sermet (1974) studied groups of anxious and nonanxious dental patients, finding a greater incidence of previous hospitalization among subjects in the anxious group. Previous hospitalization has further been associated with increased upset during anesthesia induction (Vernon, et al., 1967), greater posthospital behavioral problems (Tsigounis, 1977), and heightened upset during an injection in an outpatient clinic (Thompson, 1983). In contrast, O'Donnell (1976) reports that subjects with previous inpatient hospital experience were more cooperative during a subsequent hospitalization than inexperienced subjects, and Bolig (1980) found lower anxiety levels on discharge among children who had been previously hospitalized.

Simons, et al. (1980) found no relationship between the *number* of previous hospitalizations and children's posthospital responses. Thomson (1972), on the other hand, reports a significant relationship between the "number of prior distressing hospital experiences" and children's inhospital anxiety, though her terms are not clearly defined.

A small group of studies conducted in outpatient medical and dental settings indicate that parents' ratings of children's responses to previous health care experiences are predictive of children's reactions during later care. Heffernan and Azarnoff (1971) had parents rate the frequency of their children's previous fearful reactions to clinic visits. This rating was found to be indicative of children's anxiety on the clinic visit under investigation. Thompson (1983) found that parent assessments of children's responses to prior hospitalization and to previous medical care each correlated significantly with children's reactions to an outpatient examination.

Ratings of children's previous reactions to dental care have also been significantly associated with later dental behavior (Johnson & Baldwin, 1968, 1969). Melamed, Bennett, et al. (1983) examined the level of children's disruptiveness over a series of dental treatment sessions, finding behavioral ratings on the first session to correlate significantly with ratings on two subsequent visits.

However, this research also indicates that children became more cooperative over successive dental treatment sessions.

Aspects of Current Treatment. Nonsignificant relationships between the *duration* of children's hospitalization and their responses to the experience have been reported in several research projects (Sipowicz and Vernon, 1965; Schaffer, 1966; Simons, et al., 1980; Savedra and Tesler, 1981). However, Vernon, et al. (1966) report a tendency for longer hospitalizations to result in greater upset. Others report that aggression (Shade-Zeldow, 1976) and extroversion (Clough, 1979) increase with length of hospitalization. Menke (1972) found an association between the types of stimuli children perceived as stressful and the length of their hospital stay. However, an attempted replication of the study failed to reveal this association (Menke, 1981).

The relationship between children's physical condition or diagnosis and selected reactions has also been examined. Cormier (1975,1979) found children's diagnoses to be unrelated to their responses to hospitalization. Cannell (1970) compared children with permanent versus temporary physical disorders, finding the permanently disabled subjects to be lower on social maturity ratings. However, subjects did not differ on personality measures. Knight (1978) found no significant differences in the urinary cortisol levels of children admitted to the hospital for various short-term surgical procedures.

Two studies comparing emergency and elective admissions suggest that emergency hospitalization produces greater upset. Shade-Zeldow (1976) found emergency hospitalization to be associated with increased aggression among children. Clatworthy (1978, 1981) found that, although emergency patients were less upset on admission, they were more upset on discharge than other children. Further evidence of the psychological stress experienced by emergency admissions is provided by Roskies, et al. (1975).

The reactions of surgical and nonsurgical patients have also been compared. Sipowicz and Vernon (1965) and Vredevoe, et al. (1969) report no significant differences in the responses of children in these groups. Riffee (1981), however, documented lower levels of self-esteem among schoolaged surgical patients than among others hospitalized with medical conditions.

Finally, the effects of the treatment received by children during hospitalization have been examined in a limited number of studies. According to Rose (1972), the number of stressful events experienced by children during hospitalization was unrelated to the coping behaviors they exhibited. Vernon, et al. (1966) found no relationship between the degree of pain experienced by children (as estimated by admitting diagnoses) and their posthospital psychological upset. Burling and Collipp (1969) considered children's immediate responses to treatment, as assessed by changes in heart rate. They report that greatest elevations in pulse occurred during injections, otoscopy, and rhinoscopy.

Sibinga and colleagues (Sibinga, et al., 1968; Sibinga & Friedman, 1971) suggest that one category of medical treatment, that involving immobilization or sensory restriction of young children, has a profound effect on their later development, inhibiting intellectual functioning and language development. However, methodological problems in these studies limit their interpretation (see Chapter 4).

SUMMARY

Four categories of factors possibly contributing to the immediate or posthospital psychological upset of children have been examined in this chapter: sociodemographic factors, interpersonal factors, intrapersonal factors, and health care experience factors. Of the *sociodemographic* variables considered, relationships between children's age and emotional distress have been most consistently reported. In particular, the research indicates that children from approximately one to three or four years of age are most vulnerable to upset, both during treatment and in the period following hospitalization. There is also limited evidence that children's birth order may affect their level of upset, with first-born or only children being more upset than others. Significant sex or social class differences in children's responses to health care have been seldom reported.

The research concerning *interpersonal factors* indicates that the nature of children's relationships and interactions with their parents or health care personnel affects their responses to the treatment received. Parent presence, either through rooming-in or remaining with children during procedures, has been associated with significant alterations in indices of psychological upset. The meaning of a portion of these changes occurring during the period of health care (e.g., increased crying or aggressive behavior) has been subject to debate. Nevertheless, research examining the posthospital effects of rooming-in has consistently documented the benefits of parent contact.

A relationship between parent anxiety and children's responses to treatment has been reported in dental clinics, outpatient medical settings, and, less often, in inpatient pediatric units. However, this association appears to be weaker among patients with prior experience in the health care setting, and is modifiable through interventions directed toward parents or children.

Also associated with upset manifested by patients in medical and dental settings is parents' preferred manner of disciplining their children. In general, the research addressing this issue reports greater emotional distress among children whose parents are either overly permissive or, at the other extreme, use punishment and force, rather than positive reinforcement or modeling behaviors, to obtain cooperation.

A final interpersonal factor associated with children's reactions during treatment is the style of communication used by health care personnel in their dealings with children. Research in medical settings suggests that a friendly, empathic, child-centered approach to interactions results in a more positive response from children. Patient's fearful responses in dental settings have been reduced by dentists' use of unambiguous directions and positive reinforcement of children's behavior.

Intrapersonal variables considered in this chapter include children's unfamiliarity with the health care setting, their prehospital emotional adjustment, and personality characteristics. Evidence that unfamiliarity contributes to children's immediate and posthospital upset is found in the preparation research, which has repeatedly documented the benefits of providing children with information about their treatment. Indeed, a limited number of studies have documented a direct relationship between the amount of information children have about a medical event and their upset in response to it. Children's emotional adjustment prior to admission has been directly associated with their upset during hospitalization and following discharge, however data on specific personality characteristics are too limited and fragmentary to be readily summarized.

The final category of factors reviewed consists of *health care experience* variables. The effects of a previous hospitalization on children's responses to a subsequent admission have been examined with conflicting results. A portion of the research indicates that previous hospital experience is associated with greater upset during subsequent care, while other studies suggest that experienced patients exhibit less distress. Perhaps more predictive of children's response to a subsequent hospitalization is the adjustment demonstrated during an earlier admission, rather than the mere experience of previous inpatient care. Research in medical and dental settings alike has documented a significant relationship between children's reactions to prior treatment and their responses to the present events.

Finally, examination of specific aspects of children's current treatment has produced few significant findings. There is some evidence that longer hospitalization results in increased upset. However, relationships between upset other factors such as amount of pain, or number of stressful procedures experienced, have rarely been investigated. When examined, these relationships have been nonsignificant. Few differences in psychological upset among patients with varying diagnoses are reported in the literature. There is, however, some indication that children admitted to the hospital under emergency circumstances experience greater upset than patients hospitalized for elective procedures.

Chapter 3

CHILDREN'S CONCEPTIONS OF HOSPITALIZATION, ILLNESS, AND MEDICAL CARE

Children's conceptions of hospitalization, illness, and medical treatment have been of longstanding interest to health care researchers. The literature reviewed by Vernon, Foley, Sipowicz, and Schulman (1965) suggests that young children view hospitalization and illness in terms of punishment, mutilation, death, and abandonment. The predominant position of investigators conducting this early research was that misconceptions of this sort contribute to children's psychological upset during and after the period of hospitalization. Despite the prevalence of this belief, Vernon, et al. note that, "there has been relatively little discussion of the ways in which interpretations of hospitalization and illness contribute to psychological upset" (p. 79). Furthermore, other than clinical accounts, there is virtually no empirical evidence that misconceptions of hospitalization, health and illness result in psychological upset.

Research conducted since 1965 has continued to examine and document children's health care concepts and knowledge, including the misconceptions characteristically expressed. In this chapter, research pertaining to four general areas will be reviewed. The first of these concerns children's belief that illness and medical treatment represent punishment for their actual or imagined transgressions. The prevalence of this belief has been examined in populations of healthy children and among those who are ill or hospitalized. Although it has been suggested that children's tendency to interpret illness or medical care as punishment may be influenced by their health status, with hospitalized children, for example, being more likely to invoke punishment explanations

(Brodie, 1970, 1974), little research has directly compared the beliefs of children in these differing conditions.

A second area to be considered is the normative, developmental change that occurs in children's health care conceptualizations. Among the age-related changes reported in the literature are a decline in punishment explanations, an increase in the complexity of strategies used by children to recognize and describe states of health and illness, an increase in children's knowledge of internal body parts, and a stage-like progression in the sophistication of children's causal explanations of illness. Also examined has been the relationship between changes in children's health care conceptualizations and their cognitive development in other content domains. Results of studies examining this relationship are in conflict as to whether health causality concepts progress in unison with general cognitive development, or emerge somewhat more slowly.

A third topic addressed is the potential impact of children's medical status on their concepts and knowledge of health care. Research based on a Piagetian framework suggests that hospitalization or chronic illness may affect the level of one's illness causality explanations, either accelerating development through increased contact with the subject matter, or interfering with this progression as children avoid the emotionally charged topic. Another group of studies indicate that, regardless of the effects on conceptual sophistication of causal explanations, the experience of hospitalization or illness may increase children's objective knowledge of specific health topics.

The final portion of this chapter is devoted to consideration of research investigating children's understanding of several health care phenomena. Included in this discussion are studies concerning children's concepts of medical procedures and instruments, medical personnel, isolation technique, and research hospitalization.

ILLNESS, HEALTH CARE, AND SELF-CAUSATION

Studies prior to 1965 repeatedly documented a common childhood belief that illness is the product of one's own actions (Beverly, 1936; Richter, 1943; Gips, 1956; Gellert, 1961). The nature of the real or imagined act causing the illness may be children's overt misbehavior or, alternately, their failure to follow a recommended course of action (e.g., going outside without one's coat). The perception that one is responsible for illness may lead to the further interpretation, frequently expressed by children, that illness represents a form of punishment. Similarly, the treatment associated with illness (painful, intrusive procedures in particular) may also be viewed as retribution.

The majority of the pre-1965 studies documenting these perceptions were conducted with samples of hospitalized children. The question thus arises whether feelings of self-causation and punishment may be limited to children who are ill or whether healthy, nonhospitalized children will display the same beliefs. However, before considering this question and the literature on healthy children's beliefs, the research pertaining to hospitalized children's concepts of illness and health care as punishment will be reviewed.

Hospitalized Children's Views of Illness as Punishment

Of the studies conducted since 1965 assessing hospitalized children's perceptions of illness as punishment, two indicate that illness, as well as its accompanying treatment, is often viewed as retribution, especially by younger children (Peters, 1975; Brewster, 1982). In the first of these studies, Peters (1975) interviewed 24 hospitalized children, eight through ten years of age, concerning their conceptions of illness causality and treatment. Children were shown a series of six pictures containing cues designed to elicit comments pertaining to illness and were asked to tell stories about the pictures. The content of these stories was analyzed to determine the identity of the agent causing the illness, the intent of that agent, and the action responsible for the illness.

Of those children identifying a causal agent, sixty percent indicated that the ill character in the story was responsible for his or her own illness. However, sex differences in designation of causal agents were apparent. Girls were more likely to attribute the illness to the character's own actions than were boys, with boys more frequently implicating other persons or environmental factors.

According to Peters, analysis of the content and wording of the stories indicates an acceptance of self-causation and "a pervasive implication that illness results from disobedient or imprudent behavior" (p. 76). Treatment of illness was also frequently interpreted by children as a form of retribution. In nearly half of the references made to treatment, children indicated, either explicitly or implicitly, that the intent of the treatment agent was punitive or hostile. Despite the relatively narrow age range of subjects considered by Peters, age differences are apparent. Younger children were more likely to view illness as self-caused, and to view treatment as punitive, than were older children.

Brewster (1982) investigated the illness conceptualizations of hospitalized, chronically ill children, five to twelve years of age. In general, children less than seven years old were found to view illness as resulting entirely from human action, being a product of one's wrongdoing. Furthermore, when asked to give the purpose of medical procedures, children of this age typically stated that treatments were performed as punishment for misbehavior.

Somewhat different results are reported by Pidgeon (1967), who interviewed children three to seventeen years of age, hospitalized in an isolation unit, concerning their understanding of isolation technique. Children's responses were classified as *precausal, mixed,* or *causal,* with precausal responses consisting of exclusively psychological or moral reasons for isolation (e.g., that the child was being confined for misbehavior). Pidgeon found only 33 percent of the children in the youngest age group (3 to 7 years) to offer precausal explanations, a proportion smaller than expected. The percentage of children providing precausal explanations declined with age.

Healthy Children's Views of Illness as Punishment

Brodie (1970, 1974) suggests that, since studies on children's health care concepts had been predominantly conducted with ill or hospitalized children, the feelings of guilt and anxiety documented in that research may be specific to children in health care settings and inapplicable to healthy subjects. In particular, factors such as the nature of illness, separation from parents and home, and the unfamiliar elements of the medical environment and procedures may lead ill or hospitalized children to interpret their condition as punishment.

To determine whether healthy children also interpret illness in this manner, Brodie examined groups of nonhospitalized first, third, and fifth graders. Each child responded to a general anxiety measure and to a series of questions assessing their perceptions of: 1) illness as punishment, 2) parental reaction to illness, and 3) illness as a disruptive force in children's lives. In the assessment of illness causality, subjects were asked whether specific forms of disobedience, such as telling lies, fighting, or playing too much, can result in children's illness.

The majority of children in each age group rejected the conception of illness as punishment. Moreover, most reported no parental displeasure during periods of child illness, nor did they feel that illness was a disruptive force in their personal lives. Brodie interprets these findings as evidence that healthy children and hospitalized children have fundamentally different perceptions of illness. This conclusion is suspect, however, since a direct comparison was not made with a similar group of hospitalized subjects answering identical questions.

Though Brodie found little evidence of widespread acceptance of illness as punishment among her schoolaged subjects, other research with healthy subjects suggests that such beliefs are common, at least among preschool children. For example, Kister and Patterson (1980) interviewed children at four grade levels (preschool, kindergarten, second, and fourth grades) concerning their understanding of the concept of contagion and their use of "immanent justice" explanations to account for illness and misfortune. The concept of immanent justice derives from Piaget's (1964) writings on the moral development of children, which state that, "the younger the child . . . the stronger will be its belief in the soundness and universality of expiatory punishment" (p. 251). Young children are said by Piaget to "affirm the existence of automatic punishments which emanate from things themselves" (p. 251). Therefore, illness may be seen as one of the agents of this self-regulatory moral system.

Children interviewed by Kister and Patterson were presented with a series of questions concerning a contagious illness (a cold), a noncontagious illness (a toothache), and an accident (a scraped knee). Subjects were initially asked whether each condition was contagious (i.e., could one child "catch it" from another) and, if the condition were identified as contagious, whether the distance between the two people involved would affect the chances of one person catching it from the other. To assess the tendency to invoke immanent justice explanations, a series of vignettes were read, in which a child who had misbehaved subsequently contracts a contagious or noncontagious illness, or suffers an accident. Children were asked whether the misbehavior caused the illness or accident.

Nearly all children understood that some conditions are contagious. However, younger children were more likely to overextend the concept of contagion to noncontagious illness or accidents than were older children. That distance affects the likelihood of contracting a contagious illness was well understood, with a majority of children at each grade level responding appropriately. The proportion of children understanding of the role of distance in the contagion process increased with grade level.

Concerning the question of immanent justice, younger children were far more likely to view illness or accident as the result of misbehavior than were older children. Furthermore, there was a strong, inverse relationship between children's understanding of contagion and their use of immanent justice reasoning. This relationship remains, even when one partials out the effects of age. Kister and Patterson speculate that, "the decline of immanent justice thinking during childhood is caused by the child's growing awareness of the actual causes of the events (in this case, the causes of illness)" (p. 844–845). If this be the case, the authors suggest, then it may be possible to alleviate the fear and guilt experienced by children when ill by providing them with rational explanations of their condition.

Studies Examining Healthy and Ill Children

In addition to studies investigating punishment beliefs among samples consisting solely of hospitalized children (Peters, 1975; Brewster, 1982) or healthy subjects (Brodie, 1970, 1974; Kister & Patterson, 1980), a limited amount of research has examined the health care perceptions of both populations (Cook, 1975; Williams, 1979; Rutter, 1970; Rumfelt, 1980). Inclusion of both groups of children in this research should allow for comparison of the prevalence of self-blame or punishment explanations used by each, thus enabling one to determine whether such conceptions are limited to, or more prevalent among, ill or hospitalized subjects. In actuality, direct comparisons are seldom made of the extent of punishment explanations given by hospitalized and nonhospitalized subjects. Nevertheless, the research indicates that, when punishment explanations are provided by subjects for a given set of questions, they are offered by healthy, as well as hospitalized, children. This finding challenges Brodie's suggestion that healthy children interpret illness in a fundamentally different manner than do those who are hospitalized.

Among this group of studies is that of Cook (1975), which examined the causal thinking abilities of hospitalized and nonhospitalized French children, ranging in age from five to fifteen years. Children in both groups were found to give explanations of illness characterized by themes of self-causation and blame. In fact, self-causation reasoning was present in the spontaneous explanations of illness given by children at each of the age levels studied.

In a study conducted in the Philippines, Williams (1979) interviewed healthy and hospitalized children from three grade levels (first, third, and fifth grades). Among other tasks, children were asked to give the cause of an illness from which they had suffered. In analyzing these responses, Williams did not directly address the issue of self-causation. Nevertheless, the numerous examples of well-children's responses provided in the text demonstrate the presence of self-causation beliefs among subjects at each grade level. The absence from examples of hospitalized children precludes consideration of the self-causation issue in this group.

Rutter (1970) also provides evidence of children's belief in their own responsibility for illness. Groups of diabetic, scoliotic, and healthy children, eleven to thirteen years of age, were questioned concerning their feelings of responsibility for positive and negative experiences associated with mild or severe forms of illness or injury. Children's belief in self-responsibility for negative events was found to be significantly greater than that for positive events associated with the conditions in question.

In contrast to the preceding studies, which demonstrate substantial belief in the self-causation of illness and its accompanying treatment, Rumfelt (1980) found little indication that either hospitalized or nonhospitalized children considered the tasks commonly performed by nurses to be punitive. In this case, five-year-old children were shown a series of ambiguous pictures of female nurses with patients in pediatric settings. Subjects were asked to describe the actions that they believed the nurse in the picture would take.

Analysis of the implied intent of the actions described by children revealed few instances of aggression or punishment. Sixty percent of the actions were characterized as neutral, with 21 percent deemed nurturant. In only four percent of the cases were the nurse's actions interpreted as purposeful attempts to inflict pain or discomfort. Recognizing that this finding conflicts with earlier research, the author suggests that, although hospitalization may be viewed as punishment for children's misdeeds, "it does not appear that many children regard the nurse as a punishing person" (p. 20).

Summary

Of the nine studies examining hospitalized and/or nonhospitalized subjects' concepts of illness and health care, six indicate that children, especially young children, consider illness to be self-caused (Kister & Patterson, 1980; Peters, 1975; Brewster, 1982; Cook, 1975; Williams, 1979; Rutter, 1970). Moreover, the majority of these studies indicate that an act commonly perceived as causing the illness is one's own misbehavior, with the resulting condition considered to be punishment (Kister & Patterson, 1980; Peters, 1975; Brewster, 1982; Cook, 1975). In contrast, Brodie (1970, 1974) found little evidence that healthy children believe specific forms of disobedience cause illness. Furthermore, Pidgeon (1967) found that even preschool children can give causal, albeit frequently erroneous, explanations of isolation technique, while Rumfelt (1980) noted few instances in which five-year-old children perceived the intent of nurses to be hostile.

An issue raised by these studies is whether health status affects one's perceptions of illness as self-caused or punitive. Brodie contends that it does, with healthy, but not hospitalized, children in general rejecting the notion that illness is caused by misbehavior. Evidence from other studies including nonhospitalized subjects contradicts this position, indicating that healthy children, as well, frequently consider illness to be a product of one's own actions (Kister & Patterson, 1980; Cook, 1975; Rutter, 1970). One element distinguishing Brodie's research from others is that children were presented with specific misbehaviors (lying, fighting, playing too much) and were asked whether these might cause illness. Had children been asked for their spontaneous explanations, or had acts of omission been included in the list (e.g., failure to follow adult directives), self-causation explanations might have been more prevalent.

Discrepancy was also noted in documentation of children's interpretations of medical treatment. Brewster (1982) reports nearly universal acceptance of treatment as punishment among young, chronically ill children. The intention of treatment was less frequently perceived as punitive among Peters' (1975) group of hospitalized subjects and was virtually absent from Rumfelt's (1980) hospitalized and nonhospitalized five year olds. Perhaps the severity of the children's condition and the frequency of their encountering medical procedures accounts for a measure of this disparity.

AGE-RELATED CHANGES IN CHILDREN'S CONCEPTIONS OF ILLNESS AND HEALTH CARE

Children's conceptions of illness and health care are not static, but rather appear to change over time in quality and complexity, following certain broad, predictable patterns. The documentation of this gradual alteration has been the focus of a number of studies to be considered in the present section. This research addresses three major topics: 1) the decline of belief in self-causation and punishment, 2) the increasing complexity of explanations of health and illness, and 3) the progression of qualitatively different stages of health care concepts.

The Decline of Belief in Self-Causation and Punishment

Research considered in the preceding section indicates that children commonly view illness as self-caused and punitive. An age-related decline in the prevalence of this belief has been documented by several researchers. For example, in their study of healthy children, Kister and Patterson (1980) found use of immanent justice explanations of illness to decline with increasing age of the subjects. Peters (1975) also found an age-related decrease in self-causality explanations of illness among her sample of hospitalized children. Similarly, themes of self-causation and punishment, common among young, chronically ill children interviewed by Brewster (1982), were absent from the explanations of illness and treatment given by older children. Moreover, Pidgeon (1967), who reported relatively low levels of precausal explanations among children less than seven years of age (33%), found this figure to decline in older age groups. Among children seven to twelve years of age, 12.5 percent gave precausal explanations, while no child older than twelve years provided a precausal response.

Increase in Complexity of Health Care Concepts

Explanations of Illness and Health. The strategies used by children to recognize and describe states of illness and health have been examined in three studies (Campbell, 1978; Millstein, Adler & Irwin, 1981; Natapoff, 1978). To varying degrees, each provides evidence that children's understanding of these conditions grows increasingly complex with age.

Campbell (1975) interviewed 264 children (6 to 13 years of age, admitted to a pediatric hospital for short-term stays) and their mothers. The illness conceptualizations of children and mothers were assessed by asking each how they know when someone is sick. Multiple responses and elaborations were permitted. Responses were coded using a system of eleven hierarchically organized themes falling into four major categories, which are (in sequential order from least to most complex) *feeling states* (e.g., pain, soreness, "not feeling right"), *objective signs* (e.g., swollen joints, a hot forehead), *diagnoses* (e.g., "appendicitis," "chicken pox"), and *psychosocial states* (i.e., a change in one's emotional status or alteration in one's role behavior).

A significant degree of intergenerational consensus was reported. Rank order correlations of the frequency of use of the eleven theme categories were computed for mothers and younger children (six years to nine years, five months) and for mothers and older children (nine years, six months to twelve years, eleven months), respectively. Although both correlations were positive and significant, the correlation between mothers and older children was greater, indicating a developmental trend toward more adult-like responses with age. Despite the correspondence of the absolute frequency of themes used by the groups of children and adults, there was no indication that responses of individual children were related to those of their mothers.

The data further indicate that the age of the respondent is associated with increases in the total number of themes used, as well as increases in the sophistication of the themes mentioned. Within the sample of children, a positive relationship was found between age and the number of themes mentioned. Moreover, when responses of children and mothers were compared, the total number of different themes used by mothers was greater than that used by children. Definitions given by older children included higher level themes emphasizing specific diseases or diagnoses, and alterations in role behavior, while younger children tended to define illness in terms of vague, nonlocalized feelings.

A measure of conceptual sophistication was constructed by summing the frequency with which respondents mentioned each of six most advanced, or "adult-favored themes." As might be expected, children's conceptual sophistication was significantly related to age and grade level, respectively.

Millstein, Adler, and Irwin (1981) used Campbell's (1975) interview and coding system to examine the health concepts of adolescents ranging in age from eleven to fifteen years. Adolescent responses were examined for evidence of developmental trends, both by looking within the sample of adolescents and by comparing this sample with data on Campbell's groups of children and mothers. For purposes of making cross-age comparisons, the authors selected the "adult-favored" themes, examining the responses of this type given by each age group. It was found that adolescents' use of adult-favored themes did, in fact, fall between the levels reported for children and mothers. However, only two of the individual themes in the adult-favored cluster displayed the expected developmental pattern across the three age groups. As was true of the Campbell (1975) study, there was considerable definitional consensus across age groups. A coefficient of concordance indicated that, "themes most common in the concepts of illness of one group were prominent in the others; infrequently used themes occurred rarely in all groups" (p. 837).

When Millstein, et al. confined their examination to the adolescent group, the expected developmental trends failed to emerge. It was anticipated that older adolescents would provide more diverse themes than their younger counterparts. However, a significant *negative* correlation was found between age and total number of themes used. Furthermore, a small, but significant *negative* correlation was found between age and the number of *adult-favored* themes cited.

In contrast to the previously discussed studies, which were primarily concerned with subjects' definitions of illness, Natapoff (1978) examined children's concepts of *health.* Children in first, fourth, and seventh grades were asked to define health, to tell what it feels like to be healthy and not healthy, and to explain how a person knows when someone is healthy. Responses to these questions were coded using a system of 29 categories identified through pilot work. Children were also asked whether one could be part healthy and part not healthy at the same time.

Considered as a group, children were found to define health most frequently in terms of feeling good and participating in desired activities. When asked how one knows that another person is healthy, 84 percent of the children cited perceptual means of detecting this condition. Specific symptoms or the inability to engage in certain activities were commonly cited as evidence of the absence of health.

Age-related patterns were also noted. A broader range of categories were used by older subjects in response to the questions. Natapoff further observed that comments became, "more complex, thoughtful, and increasingly longer with age" (p. 997). Older children were less dependent on observable behavior of others to determine their state of health than were younger children, and were more likely to assert that people can be part healthy and part not healthy at the same time.

Understanding of Body Parts. Investigations of children's understanding of their body parts have been conducted, focusing in particular on their *internal* body parts (Porter, 1974; Quiggin, 1977; Smith, 1973; Williams, 1979), and on body parts covered by a bandage or cast (Howe, 1968; Spicher, 1982). Four of these studies address the question of age-related changes in subjects' knowledge (Porter, 1974; Smith, 1973; Williams, 1979; Spicher, 1982), in each case documenting increasing levels of sophistication with age.

Smith (1973), for example, interviewed hospitalized and nonhospitalized children in third and fifth grades, asking each to name the contents of the body, to draw the body parts they had mentioned on a human figure outline, and to describe the function of the organs identified. In addition, children were asked questions about a past or current illness. Subjects' responses were rated such that each received three scores: a *general body organ* score (based on all organs named by the child, no matter how obvious), a *major body organ* score (based on knowledge of 18 major organs), and an *illness* score (based on children's understanding of the cause of the illness they named, the organs involved, the function of the organs, the illness process, and its treatment). Smith found children's grade level, as well as the educational level of their fathers, to be positively associated with performance on all three measures.

In a partial replication of this study, Williams (1979) interviewed 229 well school children and 130 hospitalized children selected from third and fifth grades, living in the Philippines. Subjects were asked questions about their internal body parts and a past illness. As in the Smith study, children's grade level was found to influence their knowledge of body parts and illness. Other factors related to children's responses were the educational levels of both parents, and the sex of the child, with males scoring higher than females.

Porter (1974) asked 144 children from three different grade levels (first, third, and fifth) to draw internal body parts in the appropriate places on a human figure outline and to label each part. Drawings made by children at each grade level revealed a considerable degree of accuracy in depicting and naming body parts, with their abilities surpassing that demonstrated in earlier studies (e.g., Gellert, 1962).

Consideration of children's responses across grade levels indicated that the total number of internal body parts identified gradually increased with age. However, the frequency with which a given item was mentioned by subjects of different ages did not necessarily increase in a linear fashion. For example, first graders mentioned blood more often than third or fifth graders. Third graders more frequently included kidneys, lungs, muscles, tonsils, and veins in their drawings than did the other two groups. Fifth graders, on the other hand, tended to list a large number of "detailed and intricate" body parts, though perhaps omitting some of the more common ones.

Porter further categorized the individual body parts mentioned according to the body system to which each belonged. Of the nine systems considered, the frequency of children's reference to all but two increased with age. In a finding corresponding to that of Williams (1979), boys at each grade level were found to name more body parts than girls.

Porter's study was essentially replicated by Quiggin (1977), who confined her sample to 46 children of a single grade level (10 years, 8 months to 11 years, 9 months). All subjects were asked to draw and label internal parts on a body outline, following which a randomly selected subset of the children were individually questioned concerning the function of selected body structures. Quiggin reports that children's drawings and descriptions were quite accurate and suggests that medical terminology may be readily used with children of this age. As was true of the Porter (1974) and Williams (1979) studies, boys identified more body parts than girls.

A variation on the investigation of children's understanding of internal organs is provided by two additional studies addressing concepts of body parts that are covered by a cast or bandage. Howe (1968) interviewed 21 children (7 years, 4 months to 9 years, 9 months of age), eleven of whom were hospitalized for conditions requiring bandaging, with the remainder being participants in a recreation program. Selection of this narrow age range precluded consideration of age-related trends. Each subject was shown a series of pictures of children wearing bandages and was questioned concerning the reason for bandaging, the appearance of the wound under the bandage, and the eventual outcome of the injury.

Children almost unanimously indicated that the bandaging was performed to help the injured child, rather than as a punishment. However, explanations of how the bandaging benefited children were typically inaccurate, manifesting magical and prelogical thought. Furthermore, though subjects knew that the body part under the bandage had not been removed, their descriptions of the state of the injury site were often exaggerated and erroneous. Extensive damage was frequently described. Children also displayed a literal interpretation of phrases such as "a broken arm" or "a cracked head" by describing a visible cleft apparent under the bandage, which had, perhaps, been applied to bind the injured parts together. The belief was often expressed that the wound would never completely heal and would remain vulnerable to reinjury.

Spicher (1982) conducted a similar study, using children of a wider age range, thereby permitting assessment of age-related changes. Subjects of this study were nineteen children, seven to twelve years of age, hospitalized for orthopedic surgical procedures that required casting. Each was asked to describe the condition of the area under his or her cast and then to draw it on a body outline. Children were further asked to describe the appearance of the area when the cast would be removed and what it would be like one year later. Spicher found little evidence of the distorted perceptions of the covered sites or vulnerability to future injury reported by Howe.

Several age-related differences were apparent in the descriptions and drawings provided by children. For example, younger children (i.e., those 6 to 8 years of age) less often mentioned skin color or skin condition than did older subjects (9 years of age or older). Drawings of older children were more likely to include the incision and were more frequently rated as being moderately complex than were those of younger subjects.

Summary. The studies reviewed in the preceding sections indicate that children's health care concepts become increasingly complex with age. Natapoff (1978) found this to be true for children's descriptions of health. Similarly, Campbell (1975) found that hospitalized children's explanations of illness became progressively more sophisticated with age, yet were less mature than those of their mothers. Millstein, et al. (1981) found the level of explanations given by nonhospitalized adolescents to fall between that of Campbell's child and adult groups. However, age-related trends within the adolescent group failed to emerge.

Of the studies concerning children's conceptions of the internal body, Smith (1973) and Williams (1979) found knowledge of body parts and illness to improve with subject's advancing grade level. Porter (1974) reported that the number of individual body parts and body systems referred to by children increased with age, as did the tendency to list detailed body parts. Spicher (1982) also noted greater detail in the drawings and descriptions of older subjects. Two additional studies pertaining to knowledge of body parts limited their samples to a narrow age range, and consequently provided no information on age-related changes (Quiggin, 1977; Howe, 1968).

Stages of Health Care Understanding

Identification of Stages. The studies just considered typically used some form of *quantitative* measure in their documentation of the complexity of children's health care concepts, recording, for example, the number of different items in each of several categories mentioned by subjects. Another group of studies has followed an alternate course, adopting a Piagetian framework for documenting *qualitative,* stage-like changes in children's explanations of illness and health over time (Bibace & Walsh, 1978, 1980; Perrin & Gerrity, 1981; Brewster, 1982). In each case, the responses of children to questions of illness causality have been classified using a hierarchical scale, with each level, or stage, of the scale characterized by patterns of thought qualitatively different from that of the others.

Bibace and Walsh (1978) developed a structured, clinical interview schedule patterned after that produced by Laurendeau and Pinard (1962) to assess children's causal thinking abilities. During the development of this instrument, 180 nonhospitalized children, ranging in age from three to thirteen years, were interviewed concerning topics such as general illness, colds, measles, heart attacks, cancer, headaches, pain, and germs. The questions typically required the child to define a specified condition and to explain its cause and cure.

Responses from the pilot interviews were analyzed and classified according to the level of cognition demonstrated: preoperational, concrete operational, or formal operational thought. Within each major stage, two substages were identified, yielding a total of six sequential levels: *phenomenism* (illness caused by remote phenomena), *contagion* (illness caused by proximity), *contamination* (illness caused by contact), *internalization* (illness located in the body), *physiological explanations* (illness due to the vulnerability of specific internal structures), and *psychophysiological explanations* (illness caused by psychological, as well as physical, factors).

Following the establishment of categories, seventy-two children in three age groups (four, seven, and eleven years) were interviewed using the instrument employed during the pilot phase. The distribution of children's scores across the six identified stages demonstrated a developmental progression in causal explanations. Seventy-one percent of the four year olds were classified as being in the contagion substage (level 2), with seventy-five percent of the seven year olds in the contamination substage (level 3) and seventy-one percent of the eleven year olds in the physiological explanation substage (level 5).

An additional 72 children (also four, seven, and eleven years of age) were interviewed by Bibace and Walsh (1980). Results of this research essentially replicate the earlier findings, except that the substage occupied by a majority of the eleven year olds was internalization, rather than physiological explanations.

The authors contend that their research is of value in helping health care professionals to understand the cognitive principles underlying children's concepts of illness and health. This knowledge, it is said, will allow individuals to provide more meaningful reassurance to patients and to design educational interventions appropriate to children's level of conceptualization.

Another Piagetian-based system of categorizing children's health care concepts was developed by Perrin and Gerrity (1981). A total of 128 nonhospitalized children in kindergarten, second, fourth, sixth, and eighth grades were asked a series of questions concerning the causes, treatment and prevention of illness. In addition, questions designed to assess children's general cognitive level were presented. Topics included in the latter assessment were conservation, transformation, interrelationship among parts, physical causality, and abstract thinking.

Children's responses were analyzed using a coding system designed to be applicable across content domains and reflecting sequential movement from global to concrete to abstract explanations. These three major categories of responses, roughly equivalent to Piaget's preoperational, concrete operational, and formal operational stages, are supplemented by two intermediary, transitional stages. In sequential, developmental order, the stages specified by Perrin and Gerrity are *global responses* (circular, magical, superficial explanations of illness), *concrete rules* (symptoms, actions, or situations associated with illness), *internalization and relativity* (increased generalization), *generalized principles* (greater delineation of causal agents), and *physiologic processes and mechanisms* (illness described in terms of internal body organs or systems). Similarities between this system and the previously described categories of Bibace and Walsh (1978, 1980) are apparent.

Children's scores for illness questions were found to increase with advancing grade level, despite a wide range of illness scores at any given age. Analyses of individual questions indicated that some were consistently more difficult than others. For example, cognitively more advanced responses were provided for a question concerning the purpose of hospitalization than for questions of the causes or treatment of illness. Furthermore, an item concerning the *prevention* of illness elicited responses consistently lower than those of other questions.

Perrin and Gerrity concur with Bibace and Walsh (1978, 1980) that their research has implications for educational intervention. Recognition of children's cognitive abilities may enable health care educators to provide explanations at a comprehensible level, perhaps no more than a single step above their present level of understanding, as suggested by Turiel (1969). However, Perrin and

Gerrity also observe that adults' abilities to recognize the conceptual capacities of children is limited.

The inability of clinicians to gauge accurately the conceptual abilities of children was illustrated in a subsequent study by Perrin and Perrin (1983). In this research, examples of children's responses to questions concerning health and illness were submitted to physicians, nurses, and child development students, who were asked to estimate the ages of children supplying each answer. Considerable discrepancy between children's actual and estimated ages were apparent, with ages accurately identified (within one year) for fewer than 40 percent of all items. Respondents tended to overestimate ages for responses provided by young children (4 to 7 years of age), while underestimating those of older children (12 to 15 years of age).

In contrast to the studies of Bibace and Walsh (1978, 1980) and Perrin and Gerrity (1981), which examined *nonhospitalized* children's concepts of health and illness, Brewster (1982) investigated the conceptualizations of hospitalized children, selecting a group of fifty chronically ill children, ranging in age from five to twelve years. Children were presented with questions concerning illness causality and their perceptions of medical personnel and procedures, as well as three general cognitive tasks (conservation, physical cause and effect, and social role perspective). Scores for each task were assigned, based on a scale of 0 to 6 points, with higher scores representing more mature responses.

As expected, children's concepts of illness causality and of the intent of medical procedures became increasingly objective and complex with age. Two parallel patterns, each containing three stages were identified. First, for questions of illness causality, children in *Stage 1* are said to view illness as resulting entirely from human action, being a product of one's wrongdoing. In *Stage 2*, children believe in univariate physical causality. That is, all illness is thought to be caused by one agent, typically germs. Finally, in *Stage 3*, children acknowledge that illness can have multiple, possibly interacting causes.

During *Stage 1* of the understanding of the intent of medical procedures and the role of personnel, children believe that medical treatment is a form of punishment. Children in *Stage 2* can accurately infer the medical intent of procedures, but believe that medical personnel will only know that children undergoing procedures are in pain if they scream or cry. Finally, both intentions and empathy of medical personnel are accurately inferred by children in *Stage 3.*

Relationship between Health Concept Stages and General Cognitive Functioning. In addition to documenting the progression of children's understanding of health and illness, researchers have investigated the relationship between conceptual development in this domain and children's general cognitive growth. Two primary issues have been addressed. The first and most basic question considered is whether a significant relationship, in fact, exists between the development of children's health concepts and their general cognitive functioning. Also of interest is whether the existence of such a relationship implies that health causality concepts develop simultaneously with those of other content areas, or perhaps emerge somewhat later.

Simeonsson, Buckley, and Monson (1979) considered the first of these issues. Specifically, the development of of illness causality concepts among hospitalized children was related to their physical and social concept development. Sixty children, four through nine years of age, were given a Piagetian conservation task and a social role-taking task, and were also asked a question concerning physical causality ("What makes clouds move?"). Finally, a series of questions concerning illness causality concepts was presented. Responses to individual illness questions were assigned scores corresponding to one of three conceptual stages defined by Elkind (1967): global or undifferentiated, concrete, or abstract.

Developmental trends were evident for four of the six illness causality questions, with older children giving more advanced responses. Furthermore, children's total illness causality scores were directly related to their conservation and physical causality scores, and inversely related to their levels of egocentrism. These correlations remained significant even after partialling out the effects of age.

Carandang, Folkins, Hines, and Steward (1979) also considered the question of correspondence between conceptualizations of illness and general cognitive functioning, in this case using a sample of nonhospitalized children. Subjects identified as concrete operational, transitional, or formal operational (as determined by Piagetian conservation tasks) were presented with questions concerning illness causality and treatment. Responses were coded using an adaptation of Bernstein and Cowan's (1975) Origin of Babies Scale. As was true of the Simeonsson, et al. (1979) study, a significant relationship was noted between general cognitive level and children's illness conceptualizations.

Neuhauser, Amsterdam, Hines, and Steward (1978) similarly found the sophistication of children's health care concepts to increase across cognitive levels. Twenty-four children, rated as being either preoperational or concrete operational on the basis of their performance on a Piagetian conservation task, were interviewed concerning their concepts of illness and healing. Concrete operational children used more *internal* cues for recognizing illness and health, and had more accurate perceptions of healing, than did the preoperational subjects.

Two of the previously discussed studies also discovered a correspondence between development of health care concepts and cognition in other content domains. Perrin and Gerrity (1981) noted that illness causality concepts were highly correlated with performance on general cognitive tasks, including conservation of mass, transformations, interrelationships among parts, physical causality, and abstract thinking. Questions concerning physical causality ("Why do clouds move?" "Why does night come?") were most highly associated with illness causality questions among subjects in all grade levels. Brewster (1982) found significant, positive intercorrelations among all five cognitive tasks administered to her sample of chronically ill children (with the cognitive tasks being conservation, physical cause and effect, social role perspective, illness causality, and concepts of medical personnel and procedures).

Though a significant association may exist between development of health care concepts and other content domains, the correspondence between areas may not be exact. In fact, there is some suggestion that health care concepts may emerge more slowly, or lag behind, general conceptual development. Among those investigating this possibility was Cook (1975), who compared the causal thinking abilities of hospitalized and nonhospitalized French children, ranging in age from five to fifteen years. Children were asked to discuss the causes of two phenomena, rain and physical illness. Two methods of eliciting responses were used with each child. In the first portion of the interview, *spontaneous* explanations of the phenomena were obtained through nondirective probing. This was followed by a highly structured interview format designed to assess children's ability to give mature causal explanations. Cook anticipated that children's spontaneous explanations of illness would be less mature than their discussions of rain, despite children's *ability* to give equally mature responses to questions in both categories.

Spontaneous explanations of illness were, in fact, found to be less mature than corresponding responses for rain, with illness explanations characterized by themes of self-causation and blame. As previously mentioned, self-causation reasoning was present in children's spontaneous explanations throughout childhood. Cook speculated that adherence to this view of illness may be emotionally rewarding since it allows children a measure of psychological control over an anxiety-producing event.

Perrin and Gerrity also indicate that, despite a strong correlation between illness causality and physical causality concepts, illness concept development may lag somewhat behind. No child in their sample received a higher score for illness causality than for physical causality questions. The authors contend that these findings are, "consistent with Piaget's observation that development proceeds at variable rates depending on both the child's experience with the phenomenon and the affect connected with it" (p. 848). They further suggest that investigations with chronically ill children be conducted to determine whether extensive contact with illness might increase children's conceptual understanding or, on the other hand, whether heightened affect regarding illness might interfere with conceptualization in this domain.

Brewster's study of chronically ill children addressed this issue. It was predicted that children's responses would be influenced by the degree of affect associated with the content of each question. The author felt that questions with high affect content (in this case, those concerning children's own illness) would elicit less mature responses than items demanding similar cognitive skills, but having low affect content. Thus, illness causality and intent of treatment questions were respectively compared with physical causality and social role tasks.

Differences between the high and low affect tasks were not found, although a number of children (older children in particular) did raise egocentric or magical themes in conjunction with more advanced explanations of their illness or treatment. In an interpretation similar to that of Cook (1975), Brewster suggests that children may retain egocentric concepts concerning their conditions, even when they "know better," as a defense mechanism. Citing the work of the Gardner (1969), Brewster speculates that feelings of guilt and self-causation may help the child to defend against a sense of helplessness engendered by chance occurrence of the disease process.

THE INFLUENCE OF ILLNESS OR HOSPITALIZATION ON CHILDREN'S HEALTH CARE CONCEPTS

Impact on Cognitive Level

Studies reviewed in the preceding section suggest that health care concepts may emerge somewhat later than concepts in other content domains and that a factor possibly affecting the rate of this development is the status of children's health. Perrin and Gerrity (1981), who interviewed healthy children, detected a lag of this sort in the development of health concepts. On the other hand, Brewster (1982), who examined chronically ill children, found no difference in the level of children's competence whether performing illness-relevant or illness-irrelevant conceptual tasks. Nevertheless, spontaneous comments of children interviewed by Brewster indicate that they retained egocentric, magical beliefs.

Few studies have directly evaluated the potential impact of illness or hospitalization on children's health care concepts by comparing affected and nonaffected subjects. Among those making such a comparison are Cook (1975), who examined the effects of hospitalization, and Myers-Vando, Steward, Folkins, and Hines (1979), who considered the impact of an illness—congenital heart disease.

As previously mentioned, children in Cook's sample gave spontaneous and structured responses to questions concerning the causes of illness and rain. It was hypothesized that hospitalized children would give less mature spontaneous explanations of illness than would healthy children. Results indicate that children's state of health not only affected their explanations of illness, as had been hypothesized, but their spontaneous explanations of *rain* as well. For both phenomena, hospitalized children provided less mature causal explanations. Cook speculated that the source of this cognitive immaturity may differ depending on the age of the child. While less advanced responses may be considered adaptive among older children, in younger subjects such responses may represent a regressive reaction to stress.

Myers-Vando, et al. (1979) interviewed twelve children (8 to 16 years of age) who were chronically ill with congenital heart disease. Their responses to a physical causality task and an illness causality questionnaire were compared with those of a group of healthy subjects matched on age, sex, social class, and ethnicity. Ill subjects recorded lower scores than healthy children on the physical causality task—a finding similar to that reported by Cook for hospitalized children. However, unlike the hospitalized subjects in the Cook study, chronically ill children did not differ from healthy control subjects on their illness causality concepts.

The results reported by both Cook (1975) and Myers-Vando, et al. (1979) concerning the depressing effects of hospitalization or illness on children's general cognitive functioning are corroborated by Rieveschl (1979). In this case, the spatial and affective role-taking skills of a group of tonsillectomy patients were assessed before hospitalization, in the hospital before surgery, and after discharge from the hospital. Their scores on these measures were compared with those of a group of nonhospitalized subjects. Some regression and disorganization of skills was apparent among subjects of both groups. However, hospitalized children manifested more regression and disorganization in spatial role-taking skills during hospitalization, and in affective role-taking skills after hospitalization, than nonhospitalized subjects tested at comparable intervals. The extent of the regression was described as "shallow," seldom consisting of loss of more than a single substage of measurement.

Though the effect of hospitalization or illness on one's *own* illness causality concepts remains in question, an additional study indicates that the state of health of one's *sibling* may affect the rate of development of these concepts (Carandang, Folkins, Hines, & Steward, 1979). Adopting a systems theory approach, the authors suggest that chronic illness in a family inevitably affects all other members. Well siblings, in particular, might be affected since the emotional resources of the family are likely to be diverted toward the chronically ill individual. This diversion of support and understanding, as well as a general increase in stress within the family, may affect the cognitive performance of well siblings.

Half of the subjects in the Carandang, et al. study were siblings of diabetics, with the remaining half having healthy siblings. Subjects in these two groups were matched on sex, grade level, socioeconomic status, and general conceptual abilities (as assessed by Piagetian conservation tasks).

A majority of the children were found to answer illness questions on the same level as their pretest conservation performance. Among those scoring at a different level, half scored higher and half lower. Children with diabetic siblings recorded illness scores lower than their pretested conservation levels significantly more often than did subjects with well siblings. This effect was especially prevalent among children initially classified as formal operational.

The authors offer three possible explanations for lower levels of illness conceptualization among children with ill siblings. First, the long-term stress accompanying chronic illness may act as an "intrusion factor," preventing children from applying their most advanced cognitive structures to a given content area. Second, children with chronically ill siblings may experience an "information deficit." Although much information concerning the condition of the ill child and the specifics of illness management may be available to these children, more abstract discussions of illness may be avoided by family members. Parents, in particular, may avoid such discussions to control their own anxieties about the illness. Finally, siblings of diabetic children attaining the formal operational level may, for the first time, become aware of the greater implications of the disease. For example, they may fear that they, too, will contract this genetically-linked condition, or that they may pass it on to children of their own. Confronted with this new awareness, the authors speculate, some children may respond with avoidance of the subject.

Impact on Knowledge of Health and Illness

Although illness and hospitalization have, in certain instances, been associated with reduction in levels of health care conceptualization, there is some indication that experience with illness may increase or alter one's *knowledge* of specific elements of medical care. For example, Smith (1973) found that numerous or prolonged experiences with illness were associated with greater knowledge of illness and body organs. In addition, Smith (1973) and Williams (1979) each report that hospitalized children knew more about illness than did well children, but that the two groups did *not* differ in their knowledge of internal body parts (a finding also reported by Quiggin, 1977).

The hospitalized children in Williams' study (which was conducted in the Philippines) were said to have attributed illness causation to germs or to contagion, or, in the case of an accident, to have described events resulting in the injury. Well children, on the other hand, cited natural phenomena, such as heat, cold, or wind as causal agents. Hospitalized subjects' concepts of *treatment* were also found to be more advanced than those of well children. Williams argues that the explanations provided by well children reflect the phenomenalistic beliefs of causes and cures prevalent in their culture. Children who experience hospitalization are given objective information concerning the causes and treatment of illness—an intervention that may help to correct their misconceptions.

Spicher (1982) and Rumfelt (1980) each provide further evidence that the experience of medical treatment or hospitalization may alter one's knowledge of health care. In her study of children's understanding of their covered postoperative sites, Spicher found that subjects who had experienced prior casting gave greater and more detailed information about their present cast site. Rumfelt compared hospitalized and nonhospitalized five-year-old children's perceptions of the nursing role, finding more limited, stereotypical views of nursing among children who had never been admitted to the hospital.

The relationship between children's health history and the complexity of their definitions of illness was examined by Campbell (1975). Rather than observing a simple relationship between these two variables, an association mediated by age was found. Specifically, *younger children* whose health status, according to maternal report, was *worse* than that of their parents, displayed lower conceptual sophistication. However, among *older children* the reverse was true. Poorer health status relative to parents was associated with higher conceptual sophistication.

The effects of impending stressful procedures on children's conceptualizations were also examined by Campbell. Children facing procedures deemed to be "quite anxiety producing" displayed heightened emotionality, according to nurses' ratings. Nevertheless, the prospect of forthcoming stressful procedures did not affect the conceptual sophistication of children's responses.

CHILDREN'S CONCEPTS OF OTHER HOSPITAL-RELATED PHENOMENA

In addition to concepts of illness and health, children's understanding of a number of other topics relevant to hospitalization have been examined. The subject matter of these studies include concepts of medical procedures and instruments, medical personnel, isolation technique, and research hospitalization.

Concepts of Medical Procedures and Instruments

Studies of children's concepts of health and illness have infrequently and, for the most part, only tangentially considered children's understanding of medical instruments and procedures. For example, Bibace and Walsh (1978, 1980), Perrin and Gerrity (1981), Carandang, et al. (1979), Simeonsson, et al. (1979), and Neuhauser, et al. (1978) each asked children to explain how people recover from illness, but none of these studies specifically focused the attention of respondents on particular vehicles of treatment, such as injections or medicine.

Systematic discussion of children's perceptions of their treatment is rare. Two exceptions to this pattern are found in the previously discussed work of Peters (1975) and Brewster (1982). Peters reports frequent use of punishment themes in children's explanations of treatment, even among subjects who recognize a helpful intent behind the care provided. Brewster found that chronically ill children, five and six years of age, typically viewed treatment as punishment, but that older children were increasingly able to infer the accurate intention of medical procedures, eventually perceiving the quality of empathy in medical personnel as well.

Three additional studies with nonhospitalized subjects have specifically examined children's understanding of medical instruments and procedures (Steward & Regalbuto, 1975; Bernheimer, 1981; Thompson, 1983). Steward and Regalbuto (1975) interviewed children in kindergarten and third grade. Each child was presented with a syringe and a stethoscope and told to pretend that he or she was a doctor. While children played, they were asked to explain what they were doing and why those actions were performed.

All children were able to identify the stethoscope, although the two age groups differed in their understanding of its function. Kindergartners typically responded that the stethoscope's function is to determine whether or not one's heart is beating. Third graders recognized that the stethoscope is used to examine certain qualities of the heartbeat, rather than merely to detect its presence.

All but one child recognized the syringe, though the reason for using this instrument was not readily apparent to kindergartners. Many in this age group who demonstrated familiarity with injections did not know why they were given. Significantly more third graders identified the function of shots as curing or preventing illness than did the kindergartners. Furthermore, third graders frequently asserted that syringes contain medicine, while those in the kindergarten group (whose concept of medicine was reportedly restricted to orally ingested medications) denied that this was so.

Bernheimer (1981) investigated the perceptions of children (ages 5 years, 10 months to 6 years, 10 months) concerning routine health care, relating those perceptions to children's coping behaviors during a physical examination. The majority of children were found to have a "medically correct" understanding of procedures, recognizing their evaluative nature. However, the amount or type of knowledge possessed by children was unrelated to a summary score of their behavior across several events during the examination.

Bernheimer's results were partially replicated by Thompson (1983), who interviewed five-year-old children prior to their "kindergarten" physical examination. Children were asked to identify and give the function of a doctor, a shot or injection, and a series of other medical instruments to be used during their examination. Responses indicated a high degree of familiarity with the medical items, with more than ninety percent of the children identifying the doctor, stethoscope, tongue blade, and blood pressure cuff. The only item identified by fewer than seventy percent of the respondents was the otoscope. The majority of those children designating a function for the stethoscope, otoscope, reflex hammer, tongue blade, and blood pressure cuff accurately asserted that these instruments were for evaluation of one's condition. In contrast, the primary function of doctors and injections was considered to be *treatment* of an existing illness or injury. Increased ability of children to identify items and to offer a function for each was associated with reduced upset during the physician's examination.

Concepts of Medical Personnel

Steward and Regalbuto (1975) briefly discuss children's conceptions of doctors. The kindergartners interviewed almost unanimously denied having visited a doctor, although subsequent conversation with the children revealed that each had experience with doctors and medical settings. Nevertheless, the authors report that kindergartners "did not associate doctors with health or illness" (p. 149). Third graders, on the other hand, freely discussed their health care experiences, citing instances of contact with doctors for both treatment and prevention of illness.

The Steward and Regalbuto findings concerning kindergartners differ from those of Thompson (1983) who reports that 95 percent of the five year olds in the sample (interviewed approximately one week prior to a physical examination) defined doctors in terms of treatment, evaluation, or prevention of illness. Children's awareness of the impending medical visit and the more directive format of the interview may account for the discrepancy.

Two studies have examined children's perceptions of the role of nursing personnel (Hymovich, 1973; Rumfelt, 1980). Hymovich (1973) interviewed surgical and nonsurgical patients (4 to 8 years of age), as well as the nurses caring for them, to measure subjects' perceptions of the *instrumental* (medical caregiving) and *expressive* (emotionally supportive) components of the nursing role. Also assessed were children's ability to view the nursing role from the nurse's perspective, and the nurses' perceptions of their own "nursing style."

Though Hymovich had anticipated that surgical patients would perceive nursing as more instrumental than would the nonsurgical patients, no such difference was found. Furthermore, the expectation that children would view the nursing role as less expressive than would the nurses themselves was true only for older subjects. Those between seven and eight years of age saw the role of nursing as more instrumental than did younger children. Patients were largely unable to adopt the nurses' perspective in viewing the role of nursing.

Rumfelt (1980) used two instruments to assess hospitalized and nonhospitalized five-year-old children's perceptions of the role of nursing. The first instrument consisted of a set of 37 cards depicting various items and articles of apparel. Children were shown each item and asked whether a nurse who cares for children would need it.

The responses of hospitalized and nonhospitalized children did not differ greatly, although, as mentioned above, some perceptions of the hospitalized group appear to have been modified by their medical experience. For example, fewer hospitalized children said that nurses need a traditional white cap or a glass thermometer than did nonhospitalized subjects. The author notes that nurses in the research hospital setting wore no caps and used digital thermometers. The responses of children in both groups indicate that they were aware of the nurturant role of the nurse and also that nurses have lives outside of the clinical setting.

Rumfelt further presented a series of ten ambiguous pictures of female nurses with children in pediatric settings. Children were instructed to look at each picture and describe the nurses' actions. Responses were classified according to the nature of the action described by subjects, as well as the implied intent of that action.

The majority of children's responses described clinical actions (i.e., requiring the use of specialized skill or knowledge). Sixty percent of these responses were given by nonhospitalized children. Furthermore, a majority of the responses describing nurses as giving injections came from subjects in the nonhospitalized group. Rumfelt speculates that nonhospitalized children's lack of medical experience may have been responsible for their stereotypical views. No child in either group described a nurse as playing with children.

Analysis of the *implied intent* of nurses' actions in children's descriptions revealed few instances of aggressive or punitive intent. Sixty percent of the actions were described as neutral, with 21 percent deemed nurturant. In only four percent of the cases were the nurse's actions considered to be purposeful attempts to inflict pain or discomfort.

Concepts of Isolation Technique

Pidgeon (1967) interviewed fifty children, ranging in age from three to seventeen years, who were hospitalized in an isolation unit. Children were asked to explain why nurses wear gowns when entering their room, why there were no other children with them, and why they could not leave. Responses were scored for accuracy, with those indicating an "awareness of one or more principle basic to isolation" (p. 22) scored as correct, while responses showing no such awareness were incorrect. In addition, explanations were classified as *precausal* (providing exclusively psychological or moral reasons for isolation), *causal* (giving physical or mechanical reasons), or *mixed* (combining precausal and causal reasoning).

As would be expected, the highest percentage of incorrect answers occurred among the youngest children. Seventy-one percent of the children three to seven years of age gave incorrect responses to at least two of the three questions regarding isolation. Among children five to twelve years, this figure dropped to 23 percent, while only eight percent of the children twelve to seventeen years old gave two or more incorrect answers.

A similar age-related pattern was evident in the types of reasoning used by children. Thirty-three percent of the explanations given by children in the youngest age group were precausal. Only 12.5 percent of the children seven to twelve years of age, and none of those in the oldest age group, gave precausal explanations.

Pidgeon notes that the percentage of precausal responses given by children was smaller than expected, indicating that medical treatment is not universally viewed in moral terms by young children. Despite the relatively small proportion of precausal explanations, misconceptions concerning isolation were common. For example, gowning was described as a means of keeping clothes from getting wet or dirty. Separation from other children was viewed as a method of limiting the patients' disturbance due to noise or crying of other children. Furthermore, the purpose of confinement was, according to some children, to keep the patient from getting lost or cold.

Concepts of Research Hospitalization

Prompted by the increasing necessity to obtain informed consent prior to participation in medical research, not only from parents, but also from children capable of granting it, Schwartz (1972) examined children's capacity for understanding "research hospitalization." The sample consisted of 36 children, four to seventeen years of age, hospitalized at a clinical research center, most of whom were admitted with a diagnosis of short stature. The intent of the admission was not therapeutic. Rather, subjects were hospitalized for study to contribute to the general medical knowledge concerning their condition.

Patients and families were prepared for hospitalization by a physician beginning six months to one year prior to the event. Families visited the hospital before admission and met members of the staff, including a social worker who discussed "research hospitalization" and gave parents further suggestions for preparing their children for the experience. Although the extent of the information given to children by parents was not known, Schwartz notes that each child was present more than once during discussions of research hospitalization and had made at least one visit to the setting prior to admission.

All children were interviewed by a child psychiatrist within 48 hours of admission and again between the seventh and tenth day of their two- to three-week hospitalization. During these interviews, children's understanding of the purpose of the hospitalization and procedures was ascertained. None of the seventeen children under eleven years of age understood that the hospitalization was related to research. Only six of the nineteen children over eleven years expressed awareness of the research nature of their hospitalization. Five of the six children expressing this awareness were said to have demonstrated symptoms of extreme anxiety. Schwartz suggests that, "it is only after the age of 11 that a child may be aware of being a research subject, and that such awareness may result in overwhelming anxiety" (p. 592).

The inability of children to comprehend the meaning of research hospitalization is not surprising in light of the results of an earlier study conducted by McCollum and Schwartz (1969). In this instance, 140 parents were interviewed prior to the admission of their children to a clinical research center concerning their understanding of the hospitalization. Despite previous discussions with medical personnel concerning the nature of the admission, more than 40 percent of the parents (N = 61) displayed no awareness that their child's hospitalization was for purposes of research.

Chapter 4

RESEARCH ON SPECIFIC PROCEDURES AND ENVIRONMENTS

The stated purpose of much of the research reviewed in this volume is to examine the psychological impact of "hospitalization" on children and their families. Hospitalization, of course, is not a unitary construct, but rather is composed of differing combinations of conditions, events, and environments that interact with the personal and social characteristics of children. Studies considered in the present chapter pertain to two such categories of elements believed to influence children's psychological state: specific procedures commonly experienced by hospitalized children, and the environments in which children receive care. Research documenting children's reactions to medical procedures and treatment (including injections, restraint, rectal temperatures, binocular bandaging, anesthesia induction, and cardiac catheterization) and to hospital settings (such as the intensive care unit, recovery room, isolation units, and emergency room) are reviewed. Whenever applicable, data on parents' responses to procedures or environments and on the effectiveness of interventions intended to minimize emotional distress are also considered.

HOSPITAL PROCEDURES AND TREATMENTS

Injections

One of the most frightening and ubiquitous events experienced by young hospitalized children is the injection. In their classic 1952 study, Jessner, Blom, and Waldfogel interviewed 143 children hospitalized for tonsillectomy surgery, identifying the principal focus of anxiety for each child. Within each of four age groups studied, an appreciable number of children (ranging from 6 to 20% of each group) identified fear of needles as their *primary* source of anxiety. Among children under five years of age, fear of needles was mentioned as frequently as was fear of the operation itself.

Research published since 1965 has considered the injection in several ways. For example, the procedure has been viewed as representative of stressful events occurring during a child's hospitalization. Therefore, observation of children's responses to an injection has served as an indicator of upset, most often to assess the effects of preparation programs (e.g., Wolfer & Visintainer, 1975, 1979; Visintainer & Wolfer, 1975; Schwartz, et al., 1983). Studies addressing injections in this manner are considered more fully in Chapter 10. Other researchers have investigated the administering of injections to identify factors associated with children's upset during the procedure (Thompson, 1983) or to examine interventions designed to help children cope with the event (Torrance, 1968; Vernon, 1974; Eland, 1981; Fernald & Corry, 1981). A final study reviewed in this section evaluates the correspondence between children's self-report of pain experienced during an injection and their behavioral responses (Hester, 1979).

Factors Associated with Upset During Injections. In conjunction with a study examining five-year-old children's responses to an outpatient physical examination, Thompson (1983) obtained data on children's behavior during, and on their heart rate immediately after, an injection. Reactions during the injection were unrelated to measures of children's general knowledge or concepts of health care and illness, with one exception. Greater tendency to interpret illness as punishment was associated with increased behavioral upset in response to the injection. In addition, increased time spent in the waiting room prior to examination, and parent anxiety during the examination, were positively correlated with children's heart rate following the injection.

Since nearly one quarter of the sample had, at some point, received inpatient medical care, the possible influence of a past hospital admission on children's reactions to the injection was examined. Both the occurrence of, and children's reactions during, the prior hospitalization were significantly related to subjects' current upset. Children who had been previously hospitalized displayed higher levels of behavioral upset during the injection than subjects never hospitalized. Moreover, children previously hospitalized under *emergency* circumstances showed more behavioral upset in response to the injection than did children hospitalized for elective surgery.

The possible influence of sex, age, and birth order on children's responses to injections have also been considered. Neither Eland (1981) nor Thompson (1983) report significant sex differences, though Torrance (1968) found females to be more upset during the procedure than male subjects. The latter finding may have been affected by subjects' age, since females participating in the study were younger than males. However, when Torrance directly considered the age factor (comparing the reactions of older and younger subjects among a sample ranging from 3 to 7 years) no significant differences were found. Vernon (1974) considered the importance of birth order, finding early born subjects to be more upset prior to injection than later born subjects. This difference was not evident during the administration of the injection.

Approaches to Reducing Upset During Injections. The amount of upset experienced during an injection is potentially modifiable through alterations in technical aspects of the procedure or through preparation of children for the event. Research has addressed both of these approaches. For example, Torrance (1968) compared the reactions of children (3 to 7 years of age, hospitalized for minor elective surgery) to injections given with an ordinary syringe (N = 20) versus an automated jet spray apparatus (N = 21). Behavioral observation and data on children's heart rate before, during, and after the procedure revealed few differences in reactions attributable to the method of injection.

Eland (1981) examined the effectiveness of a skin coolant, Frigiderm, on children's subjective assessments of their pain during an injection. It was believed that the coolant would reduce children's pain by altering the ability of small nerve fibers to transmit pain messages. Half of the forty children in the sample had the coolant sprayed on their skin prior to the injection. The injection site of the others was sprayed with aerosol air instead. Significantly less pain was reported by children receiving the coolant.

The effects of the type of explanation given to children immediately before the injection were further assessed by Eland. Half of the children in each spray group were told that the spray would feel cool and would help reduce the pain of the shot. The others were merely told that something would be sprayed on their skin. No effect was found for type of introductory message given to children.

Two manners of approaching and interacting with children prior to an arm venipuncture or fingerstick were contrasted by Fernald and Corry (1981). Thirty-nine children, three to nine years of age, were randomly assigned to either the *empathic* or *directive* treatment condition. Subjects in each group were approached by the same male laboratory technician, who introduced himself and briefly explained what would happen during the procedure. Following this basic explanation, children in the empathic group were informed that the procedure was not intended as a punishment, that it might hurt, and that they could cry if they wished. The technician also commented on the sensations the children might experience. All information was given while the technician knelt down to the child's eye level. Children were encouraged to participate in the procedure, by holding an empty syringe or drying alcohol from their skin with a cotton swab. Subjects in the directive group, on the other hand, were essentially told to be brave, not cry, and remain still. No effort was made to involve these children in the process.

Observations of children's behavior during the procedure were made, though it is unclear whether this was done by the technician conducting the procedure or an independent observer. The authors report that empathic group children displayed lower levels of crying, negative remarks, wincing, and refusal to comply than did subjects in the directive group. Furthermore, in response to questions asked after the procedure, directive group children more frequently expressed anger toward the technician and the belief that he had intended to hurt them.

In a study of the preparation of children for injections using a filmed modeling approach, Vernon (1974) randomly assigned thirty children (four to nine years of age, hospitalized for minor surgery) to one of three groups. Children in the *no-pain-movie* group viewed a film in which a series of children received injections with no apparent fear or discomfort. Those in the *pain-movie* group saw a film similar to that of the first group, but in which children exhibited transitory, moderate reactions to the injection. *Control* group subjects saw neither film. Children viewing either of the modeling films did so in their own homes the evening before admission to the hospital, approximately 36 hours before receiving an injection.

Children's behavior was observed and rated prior to and during administration of the injection. Though the groups did not differ immediately before the injection, significant differences in upset were noted during the procedure. Subjects in the pain-movie group manifested the least distress, while the upset level of children who had viewed the no-pain movie was greatest, exceeding even that of control group children. Vernon interprets these results as evidence that "modelling that conveys accurate information about the nature and/or timing of a painful stimulus can ameliorate pain, while modeling that conveys inaccurate information can increase pain" (p. 787).

Self-report of Pain During Injections. Self-report measures have been frequently used to assess children's perceptions of fear, upset, or discomfort under specified conditions (e.g., see Melamed & Siegel, 1975; Johnson, Kirchhoff, & Endress, 1975; Eland, 1981). The nature of the relationship between children's subjective assessments of the pain experienced during an injection and their behavioral manifestations of discomfort were examined by Hester (1979), who selected two separate self-report measures for consideration: Eland's (1974) Projective Tool (an instrument different than that used by Eland, 1981) and a Poker Chip Tool developed by Hester for this project.

The 44 children sampled ranged in age from four to seven years and were classified as preoperational thinkers on the basis of Piagetian tasks. Vocal, verbal, facial, and motor responses of the children were observed during an outpatient immunization, following which the subjective assessments of pain were administered. The Eland Projective Tool consists of four pictures of an animal experiencing painful events with which children would be familiar.

Subjects are asked to order these pictures from least to most painful, then to insert a picture of the same animal receiving an injection in rank order with the others. Children's ranking of the injection picture constitutes their pain score. The Poker Chip Tool consists of four white chips that the children are told correspond to "pieces of hurt." Children are asked to select the number of chips corresponding to the degree of pain they experienced during the injection.

Significant rank order correlations were found between the Poker Chip Tool and all four types of behavior observed, although only two of these correlations (those with vocal and verbal behaviors) were in the expected direction. Observed ratings of facial and motor behavior were *inversely* related to children's subjective assessments of pain. The Eland Projective Tool was found to correlate positively with children's vocal behavior and negatively with their facial behavior, while correlations with verbal and motor responses were not significant. Nonsignificant relationships were also reported between the two subjective measures of pain in response to an injection. Hester suggests two explanations for the unanticipated findings concerning facial and motor responses. Either these behaviors are invalid indices of pain for subjects of this age, or "the motor and facial expression may be gating mechanisms used by children to abate pain" (p. 253).

Immobilization

Restrictions of the physical activity of hospitalized children through casting, application of splints, or the restraining of limbs to minimize interference with medical equipment has been implicated in the disturbance of children's emotional, cognitive, and physical development. For example, Williams (1973) suggests that, "Restriction of a child's motility activates varying degrees of aggressive and regressive reactions, ranging from severe lethargy to restlessness or hyperactivity, to a full-blown rage-like reaction as the child attempts to cope with the hampering of his instinctual drive" (p. 233). Similarly, Becker (1975) contends that, "The evidence is as strong as it is convincing that immobilizing experiences of whatever nature and prescribed for whatever reason have the potential for a significant and dramatic interference with a host of interpersonal relationships which may be necessary for the acquisition of basic learning skills, indeed including speech," (p. 256). Dowd, Novak, and Ray (1977) note the adverse physical consequences of restraint, citing evidence that immobilization results in loss of muscle strength and excretion of essential electrolytes.

There can be little doubt that physical restraint is distressing, especially to children who are too young to understand its function and are likely to misinterpret its use. Holt (1967, 1968) conducted a series of interviews with children who, five years earlier, had been hospitalized as preschoolers. Subjects who recalled being restrained, including confinement to bed, considered this to be among the most disagreeable aspects of their hospital experience. Holt reports that when, in the course of interviews, children recalled hospital personnel "with negative affect, restraint was the theme" (1968, p. 65). Barnes (1975a, 1975b) found misunderstanding or exaggeration of the use of restraints to be common among children hospitalized in an intensive care unit. Unfortunately, the research literature since 1965 documenting the emotional or developmental effects of immobilization is sparse. Moreover, the few studies that exist are limited by methodological problems.

Two studies conducted by Sibinga and colleagues suggest that immobilization at an early age is associated with delays in intellectual and language development and with difficulties in speech articulation. In the first of these studies, Sibinga, et al. (1968) considered thirty children with phenylketonuria (PKU). Parents of the subjects were interviewed to ascertain whether their children had been immobilized, isolated, or physically restricted prior to three years of age. Investigators made special inquiries about procedures used by parents to control behaviors such as indiscriminate eating, hyperactivity, head-banging, or nail-biting. On the basis of these interviews, children were assigned to either the "stress" (i.e., immobilization) group or the control group. The characteristics of the groups were then compared.

Fourteen of the sixteen stress-group children had been previously hospitalized, compared to only three of the fourteen children in the control group. Subjects in the stress group were found to manifest more severe and frequent symptoms of emotional disturbance than control group children and to have significantly lower scores on measures of intelligence, language comprehension, and interpersonal relations.

While Sibinga, et al. suggest that the immobilization is responsible for these differences, this contention is suspect. The stress group is distinguished from the control group by several, possibly interrelated characteristics (e.g., higher rate of hospitalization and greater emotional disturbance) in addition to the history of immobilization, all of which may simply be indicators of greater severity of children's medical condition. Confounding of these factors makes unambiguous attribution of test score differences to prior immobilization unwarranted.

Methodological problems also limit interpretation of a subsequent study by Sibinga and Friedman (1971). Seventy-one children who had previously experienced immobilization were considered. Through interviews with parents, investigators determined whether children had experienced speech delays or articulation problems. The neurological status of the children was also assessed, with children categorized as having no brain damage, questionable brain damage, or clear brain damage. Language delay and articulation problems were noted in at least 55 percent of the children in each neurological group. However, given the method of sample selection, this high incidence of problems is hardly surprising. Most children participating in the study were identified after visiting a clinic for evaluation of speech or emotional problems, or were siblings of children undergoing such evaluation.

Though the potential problems of motor restriction have not been rigorously documented, some attempts have been made to modify the use of restraints. For example, Dowd, et al. (1977) describe a program consisting of preparation of children for restraint, removal of restraints every two hours for ten minutes, changing of children's position before replacing restraints, and the providing of stimulation while children are immobilized. The authors made informal observations of 29 children immobilized for a variety of reasons. During periods of immobilization, children less than eighteen months of age cried and fought their restraints. Older children also cried when restrained, though they displayed less struggling behavior. When restraints were initially removed from infants, they remained temporarily immobile, as if unaware of the removal. However, as the infants experienced several cycles of release and reapplication of restraints, they became more active upon release and demonstrated more upset with subsequent restraint. Protests of toddlers and preschoolers, on the other hand, decreased with successive release and restraint cycles. During the periods of release, none of the children attempted to disturb tubes or suture lines.

Rectal Temperatures

Only one research project specifically investigated children's responses to rectal temperatures. In this study, McCaffery (1971) examined the effects of a preparation experience on children's behavior during the procedure. Temperatures of the 27 children (30 to 54 months of age) were taken twice per day for three days. On the first day, children were provided with no preparation or play prior to the procedure. On each of the remaining two days, children in an experimental condition received preparation from a nurse who demonstrated the process with the use of a doll and allowed the children to take the doll's temperature. Control group children participated in a play session requiring the same type of child-nurse interaction as that of the experimental group preparation. Instances of negative, passive, and positive behavior during the rectal temperature procedure were recorded by an observer. In addition, the nurse taking the temperature noted whether children's anal sphincter and/or gluteal muscles were contracted or relaxed. All children were allowed to play with a small pail and blocks during this period.

Despite an attempt to match children on factors such as age, sex, medical status, previous hospitalization, and familiarity with rectal temperatures, significant differences in behavior were noted between control and experimental group children on the first day of the study, *prior* to any intervention. Experimental group children displayed more positive and fewer negative behaviors at that time than did those in the control group. Following the institution of play and preparation interventions on the second day, the total positive and negative behaviors of the two groups approximated each other.

Differences in specific behaviors were, nevertheless, noted from the pre- to post-intervention sessions. For example, the experimental condition was found to be effective in reducing muscle contraction, and in decreasing children's negative verbal responses and their tendency to pull away from the experimenter. The control condition, on the other hand, was found to reduce the frequency of children's calling for parents. Overall, behaviors noted most often among children during the procedure were (in decreasing order of frequency) lying still without resistance, playing, and crying or screaming.

Binocular Bandaging

Through incidental observations, Riddle (1972) came to believe that hospitalized children wearing binocular bandages exhibit a characteristic pattern of behavior, which she described as "passively compliant." To assess the accuracy of this impression, the communicative behaviors of five children (7 to 12 years of age, hospitalized for eye trauma necessitating the wearing of binocular bandages for a minimum of four days) were investigated. The author visited the subjects daily during their hospitalization, conducting unstructured interviews. In addition, observations were made of children's nonverbal behavior and of their interaction with hospital personnel and other children.

Children's communication with unfamiliar people while wearing bandages was characterized as restricted, and was "distinguished by lack of verbal spontaniety, a limited use of gestures to enhance verbal information, and a frequent use of movements as a substitute for verbal responses" (p. 348). The author attributes this behavior to children's inability to make eye contact or to gain visual feedback—a situation that limits their knowledge of the identities, intentions, and actions of people in their proximity.

In contrast to their behavior with strangers, children displayed more spontaneous, expressive communication when with the investigator by the third day of her visits. Following removal of bandages, children exhibited active, social involvement with, and inquisitiveness about, others in the hospital environment. None of the children were found to experience mental confusion or perceptual disturbances—conditions occasionally reported among adults wearing binocular bandages.

Anesthesia Induction

Among the threatening procedures encountered by pediatric surgical patients is the induction of anesthesia. Fears and misconceptions concerning the involuntary loss of consciousness are often compounded by situational factors, such as separation from parents prior to induction, exposure to unfamiliar equipment, and the approach of strangers in medical apparel. The research literature includes descriptive information on children's responses to anesthesia induction (Bothe & Galdston, 1972; Davenport & Werry, 1970; Hanna & Sherlock, 1983), as well as data on factors potentially associated with children's immediate or posthospital psychological responses to anesthesia such as the presence of parents before or during induction (Kay, 1966; Vernon, et al., 1967; Schulman, et al., 1967; Lee & Greene, 1969), preparation of children for the procedure (Vernon, 1973; Vernon & Bailey, 1974), differences in approaches used by medical personnel (Meyers & Muravchick, 1977; Schulman, et al., 1967; Vernon, et al., 1967), and children's birth order (Vernon, et al., 1967).

Responses to Anesthesia. Bothe and Galdston (1972) considered the responses of fifty children to the induction of anesthesia. Subjects (who were 4 to 14 years of age, hospitalized for minor surgical procedures) were interviewed the night before, the morning of, and the day after surgery concerning their understanding and perceptions of events associated with anesthesia. In addition, observations of children's behavior were made during induction and upon emergence from anesthesia. Two-thirds of the subjects were said to manifest signs of obvious apprehension while in the area outside of the operating room. During the induction procedure, most children were reported to regard the anesthesia mask with caution. Nevertheless, the incidence of difficult inductions (characterized by open crying, shouting of objections, or physical resistance) was relatively low, occurring in only seven children (or 14% of the sample). This finding corresponds to data provided by Lee and Greene (1969), who found that 14.6 percent of their sample (in this case, a somewhat younger group of children, 1 to 8 years of age) cried upon arrival at the operating room. Davenport and Werry (1970) report that fewer than six percent of their sample (1 through 15 years of age) experienced "real difficulty" with induction.

The incidence of disturbance during emergence from anesthesia was similarly low, according to Bothe and Galdston. Only five children (10% of the sample) emerged from anesthesia with obvious, agitated physical behavior. In no instance did this behavior persist longer than twenty minutes, nor could children reacting in this manner recall the experience when questioned about it the day after surgery.

Hanna and Sherlock (1983) also report that events in the immediate postoperative period are recalled by children with less frequency than those occurring prior to surgery. Of the fifty children who were asked to describe what they remembered about their surgery, 76 percent recalled a preoperative injection, 86 percent the ride to the operating room, and 68 percent the arrival in the operating suite. However, only 36 percent of the children described waking up in the recovery room and 30 percent mentioned the ride back to the ward following surgery. Recall of the induction procedure itself varied with the type of anesthesia given. Eighty percent of the children having intravenous induction remembered insertion of the needle, but only 35 percent having inhalational induction recalled the anesthesia mask. Few children spontaneously expressed fears associated with the events of surgery or anesthesia.

Effects of Age. An early study of children's reactions to tonsillectomy and adenoidectomy surgery, conducted by Jessner, Blom, and Waldfogel (1952), indicated that subjects' fear of the impending loss of consciousness through anesthesia increased with age, becoming the primary focus of anxiety among surgical patients ten to fourteen years old. The relationship between children's *age* and their behavioral responses to anesthesia has been examined in several studies conducted since 1965, with this research yielding inconclusive results. Bothe and Galdston (1972) provide observational data corresponding to the subjective responses reported by Jessner, et al., noting that children who resisted anesthesia induction tended to be among the older subjects in a sample ranging from four to fourteen years. In contrast, studies limiting their samples to children seven years of age or less have documented more behavioral disturbances among younger children. For example, Lee and Greene (1969) report a greater incidence of crying among children under five years of age than among those five or older. Vernon, et al. (1967) found two- to three-year-old children to be significantly more upset during the first minute of anesthesia induction than four- to five-year-old subjects.

If taken together, these studies could suggest the existence of a U-shaped relationship between age and the behavioral upset associated with anesthesia. However, the research currently available does not permit assessment of this possibility. The only study of children's responses to anesthesia that has considered a sample of sufficiently wide age range to meaningfully examine this relationship presents no information on the impact of age (Davenport & Werry, 1970). The sample used by Bothe and Galdston spanned a ten-year period, but included no children less than four years old. In the absence of a well-designed observational study including children from early preschool years through late schoolage and early adolescence, the precise influence of age on children's responses to anesthesia remains speculative.

Effects of Parent Presence. The effect of *parent presence* during anesthesia induction has also been investigated. Kay (1966) found that children accompanied by parents (especially children one through six years of age) were less upset in the anesthesia area than unaccompanied patients. Vernon, et al. (1967; also reported in Schulman, et al., 1967) similarly observed less upset among children immediately prior to induction ($p < .10$) and during the final minutes of induction ($p < .01$) when parents were present for the procedure. Neither Kay (1966) nor Vernon, et al. (1967) report significant posthospital differences between accompanied and unaccompanied children. Lee and Greene (1969) observed an elevated level of crying upon arrival at the operating room among children whose parents had roomed-in the night before surgery. However, this finding is confounded with age effects, since children of rooming-in parents were younger than subjects whose parents chose not to room-in.

Effects of Preparation. The effectiveness of *preparation* for anesthesia induction on children's responses to the procedure was examined by Vernon (1973; also reported in Vernon & Bailey,

1974). Experimental group subjects, who had viewed a film depicting four children calmly undergoing anesthesia induction, were less upset than control subjects immediately prior to, but not during induction. The posthospital behavior of experimental and control group subjects did not differ significantly one week after discharge from the hospital. However, when assessed again three weeks later, children prepared for anesthesia through use of filmed modeling exhibited significantly less behavioral upset than subjects given no preparation. Other research evaluating preparation of children for surgery has documented increased cooperation and reduced levels of resistance or upset prior to anesthesia induction (Visintainer & Wolfer, 1975; Wolfer & Visintainer, 1975, 1979; Schwartz, et al., 1983).

Variations in Induction Techniques. Meyers and Muravchick (1977) contrasted the effects of differing styles of anesthesia induction on children's posthospital behavioral responses. Forty-eight of the subjects in the sample (all of whom were 1 through 8 years of age) were visited the night before surgery by an anesthesiologist who briefly explained the induction procedures. Preoperative medications were given to these subjects more than an hour before anesthesia induction. Twenty-four of these children were asleep upon arrival at the operating room and were anesthetized without being awakened. The other 24 (who were awake upon arrival) received anesthesia from medical personnel who elicited children's cooperation with the procedure or provided them with distractions.

A third group of 37 subjects received no preoperative visit from an anesthesiologist. All children in this group were premedicated by the surgeons and anesthetized while awake. Within a month after discharge from the hospital, parents of subjects in these three anesthesia groups, as well as parents of a control group of 37 pediatric inpatients who had not received anesthesia, completed a questionnaire on their children's posthospital behavior.

Although systematic observations of children's behavior during induction were not made, the authors report that subjects who had received no preoperative visit were often frightened and upset during the anesthesia induction and frequently required restraint. Nevertheless, comparisons of the total number of behavioral disturbances manifested by subjects failed to reveal significant differences in upset among the four groups. In fact, the only significant difference noted occurred within the group of subjects who had received the preoperative visit. A larger percentage of children in this group who had been anesthetized while asleep manifested no posthospital behavioral difficulties than subjects who were awake during anesthesia induction.

Data provided by Vernon, et al. (1967; also reported in Schulman, et al., 1967) suggest that children's immediate reactions to anesthesia induction may be influenced by the manner of the medical personnel performing the procedure. Ratings of children's mood during the first minute of induction were found to vary significantly among groups of patients treated by different anesthetists. The subjective impression of an observer who rated children's behavior was that the variation in patient responses reflected the attempts of individual anesthetists to establish rapport with children prior to anesthesia induction.

Birth Order. A final factor considered in the literature, children's *birth order*, appears to be unrelated to patients' responses to anesthesia. Vernon, et al. (1967) found no significant differences between early born and later born subjects' immediate responses to anesthesia or their posthospital behavior. Also unrelated to birth order was the effectiveness of preparation for anesthesia.

Cardiac Catheterization

A commonly performed diagnostic procedure receiving some attention in the research literature is cardiac catheterization. Concern over children's responses to this procedure arises since patients are typically conscious during portions of catheterization and are, therefore, exposed to stimuli in surgical areas that patients receiving general anesthesia may avoid. Moreover, information obtained during catheterization may indicate the need for surgery. An unpleasant experience during this diagnostic procedure may negatively affect children's responses to subsequent hospitalization. The research reviewed in this section considers children's psychological responses to the procedure (Youssef, 1981; Aisenberg, Wolff, Rosenthal, & Nadas, 1973) and the effectiveness of a preparation intervention (Cassell, 1965; Cassell & Paul, 1967).

The coping behaviors of ten schoolaged children hospitalized for catheterization were observed by Youssef (1981) during four periods: on admission, during an echocardiogram, during the catheterization itself, and upon discharge. The most frequently observed coping behaviors were the *orienting* of oneself to the situation (predominant in all periods, except at discharge) and *seeking support* from oneself or others (common during both medical procedures). Less evident were children's attempts to *avoid* necessary activities or their *expression of feelings*. Few of the behaviors exhibited by children indicated *loss of control* (e.g., whimpering, crying, screaming, etc.). However, nearly all observed instances of loss of control behavior occurred during the catheterization procedure (see Chapter 2).

Aisenberg, et al. (1973) examined the psychological impact of cardiac catheterization on fifty children between four and fifteen years of age. Data on children's responses were obtained through direct observation on the ward and during catheterization, through interviews with patients and parents, and through psychological tests administered to the subjects. Though children received premedication prior to catheterization, none of the procedures was performed under general anesthesia. Four children slept throughout the catheterization, and nine remained awake, with the other 41 patients fluctuating between sleep and waking states.

No measurable psychological changes were found in twelve of the patients following catheterization. Three children were judged to be improved following the hospitalization, with a positive response indicated by developmentally more mature responses to psychological assessments and greater social adaptation after the catheterization than before. The remaining 35 children exhibited negative responses. Among the commonly observed changes were increases in physical and verbal aggression, behavioral regression, attitudinal and affective changes, and increased anxiety. Negative reactions were found to be age-related, decreasing in frequency among older subjects.

Preparation of children for cardiac catheterization has been examined by Cassell (1965; also reported in Cassell & Paul, 1967). Prior to catheterization, half of the forty subjects observed were allowed to play through the procedure using puppets and miniature medical equipment, while the others received no experimental intervention. Observations indicated that children receiving preparation were less upset than control group children during the catheterization procedure. However, no differences were noted in the behavior of experimental and control subjects on the day of discharge, nor did parents report differences in children's behavior on return home. Nevertheless, experimental group children expressed a greater willingness than control group children to return to the hospital after discharge, should it be necessary.

SPECIFIC HOSPITAL ENVIRONMENTS

Reactions exhibited by children and parents in the hospital may be partially attributable to the context in which care is provided. Among the specific areas of the hospital receiving research attention because of their potential for producing or exacerbating upset are the intensive care unit, the recovery room, isolation units, and the emergency room.

Intensive Care Units

Concern has been frequently expressed for the emotional well-being of children hospitalized in the intensive care unit (ICU). Aside from the serious nature of the condition necessitating admission to the ICU, children in such units are believed to be at risk for several reasons. The environment is foreign, typically intense, and, paradoxically, capable of providing children with overstimulation (e.g., from continuous lighting, sounds from monitors, nursing activities) or sensory deprivation (limited activities, little change in the physical setting). Moreover, children in the ICU may passively observe a variety of illness conditions, treatments performed on others, and possibly the death of fellow patients, all with little or no explanation. Further concern for children is based on studies of adult postoperative cardiac patients, which indicate that a condition of transient delirium in the intensive care unit (sometimes referred to as ICU syndrome) is not uncommon. In the present section, research concerning the hospitalization of children in intensive care units will be reviewed, including studies on children's reactions in the ICU, their recall of the experience following discharge, the effects of play interventions designed to alter children's behavior in the unit, and the responses of parents to an ICU experience.

Children's Reactions in the ICU. Periods of delirium have been frequently observed among adult patients in the intensive care unit following cardiac surgery, though the etiology of this condition is unclear. Kaplan, Achtel, and Callison (1974) list several factors as possibly contributing to this so-called ICU syndrome, including neurological deficits resulting from surgery, the amount of time blood flow through the heart is bypassed during the operation, and conditions related to the ICU experience itself, such as sleep disruption or stimulus deprivation.

Despite the frequent occurrence of this condition among adults, instances of delirium among children appear to be less common. In their review of the literature on postcardiotomy psychosis, Lasater and Grisanti (1975) uncovered virtually no evidence of ICU syndrome among children under fourteen to sixteen years of age. For example, Kornfeld, Zimberg, and Malm (1965) found no psychiatric complications among twenty children undergoing surgery to correct congenital defects. Kaplan, et al. (1974), on the other hand, observed transient delirium postoperatively in five of 58 cardiac patients, seven to fourteen years of age. Though the incidence of ICU syndrome among children may be low, reports of its occurrence are not limited to cardiac patients. May (1972), for example, examined the responses of patients in a pediatric intensive care unit, hospitalized for various conditions, and found their reactions to be "surprisingly mild," although many children were observed to have "fluctuating degrees of delirium" (p. 78).

In addition to recording instances of delirium among pediatric patients, researchers have examined other reactions manifested by children hospitalized in the ICU. Cataldo, Bessman, Parker, Pearson, and Rogers (1979) observed the behavior of 99 ICU patients (two days to 22 years of age) admitted for medical and surgical conditions. Using a time sampling technique, observers recorded data concerning children's waking state, position, verbalizations, eye contact, activity, and affective state. Information on caregiver verbalizations and the number and identity of persons at children's bedside was also obtained.

Fifty-four percent of the children were said to be either sleeping, in a coma, or in a medically induced state of unconsciousness, with eleven percent awake and thirty-five percent alert, as well as awake. Among the children judged to be awake and alert, substantially more negative affect (33% of all observations) was noted than positive affect (3%), with a majority of children displaying "neutral" affect (58%). Verbalizations by awake and alert children were rare, occurring in only eighteen percent of the observations. The modal form of eye contact, recorded in 37 percent of the observations, was described as "staring into space, scanning the room, or not attending to anything specific" (p. 88). Nonengagement in activities was noted in 54 percent of the observations, though in a second portion of the study, to be discussed below, the authors found the passive behavior of awake and alert patients to be modifiable through a program of planned play activities.

Carty (1977) investigated the behavioral responses of five preschool-aged children before, during, and after hospitalization in a pediatric intensive care unit. Data were collected through direct observation of children and through parents' assessments of their children's social maturity. Prior to entering the ICU, all children were found to have a social age at or beyond their chronological age. Though only one child displayed significantly high levels of anxious behavior before admission to the ICU, three of the five children (each of whom had been admitted to the ICU following a *surgical* procedure) manifested elevated levels of anxious behavior throughout their ICU stay. Of the children admitted with *medical* diagnoses, one displayed significant anxiety only on the first day in the ICU. The other medical patient (in the unit for only 24 hours) recorded levels of anxiety behavior considered to be within normal limits. With the exception of blood drawing, children were found to generally tolerate the majority of procedures performed on them while in the ICU, possibly crying, but not physically resisting. All five children, however, cried and resisted blood tests. None of the subjects displayed delirium while in the unit.

Upon return home, three of the five children (again, those having surgery) were found to have regressed in social age, while the two medical patients, who were also the youngest in the study, increased in social maturity. All children exhibited some disturbance of sleep patterns. Among other behaviors observed in a minority of the subjects were regression in toilet training, increased thumb sucking, hostility toward mothers, and increased discipline problems.

Levels of Consciousness and Recall of the ICU. Barnes (1975a, 1975b) examined children's responses to hospitalization in the intensive care unit using direct observation, interviews, and children's drawings. Thirteen children, six to thirteen years of age, hospitalized for heart surgery, were included in the sample. The nurse-investigator, who had prepared children for surgery and given them nursing care, observed each child for approximately four hours per day while in the ICU. Observations of children's general appearance, alertness to phenomena, movements, nonverbal responses and verbalizations were made in note form and subsequently transcribed into narratives. Two to four days after discharge from the ICU, children were asked to draw a picture of the unit and were later interviewed concerning their drawings.

Transcripts from observations and interviews were considered together. Within both sources of data, the investigator identified discrete units of behavior, with a unit defined as "a verbal or motor expression by the child that refers to one Intensive Care Unit phenomena or has its stimulus in the intensive care room" (Barnes, 1975a, p. 234). Units of behavior were coded for the types of phenomena referred to (treatments and procedures, persons, events, furnishings, or general phenomena) and for the level of consciousness exhibited in each unit. Level of consciousness categories included *alertness* (accurate understanding of phenomena), *distortion* (exaggeration or misunderstanding), *fantasy* (imagined responses), *affective memory* (responses referring to emotional experiences occurring prior to hospitalization), and *dreams.*

The majority of children's responses referred to treatments or procedures (55.5%), followed by references to persons (15.0%), events (12.3%), furnishings (12.2%), and other phenomena (5.0%). Analysis of the level of consciousness of children's responses indicated a high degree of accuracy in their perceptions, with 60.7 percent of all responses classified as alert. Nevertheless, 35 percent of the responses were said to be distorted. Misunderstandings or exaggerations were frequently present in children's discussions of pain, death, and use of restraints.

The Effects of Play on Children's Behavior in the ICU. Two related studies have examined the effects of the introduction of play activities on the behavior of children hospitalized in the ICU (Cataldo, Bessman, Parker, Pearson, & Rogers, 1979; Pearson, Cataldo, Turemann, Bessman, & Rogers, 1980). Subjects in the Cataldo, et al. (1979) study consisted of eleven patients, one to twenty-one years of age. Children were exposed to one of three experimental protocols, each consisting of three five-minute segments during which toys were either not available, were available with the supervision of a child life specialist, or were available by themselves. Affect, eye contact, interaction with materials, and the appropriateness of children's behaviors were observed and recorded during each segment.

The introduction of supervised play activities (following a period when toys were unavailable) resulted in increases in positive affect, appropriateness of behavior, and children's involvement with the environment. A corresponding decrease in children's attention to activities or people in their proximity was noted when both supervision and toys were withdrawn. A lesser decline in attention and interaction was recorded when toys were left with subjects following a period of supervised play. Moderately high levels of interaction with, and attention to, play materials were also apparent when toys were made available to children *prior* to the period of child life supervision.

Using a similar research design, Pearson, et al. (1980) observed the affect and interaction with materials of eleven ICU patients (2 to 17 years of age) prior to, during, and after a twenty-minute play intervention. All participating children had some play materials present during the preintervention period. Following the play intervention, the child life specialist conducting the session left the materials used with the child.

Substantial increases in both positive affect and interaction with materials were recorded during the intervention period. However, unlike in the Cataldo, et al. (1979) study, levels of these indices returned to baseline in the postintervention period, despite the fact that materials had been left with children. This difference is likely due to the timing of the postintervention observations.

Cataldo, et al. continued observations of children's behavior during the five minutes immediately following conclusion of the child life specialist's participation, whereas Pearson, et al. delayed the start of postintervention observations for some 30 to 45 minutes. Thus, it appears that, although children may have continued to play with materials for a time following withdrawal of supervision, the effects of the intervention were not observable after a period of delay. (See Chapter 9 for additional discussion of these studies).

Parent Responses to the ICU. Though several authors have surveyed or observed the parents of children hospitalized in intensive care units, only a limited amount of systematically presented data has resulted from this research. Harper and Varakis (1970) interviewed parents of children admitted to the adult ICU of a general hospital. Parent approval of the decision to hospitalize their children in the ICU, and of the care received while in the unit, was nearly universal. None of the parents contacted felt that the ICU experience had a lasting, adverse effect on their children. Parent comments favorable to the care received in *pediatric* intensive care units are also reported by May (1972) and by Fiser, Stanford, and Dorman (1984).

Lewandowski (1980) observed and interviewed 59 parents of children hospitalized in the ICU following open-heart surgery, in order to identify conditions perceived by parents as stressful and to assess their means of coping with the events. Among the elements found to cause the greatest stress were the decision to give consent for surgery (especially when the child appeared active and healthy at the time of diagnosis), the disruption of lifestyle caused by the hospital environment, the unfamiliarity and intensity of the ICU, the sight of the children following surgery, and the possibility that surgery might result in a child's death. Coping mechanisms used by parents, such as initial immobilization, visual survey of the unfamiliar environment, withdrawal, and intellectualization, are discussed.

Rothstein (1979, 1980) examined the reactions of parents whose children were admitted to a pediatric intensive care unit for catastrophic conditions such as major trauma, Reye's Syndrome, and septic shock. Through interviews with parents, the author identified a series of phases commonly experienced. Parents were said to initially encounter a period of overwhelming shock, characterized by feelings of helplessness and lasting about twelve hours. The next phase, occurring within the first twenty-four hours of the ICU experience, consisted of "a groping for explanations" (1979, p. 130). Self-blame and invoking of religious causes for events were common during this time. The third phase, anticipatory waiting, occurred when the child's condition stabilized, but had not begun to improve. Finally, if the child were discharged from the unit, a period of elation was observed; if the child died or was left impaired, mourning began.

The process of developing an instrument for the assessment of sources of parental stress in pediatric intensive care units is described by Miles and Carter (1982). Through observations of parents in the ICU, interviews with parents and ICU nurses, and consultation with a pediatric nursing research group, 79 items representing eight dimensions of the intensive care unit experience, possibly contributing to parental stress, were identified. The eight stress dimensions included sights and sounds of the environment, children's appearance, behavior, and emotional responses, medical procedures, staff communications, staff behaviors, and parental role deprivation.

Finally, preferences of parents and nurses for the type of clothing worn by ICU personnel were examined by Gardner and Simkins (1976). Three ways of dressing were selected for study: 1) traditional white uniforms, 2) uniforms with colorful smocks, and 3) street clothes. During each experimental period, which lasted from two to three weeks, all ICU nurses wore one of the specified styles of dress. Twenty parents during each period were interviewed concerning their general attitudes towards ICU nurses, including those qualities of personnel considered helpful in reducing their worry. In addition, parents were shown pictures of nurses wearing the three styles of dress and were asked to rank them in order of preference.

Characteristics of nursing personnel identified by parents as helpful in minimizing their worries most often pertained to nurses' work habits and personal behavior, but not their manner of dress. When asked to indicate their preference for style of nursing attire, parents demonstrated a slight tendency to prefer the type of clothing worn by nurses during the experimental period in which they participated, although more than half selected the combination of uniform and smock as their first choice. Ease of identification of nursing personnel, plus the addition of an element of cheerfulness to an otherwise impersonal white uniform, were among the reasons cited for this choice. ICU nurses concurred with parents in selection of the uniform-smock combination.

The Recovery Room

The only study exclusively devoted to the pediatric recovery room is a survey of parent attitudes conducted by Dew, Bushong, and Crumrine (1977). Fifty-seven parents who were permitted to be with their children in the pediatric recovery room (RR) following surgery were questioned concerning their responses to the experience. Though 84 percent of the parents expressed nervousness during the period of surgery, 86 percent of all respondents said they felt better when seeing their child in the recovery room. Of the five parents who said that they felt worse upon first seeing their child in the RR, all but one felt better by the time they left. Eighty-eight percent of the parents thought that their presence had been helpful to their child, and all parents said they would want to visit the RR again, if the need should arise. A minority of parents (9 in all) identified specific aspects of the recovery room experience that they disliked, such as the appearance or behavior of their child and the condition of other children. Nearly all parents found the guidelines for visitation (reprinted in the research report) to be helpful.

Isolation Units

The experience of hospitalization in an isolation room or unit is qualitatively different from that of other inpatient settings. In the standard pediatric ward, and even in intensive care units, the opportunity for frequent interaction with and observation of others is available to children, even among those whose mobility is restricted. However, the requirements of isolation technique, which demand confinement to one's room and restrict access to people and possibly play materials unless strict procedures are followed, effectively impede children's movements and activities, and discourage their contact with staff members and visitors. A limited amount of research has considered children's conceptions of isolation, as well as their responses to this condition.

Children's Concepts of Isolation. Given the restrictions of isolation, one might expect that children's understanding of this type of treatment would be distorted, with young children in particular viewing the experience as a form of punishment. Pidgeon (1967) interviewed fifty children (3 to 17 years of age, hospitalized in isolation) concerning their understanding of isolation technique. One-third of the youngest group of subjects questioned (3 to 7 years of age) provided *precausal* explanations, characterized by psychological, magical, or moral reasons for the use of isolation procedures. This percentage was smaller than had been anticipated on the basis of earlier research on children's health care concepts. Nevertheless, it represents an appreciable number of children who may view isolation as a result of their own misbehavior. The proportion of children providing precausal explanations declined with age. A corresponding rise of *causal* responses (i.e., those using physical or mechanical reasoning) was noted among older patients. Finally, the *accuracy* of children's explanations (defined as an awareness of one or more basic principle of isolation) was also found to improve with age (see Chapter 3).

Children's Responses to Isolation. Three studies have considered the responses manifested by children hospitalized in isolation for specific medical conditions. Kueffner (1973, 1975) provides a qualitative description of the passage through isolation of severely burned schoolage children. Hollenbeck, Susman, Nannis, Strope, Hersh, Levine, and Pizzo (1980) examined the behavioral and physiological responses of preschool cancer patients to isolation in a Laminar Air Flow room, while Powazek, Goff, Schyveng, and Paulson (1978) compared the responses of patients (and their parents) hospitalized in two differing types of isolation settings in a cancer hospital.

Kueffner (1973, 1975) had originally intended that the focus of her study be the phenomenon of isolation, but found it difficult to separate the effects of the environment and treatment from the condition for which children were hospitalized—in this case, severe burns. Six children, six to ten years of age, isolated for a minimum of two weeks for treatment of their burns, were considered. Two of the six children were isolated alone, while the remaining four were isolated together in a special burn unit. The investigator visited each child several times per week and occasionally observed them undetected. Three stages in the hospitalization of burned children were identified. *Stage I* (termed the phase of "agony") begins with children's hospitalization and continues until they perceive their condition as improving. *Stage II* (hope) proceeds from the time improvement is noted until a date for discharge is set. Finally, *Stage III* (the period of "reorganization") extends from the time a discharge date is set until actual release from the hospital.

Among the concepts discussed by Kueffner, possibly applicable to children isolated for other conditions, is children's sense of "aloneness." The author notes that solitary isolation often appeared to be upsetting to children, who frequently exercised strategies to bring people to their proximity and keep them there. Yet at other times, it seemed as though children were not distressed by aloneness, but may actually have preferred that condition.

According to Kueffner, the literature on childhood burns suggests that children isolated alone recover more slowly than those treated together in a burn unit. It is unclear whether this is attributable to differences in the opportunity to interact with others or to the increased sophistication of service provided in the specialized units. The author suggests that the question of long-term effects of isolation alone or with others be considered.

Hollenbeck, et al. (1980) documented the reactions of four children, ranging in age from eighteen months to four years, while receiving chemotherapy for cancer in protective isolation of a Laminar Air Flow room. Physical contact with children could only be made through plastic gloves, and all persons entering isolation rooms were required to wear sterile gowns. Parental visitation was permitted, provided that isolation technique was observed.

Research observations of children were made via videotape, once in the morning and once in the afternoon, four days per week, for up to six weeks. In addition to the data on children's behavior derived from videotapes, measures of their body temperature, heart rate, respiration, and blood pressure were obtained from patient records. The behavioral data indicated that:

> During the first few weeks, children were generally physically active and engaged in a variety of vocal behaviors, such as crying and talking. Play remained relatively constant throughout the isolation period. Passivity gradually increased during isolation and declined after discharge from the Flow room (p. 6)

Examination of the physiological indices revealed that children's body temperature dropped well *below* normal during the first 24 hours after hospitalization—a phenomenon that, according to Hollenbeck, et al. has also been observed among infant monkeys separated from their mothers.

Powazek, et al. (1978) compared the reactions of 123 patients (1 to 29 years of age) and their mothers to two different types of isolation in a cancer hospital. Patients in one group, observed in standard isolation, were placed in private rooms, though occasionally two patients were assigned to one room. Parents (but no other persons) were allowed to visit one at a time, from noon until 9:00 PM. A second group of subjects, treated after the opening of a new isolation unit, were observed in a more rigidly controlled environment. In this case, each subject was assigned to a private, peninsular isolation room, separated from parents and other visitors by a glass partition. Although only hospital staff could enter these patient rooms, visitation through the glass partition (facilitated by a voice-activated intercom) was unrestricted.

Standardized questionnaires were used to assess the depression of mothers, and the state and trait anxiety levels of mothers and of patients seven years of age or older. In addition, nurses completed a checklist documenting children's anxious or depressive behaviors. Finally, parents in the strict isolation group completed a questionnaire on their attitudes toward the newer form of isolation.

Levels of maternal anxiety and depression were not significantly affected by the format of isolation. Under both conditions, mothers' trait anxiety levels were normal, although their state anxiety while in the hospital was considerably elevated. This was especially true of mothers with preschool children. About half of the mothers in each isolation condition exhibited appreciable amounts of clinical depression.

Results for patients paralleled those of mothers, with anxiety scores unrelated to the type of isolation experienced, and trait anxiety levels falling within normal limits. State anxiety measures, on the other hand, were elevated only among patients 13 years of age or older. Children seven to twelve years of age displayed normal levels of state anxiety. Patient behavior, as rated by nurses, was found to be similar under both isolation conditions. In each case, preschool children displayed anxious and depressive behaviors more frequently than did older subjects.

Parental opinions about the more rigid form of isolation varied, to some degree, with the age of the child. Those with children over six years of age registered more positive comments, while parents of younger patients had more negative and ambivalent opinions.

Emergency Rooms

For many children, experiences with hospital settings are limited to, or begin with, treatment in the emergency room (ER). Children admitted for truly emergent conditions, such as injury or sudden illness, may be at increased risk for psychological upset due to the unpredictability of the event, the lack of preparation for the experience, and possible increased anxiety of their escorts. Even when the condition of children seeking treatment cannot clearly be considered an emergency, young patients in the emergency room may be upset by observation of the medical condition of others, as well as the equipment and procedures used in their care. The research reviewed in the present section considers the reactions of children entering the emergency room and the continuing responses of those eventually admitted for inpatient treatment.

Children's Responses to Emergency Room Care. Two studies based on the same data set examined children's and parents' responses to treatment in a pediatric trauma center (Resnick & Hergenroeder, 1975; Gratz, 1977). One hundred children, three to thirteen years of age, were randomly selected for study. Children's behavior while receiving treatment was assessed using a behavioral rating list designed for the study. Medical and demographic information was obtained from patient registration forms. In addition, anecdotal records of the activities of patients, parents, and staff were kept. Boys were reported to visit the unit twice as often as girls, with this ratio remaining constant across all age groups. Peak hours of admission were found to be between 3:00 PM and 11:00 PM.

Resnick and Hergenroeder (1975) report that all but three subjects were accompanied to the pediatric trauma unit by an adult. One-third of all parents maintained some form of physical contact with their children during procedures (e.g., holding children on their laps or holding their hands). Forty-four percent of the parents were in close proximity to their children, standing within five feet of them during treatment. Another 22 percent of the adults remained in the waiting area, either at their own request or that of the staff, while their children received care.

Anecdotal data on children's verbalizations are reported. Among the concerns most frequently expressed were fear of needles or painful procedures, fear of losing control under anesthesia, and fear of mutilation. Children also expressed curiosity about the environment, sought clarification of medical terminology, and raised concerns about how the injury might affect their immediate future. Parent responses to the emergency room experience fell into five basic categories: 1) quieting the child, 2) making the child feel guilty for the accident, 3) expressing their own feelings of guilt, 4) expressing anger, and 5) displaying concern or affection.

The data gathered by Resnick and Hergenroeder (1975) were reanalyzed by Gratz (1978) in order to determine more precisely how children respond when receiving emergency room treatment and to identify factors associated with their responses. To answer the question of how children respond when in the emergency room setting, a principal components analysis was performed on the data obtained from behavioral checklists. Two primary types of responses were found: *protest* (i.e., kicking, crying, resisting, etc.) and *withdrawal* (e.g., reticence, lack of eye contact). Subsets of these behaviors were used as dependent variables in analyses to determine the types of personal, situational, or parental variables associated with children's responses.

Personal variables considered in this study were children's age, sex, past medical experiences, and verbalizations. Children's protest behavior declined significantly with age. In addition, several significant relationships between subject's verbalizations and their level of protest were found. Verbalization of fear was associated with increased protest, while expressions of curiosity or concern for the immediate future were associated with reduced protest scores. However, neither sex nor familiarity with medical environments was associated with children's protest or withdrawal.

Situational variables, such as time of day entering the ER, length of time spent there, type of injury, laceration size (if applicable), and rank of medical staff member providing the care, were largely unrelated to children's responses. However, protest scores were found to be lower among children treated after 7:00 PM and higher among laceration patients who were restrained for suturing. Withdrawal scores were higher among children experiencing head trauma (possibly a product of their injury) and lower among children coming to the ER via ambulance instead of car, although few children in the sample arrived in ambulances.

Concerning *parental variables,* neither the identity of the person escorting children to the emergency room (mother, father, or other) nor their proximity to the patient during treatment was related to children's responses. Parental behaviors of quieting the child or expressing guilt feelings were associated with increased child protest levels. Responses of parents were also found to vary with children's age. Parents of younger children demonstrated more caretaking behavior and more frequently expressed personal responsibility for the child's condition, while those of older children were more likely to assign responsibility for the injury to the child.

Admission to the Hospital via the Emergency Room. Despite the emphasis in the research literature on the hospitalization of elective surgical patients, a substantial percentage of children enter the hospital under emergency circumstances. At least one study has shown that unplanned, emergency hospitalizations constitute a majority of the admissions of children under five years of age (Stacey, Dearden, Pill, & Robinson, 1970). Concerned over the absence of research pertaining to this form of hospital experience, Roskies, Bedard, Gauvreau-Guilbault, and LaFortune (1975) conducted a pilot study to examine the reactions of children admitted to the hospital through the emergency room.

The sample consisted of sixteen children, eleven to 48 months of age, half of whom were admitted to the hospital from the emergency room. The others were admitted directly to the inpatient unit for elective procedures. Structured observations of children and parents during the first six hours in the hospital were conducted. In the case of emergency admissions, the observation period was extended, if necessary, to include at least one hour of observation after the child was transferred from the ER to an inpatient ward. In addition, parents were interviewed concerning children's prior medical experiences, circumstances leading up to hospitalization, and their perceptions of events occurring in the hospital.

Though statistical analyses were considered inappropriate due to the small number of subjects, differences reported between the two groups were deemed of sufficient magnitude to merit consideration. As would be anticipated, subjects admitted through the emergency room were more acutely ill than were the elective admissions. Less expected, however, was the difference in the health history of the two groups. While the elective admissions were typically "well" children with little or no prior hospital experience, three-fourths of the children in the emergency group had one or more previous hospitalization. Furthermore, the condition necessitating the present admission was, in most cases, not truly emergent, but was either related to, or an exacerbation of, a preexisting illness.

The emergency and elective groups of children were found to differ in the quantity and quality of stressful experiences encountered. Children in the emergency group experienced an average of eight painful procedures during the first six hours of admission, as compared to three such procedures experienced by the elective group subjects. Moreover, the types of procedures performed on emergency group children tended to be more extreme and of longer duration than those of the elective group. Nearly twice as many white-coated strangers were encountered by emergency subjects during the period of observation.

An additional factor, possibly compounding the stress experienced by the emergency group, was the compression of events into a shorter period of time. Roskies, et al. report that routine events such as the donning of hospital clothes, confinement to bed, physical examination, and the encountering of painful procedures (events experienced by the elective group over a two to six hour period) were required of emergency group children within the first fifteen minutes of hospitalization.

In addition, a more limited amount of parental support was available to emergency group children. Separation from parents occurred earlier in the hospital stay of emergency patients. Even when parents were present, less positive parent-child interaction was observed among emergency, than elective subjects. Parents in neither group, however, were found to be particularly effective in helping their children adjust to the new environment.

Play experiences were also effectively denied to emergency group children within the initial hours after arrival at the hospital. While a majority of the elective admissions brought a favorite toy to the hospital and used the playroom within the first six hours of admission, only one emergency group child brought a toy and none used the playroom.

Although it might be anticipated that the amount of preparation given to children by parents or hospital staff would differentiate the groups, with the emergency group receiving less information, such was not the case. Roskies, et al. report that, "Regardless of the type of admission, regardless of the age of the child, the almost universal pattern, with very few exceptions, was to give the child no or misleading information about the events he was to encounter" (p. 575). This was true of parental explanations before admission and of hospital staff interactions with children prior to the administering of procedures.

Chapter 5

SEPARATION AND ROOMING-IN

Vernon, Foley, Sipowicz, and Schulman (1965) have identified separation from parents as a major factor contributing to the immediate and posthospital psychological upset of preschool children. The upset reactions manifested by young children during separation, and the alterations in their behavior toward parents following separation (e.g., clinging to or following parents, or perhaps ignoring them) have been repeatedly documented. However, the elements responsible for producing this upset are imperfectly understood. It has been suggested that children form attachments to specific individuals, including, but not necessarily limited to, their parents. Separation from these recognized sources of support is said to leave children emotionally vulnerable, especially when it occurs under unusual circumstances, away from the familiar setting of home. Others, such as Branstetter (1969a, 1969b), propose that the absence *per se* of a specific individual is not the sole operative factor in producing upset. In addition, the unavailability of certain qualities or characteristics associated with the absent attachment figures must be considered. For example, when a parent is not present at the hospital, the child is denied the support of a consistent individual who can provide undivided attention and intercede on the patient's behalf with the foreign environment.

The research considered in this chapter examines the responses of children to various types of separation. Initial consideration is given to studies involving substitute caregivers, since this research is pertinent to the determination of the source of children's upset when separation occurs. Specifically, this research examines the question of whether replacement of certain characteristics of the absent attachment figure serves to reduce or eliminate children's upset. The effects of rooming-in and unlimited visitation on the inhospital and posthospital responses of children are then examined, followed by a review of research on parental presence during medical procedures. Information on two other forms of intervention designed to minimize the effects of separation, the use of care-by-parent units and voice recordings of parents played for children in their absence, are also presented. Finally, survey data on the prevalence and adequacy of services provided by hospitals to promote parent-child interactions is reviewed.

SUBSTITUTE CAREGIVERS

As mentioned above, it is Branstetter's (1969a, 1969b) suggestion that much of the upset noted among children separated from parents during hospitalization results from absence of the consistent attention, or "mothering care," attachment figures normally provide, rather than separation, in itself, from these specific individuals. To test this proposition, thirty children (14 to 36 months of age, neither acutely ill nor hospitalized for surgery) were observed. Each child was hospitalized under one of three conditions. Children in the *mother-present group* had ready access to their mothers, who remained with them at the hospital day and night. The *substitute-mother group* consisted of children whose mothers could not stay with them during the course of hospitalization, but who were assigned a caretaker who was present throughout children's waking hours. Subjects in the *mother-absent group* had no additional caretaker assigned, but were merely provided with the care normally received on the pediatric unit. Observations of children's behavior (made twice per day on four separate days) were recorded continuously on audiotape and later transcribed into narratives, from which behavioral units were identified and coded.

Branstetter found the behavior displayed by children in the mother-present and mother-substitute groups to be quite similar, with both groups demonstrating less disturbed behavior than the mother-absent group (which was described as being generally unhappy). Specifically, mother-present and mother-substitute groups displayed less crying, aggression, and withdrawal, engaged in fewer self-oriented activities, and played more than did mother-absent children. Despite the similarity between the mother-present and mother-substitute groups, certain differences were noted. For example, the mother-substitute group exhibited more dependency behavior, withdrawal, and self-orientation than the mother-present group, as well as a greater amount of play.

Subjects provided with substitute mothers were said to quickly accept the surrogate, displaying signs of attachment toward the caretaker within the first four days of admission. However, the substitute relationship did not supersede that with one's own parent, as children readily responded to mothers upon their return.

The effects of a less intensive substitute visitation program, daily two-hour visits by foster grandparents, were examined by Ziegler and King (1982). Subjects in the sample were hospitalized for a minimum of one week and ranged in age from seven months to six years. Comparisons were made of the inhospital behavior exhibited by three groups of subjects. An *undervisited group* (N = 21) consisted of children who spent less than five hours per week with visitors and who received no experimental intervention. The *parent-visitation group* (N = 20) had at least ten hours of parental contact per week (an amount equal to the time a foster grandparent would spend), though, in most cases, subjects in this group received considerably more. The *experimental group* (N = 26) had a level of visitation similar to that of the undervisited group, but additionally received the daily, undivided attention of a foster grandparent.

The authors hypothesized that the undervisited group would show the least adaptive behavior during hospitalization, and the parent-visited group the most adaptive, with the behavior of experimental group children falling between these extremes, though closer to the level of the parent-visited group. The mean scores on all five of the behavioral variables examined (vocalization, motor behavior, play, fear, and environmental responsiveness) were, in fact, lowest for the undervisited group, though significant group differences were evident only for the category of "play," with undervisited children exhibiting less play behavior than either the parent or foster grandparent groups. In addition, for three of the five behaviors, mean scores of the experimental subjects were closer to the parent-visited than to the undervisited group scores.

Despite the tendency of the data to appear in the predicted order, no significant overall group effect was evident in a multivariate analysis. The authors suggest that a more extensive intervention (on the order of that provided by Branstetter, in which substitute caregivers were nearly always available during waking hours) may be necessary to detect significant group differences.

THE EFFECTS OF PARENTAL ROOMING-IN

If separation from parents represents a threat to the emotional well-being of young children in the hospital, then efforts to minimize separation should result in a reduction of children's psychological upset. One means of reducing separation, having parents remain at the hospital throughout a child's hospitalization (a practice referred to as "rooming-in" or "living-in"), has been the subject of several research projects. Responses of children have been examined during hospitalization (Brain & Maclay, 1968; Lee & Greene, 1969; Lehman, 1975; Couture, 1976; Shanley, 1981), as well as after discharge (Brain & Maclay, 1968; Fagin, 1966, 1969; Lehman, 1975; Couture, 1976; McGillicuddy, 1976).

Research concerning the impact of rooming-in on children's inhospital reactions has produced mixed results, with studies alternately indicating that children whose parents room-in make more satisfactory adjustment than other children while in the hospital (Brain & Maclay), show greater aggression (Lehman, 1975), or possibly cry more during anesthesia induction (Lee & Greene, 1969) than children whose parents have not remained at the hospital. An additional study found no evidence of inhospital differences between rooming-in and non-rooming-in groups (Couture, 1976).

Interpretation of these studies is dependent on the meaning one ascribes to the behaviors when manifested in a specific context—in this case, when children are in the presence of parents. As discussed above (see Chapter 2), seemingly "negative" behaviors such as crying or displaying aggression may be interpreted as true indicators of upset (e.g., see Lee & Greene, concerning children's crying) or as evidence that children feel comfortable enough in the presence of their parents to express their feelings.

Studies concerning posthospital effects, on the other hand, are more uniform in their conclusions that parental rooming-in is beneficial. Greater incidence of emotional disturbance (Brain & Maclay, 1968) and regression (Couture, 1976) has been noted among children of non-rooming-in parents. Moreover, children whose parents have remained with them during hospitalization have demonstrated increases in maturity (Fagin, 1966, 1969; McGillicuddy, 1976) and reduction in postoperative complications (Brain & Maclay, 1968; Lehman, 1975).

Immediate Effects of Rooming-in and Unlimited Visitation

Four studies have examined the impact of parental rooming-in on various indicators of children's adjustment while in the hospital (Brain & Maclay, 1968; Lee & Greene, 1969; Lehman, 1975; Couture, 1976). An additional study, Shanley (1981), compared the behaviors of children who experienced either limited or unlimited maternal visitation during their hospitalization for cancer treatment.

Brain and Maclay (1968) selected subjects from a pool of mothers who had expressed willingness to accompany their preschool children (who were scheduled for tonsillectomy and/or adenoidectomy surgery) to the hospital. Mothers were randomly assigned to either room-in with their children during hospitalization (N = 101) or not (N = 96). Accompanied and unaccompanied children were hospitalized on alternate weeks.

While in the hospital, children were observed by ward personnel and by an anesthetist, who recorded observations of children's reactions during induction of anesthesia. The methods used for making observations are not specified. However, on the basis of this information, children's inhospital adjustment was classified as *satisfactory* (defined as demonstrating an awareness of their situation with no undue disturbance), *unsatisfactory* (panic, complete denial of the situation, withdrawal), or *limited* (overt signs of disturbance, but with the ability to express feelings and make a partial adjustment). Significantly more favorable adjustment was reported for experimental (i.e., accompanied) group children, with 76.2 percent considered to have made satisfactory adjustment, versus 42.7 percent for control group children.

Lee and Greene (1969) examined the behavior of children undergoing anesthesia induction, relating children's responses during the procedure to the type of contact parents had maintained with their children prior to surgery. Subjects included 144 children between one and eight years of age, hospitalized for elective surgery. Immediately after arrival in the operating room area, children were classified as being awake or asleep. Those considered awake were further classified as "calm" or "crying."

Following surgery, parents were interviewed to determine the type of presurgical contact they had had with their children. Curiously, parents were considered to have roomed-in if they had either stayed overnight in the hospital *or* had left the hospital at the child's bedtime and returned the following morning prior to surgery. In addition to rooming-in, two other categories of parental contact were considered: 1) parents leaving the hospital the previous day (presumably earlier than bedtime), but returning before the child's surgery, and 2) parents having no contact with their child before surgery.

Ratings of children's emotional state were unrelated to the type of contact they had had with their parents prior to surgery. Although Lee and Greene note that the proportion of children crying in the rooming-in group was more than twice that observed among children with no presurgical parent contact, they failed to adequately relate this difference to other characteristics of the self-selected contact groups. Crying was found to be significantly greater among the younger subjects in the sample. Moreover, the authors note that significantly more parents of young children chose to room-in than did parents of older subjects. Therefore, the increased level of crying among children of rooming-in parents may merely be a reflection of their age.

Another nonexperimental evaluation of rooming-in was conducted by Lehman (1975). In this case, 48 subjects (3 to 5 years of age) were considered, half of whose mothers had chosen to room-in. Lehman hypothesized that, although children of rooming-in mothers would display more aggressive behavior while in the hospital (a reflection of the greater security felt by these children) they would be less disturbed upon return home than unaccompanied children. To assess the question of children's inhospital aggression, questionnaires were completed by the mother and nurse of each child regarding that child's behavior. Nurses' progress notes were also reviewed for instances of uncooperative behavior. As expected, children whose mothers roomed-in displayed more aggression than did those in the non-rooming-in group. Lehman observes that this difference was found despite the fact that the amount of time mothers in either group spent with their children during waking hours did not differ significantly. Children's post-hospital physical recovery and behavioral responses were also in the hypothesized direction, though the behavioral data fell somewhat short of a conventional significance level (see posthospital effects below).

Couture (1976) considered the inhospital effects of rooming-in on children, three to six years of age, hospitalized for tonsillectomy and/or adenoidectomy surgery. The visitation patterns of parents were used to classify children as being in the *rooming-in group* (parents remained at the hospital overnight, N = 13), the *unlimited visitation group* (parents visited more than eight hours per day, N = 8), or the *limited visitation group* (less than eight hours of parental contact per day, N = 10). Observations of children's behavior on the ward were made hourly during daytime hours for ten-minute periods and were recorded in a written, running narrative form. Analysis of the data failed to reveal differences in inhospital behavior of children in the three contact conditions.

The impact of limited versus unlimited visitation on the inhospital adjustment of young cancer patients (15 to 48 months of age) was examined by Shanley (1981). Observations of seventeen children experiencing limited visitation and of another twenty subjects receiving unlimited visitation were conducted over a three-day period. The results indicate that children in the unlimited condition displayed more developmentally appropriate behavior than the limited visitation group in each of seven identified categories (mother-child interaction, separation anxiety, eating behavior, play activity, autoerotic behavior, sleep behavior, and elimination).

Posthospital Effects of Rooming-in

Studies investigating the posthospital effects of parental rooming-in have used two basic indices to assess children's responses:

their posthospital behavior (Brain & Maclay, 1968; Fagin, 1966, 1969; Lehman, 1975; McGillicuddy, 1976; Couture, 1976), and the medical recovery of children upon return home (Brain & Maclay, 1968; Lehman, 1975). Each type of response will be considered in turn.

Posthospital Behavior. In addition to their observations of children's behavior while in the hospital, Brain and Maclay (1968) interviewed mothers in their homes one month before admission to the hospital, two weeks after discharge, and again approximately four months later. Posthospital interviews addressed changes in children's behavior and physical state after leaving the hospital. Information gathered from the interviews was used to classify children as *disturbed* (if a new behavioral disorder or trait was observed) or as *undisturbed* (if no such change in behavior was reported following hospitalization). Significantly fewer children whose mothers had roomed-in were rated as disturbed after discharge from the hospital. Moreover, the duration of the disturbance experienced by children of rooming-in mothers was significantly shorter than that of control group children.

Couture (1976) provides evidence that the negative impact of hospitalization, though possibly affecting all subjects, may be greater among preschool children whose parents fail to room-in. Parents of all subjects completed a behavior adjustment scale at the time of children's admission, as well as one week and one month after discharge. The scale, which was administered to parents in a structured interview format, assessed the status of children's behavior in several domains, yielding a single adjustment score. Comparison of children's prehospital and initial posthospital adjustment scores suggests that, although children in the rooming-in and non-rooming-in groups alike showed regression in behavior, the decline among children whose parents did not room-in was more precipitous ($p < .10$). During the period between the first and second posthospital ratings, adjustment scores of both groups demonstrated a similar rate of recovery. Nevertheless, only the rooming-in group had exceeded its prehospital rating level by the time of the second posthospital parent interview, one month after discharge.

As mentioned above, Lehman (1975) proposed that, although

children accompanied by parents may be more aggressive during hospitalization (a finding supported by the data), their posthospital adjustment would be more favorable than that of unaccompanied children. Some indication of less severe posthospital upset among children of rooming-in parents was, in fact, noted. According to Lehman, responses to the Posthospital Behavioral Questionnaire (Vernon, et al., 1966), completed by parents two weeks after children's discharge from the hospital, demonstrated "a tendency toward there being fewer rooming-in children with behavioral disturbances than non-rooming-in children" (p. 42). However, as was also true of the Couture (1976) data, this difference was not significant at the conventional level of $p < .05$.

Two additional studies (Fagin, 1966, 1969; McGillicuddy, 1976) indicate that rooming-in is associated with positive changes in posthospital behavior, while failure of parents to room-in may encourage regressive behavior measurable after discharge. Fagin (1966, 1969) interviewed sixty mothers at admission and twice after discharge, gathering information on children's behavioral patterns. Half of the mothers remained with their children throughout the period of hospitalization, with the other half visiting their children daily, but not staying at the hospital overnight. Posthospital disturbances in eating, sleep patterns, and bladder control were more common among children with non-rooming-in mothers. Furthermore, significant increases in indices of maturity from the prehospital to posthospital periods were noted among subjects in the rooming-in group.

McGillicuddy (1976) examined the effects of rooming-in on the posthospital behavior of children, 14 through 48 months of age, who were hospitalized for periods ranging from two to ten days. Rooming-in and non-rooming-in groups each consisted of thirty mother-child dyads. The investigator notes that mothers in both conditions had expressed a desire to remain with their children during hospitalization, but that non-rooming-in mothers could not do so "because of hospital policy" (p. 36). Since this group was presumably hospitalized at a facility different than that of the rooming-in group, the form of parental contact experienced by children is confounded with other characteristics of the individual settings.

In addition to the two hospitalized groups, McGillicuddy included a comparably aged group of nonhospitalized subjects as another control. Parents of the hospitalized children completed a modified Posthospital Behavioral Questionnaire (PHBQ) prior to hospitalization or upon admission and again one month following discharge. Mothers of nonhospitalized children also completed the questionnaire twice with a comparable interval.

Results of the questionnaire revealed positive changes in the behavior of rooming-in children one month after discharge, with unaccompanied children manifesting increased behavioral disturbance. Specifically, subjects in the rooming-in group displayed improvements over the course of the study on the PHBQ subscales of general anxiety and regression, eating disturbance, and apathy-withdrawal. Non-rooming-in children, on the other hand, had significant negative changes in areas of separation anxiety, anxiety about sleep, aggression toward authority, and apathy-withdrawal, as well as in their overall behavioral scores. Differences between the two groups of hospitalized children were significant for all but two of the PHBQ factors, with each difference in favor of the rooming-in group. In fact, a significant difference was found between overall behavior scores of rooming-in children and nonhospitalized subjects, with the nonhospitalized group showing slight *regression* during the period of study. However, McGillicuddy attributes this difference to coincidental traumatic events experienced by three nonhospitalized children between initial and final evaluations.

Posthospital Physical Recovery. Two studies have considered the impact of rooming-in on children's posthospital physical recovery (Brain & Maclay, 1968; Lehman, 1975). In their postdischarge interviews with mothers, Brain and Maclay (1968) inquired about the status of children's health after leaving the hospital. Postoperative complications, defined as hemorrhage or infection at the site of the operation, were significantly more common among control group children (occurring in 23% of the patients) than among children of rooming-in parents (11%).

Lehman (1975) also examined the incidence of postoperative complications (e.g., hemorrhaging, vomiting, or croupy cough) among her subjects and found rooming-in to be associated with a reduction of their occurrence. Though a similar number of children in rooming-in and non-rooming-in groups had at least one such complication, multiple complications were more frequent in the latter group.

SEPARATION DURING MEDICAL PROCEDURES

Parent access to hospitalized children has increased over the past decades. Nevertheless, separation commonly occurs at specific points throughout the course of hospitalization, especially during the performance of medical procedures. The effects of parental presence on children's responses have been examined during routine hospital admission procedures (Vernon, Foley, & Schulman, 1967), the induction of anesthesia (Vernon, et al., 1967; Schulman, Foley, Vernon, & Allen, 1967), and the administration of an injection (Shaw & Routh, 1982). The results of these studies differ, though they have been generally interpreted as evidence of the beneficial effects of parental presence.

In the first of two related investigations of the effect of maternal presence during periods of hospitalization, Vernon, Foley, and Schulman (1967) assessed children's reactions while undergoing routine admission procedures, which included the undressing and weighing of the child and the taking of a rectal temperature and blood pressure reading. Thirty-two children (2 to 6 years of age, hospitalized for elective procedures other than tonsillectomy) were randomly assigned to either the accompanied or separated condition, with mothers in the latter group leaving the child's room when the procedures were conducted. Prior to performance of admission procedures, all children had engaged in a fifteen-minute period of free play during which assessments were made of their aggression and the quality of their play. A similar play session with corresponding observations was held upon the conclusion of admission procedures. Mothers of children in both groups were present during the play sessions. Ratings of children's mood immediately prior to and during procedures, as well as during both play sessions, were made using a seven-point scale. No differences in mood, quality of play, or aggression were noted between separated and accompanied children during any assessment period.

Vernon, et al., (1967) conducted a similar investigation of children's responses to the induction of anesthesia (also reported in Schulman, et al., 1967). In this instance, 32 children (between 2 and 6 years of age, admitted to the hospital the morning of their tonsillectomy surgery) were considered. Subjects were classified by age, sex, and birth order, then randomly assigned to the accompanied or separated condition, with mothers in the accompanied group remaining with their children throughout the induction of anesthesia.

Observations of children's mood were made during a fifteen-minute play session prior to induction (similar to that held in the admission study), and during three phases of the induction procedure. The *threat phase* was the period between the time mothers left their children (or, in the case of the accompanied group, would have left them) until the start of the anesthesia induction. *Impact phase A* began when the mask was placed on the child's face and lasted for one minute. *Impact phase B* followed immediately thereafter and continued until a surgical level of anesthesia was achieved.

Although children in the separated condition appeared to be somewhat more upset than those accompanied by their mothers during the threat phase, this difference failed to reach a conventional level of significance ($p < .10$). No difference in children's mood was reported during impact phase A. However, during impact phase B, children in the separated group were significantly more upset than those with mothers present. Differences in posthospital reactions between accompanied and separated children were not found.

Shaw and Routh (1982) attribute the difference found by Vernon, et al. (1967) during impact phase B to the "disinhibiting" effects of the anesthesia given to the children. Though the separated children may have been more upset than accompanied children throughout the induction process, absence of their mothers may have inhibited expression of feelings. Only when anesthesia physiologically affected the children (i.e., during phase B) was the upset of the separated children manifested.

This interpretation is, in part, the product of a study conducted by Shaw and Routh to determine the affects of mothers' presence on the behavior of children receiving an injection in an outpatient setting. In this study, children of two different ages (18 months and 5 years) were considered. Twenty children of each age were randomly assigned to either the mother-present or mother-absent group. Mothers in both conditions were present throughout most of the child's physical examination, with those in the mother-absent group leaving the room temporarily when children received an injection. Children's behavior was rated at specified points during the examination using a five-point scale. In addition, the presence or absence of six behaviors (fussing, crying, laughing, talking, playing, and covering up) was noted during every twenty-second interval.

Considering the eighteen-month-olds first, Shaw and Routh found significant differences between the behavior of mother-absent and mother-present groups during two periods of observation. A substantial amount of crying was noted among children in the mother-absent group when their mothers left the room, while none of the mother-present children cried during the corresponding period. However, during the injection itself, results were markedly different. Each child in the mother-present group received "the maximum possible negative rating, while those in the mother-absent group received a significantly less negative rating" (p. 39).

Similar results were noted among the five-year-old children. Ratings of children's behavior in the mother-present group were significantly more negative than those of the mother-absent group, both during and immediately after the injection. While eight of the ten children whose mothers were present during the injection cried, only one of the mother-absent children did so. Shaw and Routh interpret these findings as supportive of maternal presence, proposing that children under stress may actually be "more emotionally upset in the sense of physiological arousal when their mothers are absent than when they are present" (p. 41). The presence of mothers, the authors suggest, serves as a disinhibitor, which permits free expression of children's feelings much as did anesthesia in the Vernon, et al. (1967) study.

The behaviors and attitudes of parents who remained with their children during one particular type of procedure, blood drawing, were examined by Savedra (1981). Subjects of the blood drawing were sixty children, two weeks to six years of age. Forty-eight of the patients were accompanied by their mothers, with the remainder escorted by their fathers or both parents. A combination of verbal and nonverbal strategies were used by parents to help their children cope with the procedure. Though 25 percent of the parents indicated, either verbally or nonverbally, that the experience was distressing, their actions were not considered to be disruptive of the blood drawing. No relationship was found between the strategies used by parents to help their children and their children's actual behavior.

When questioned after the procedure, parents were generally positive about accompanying their children for blood drawing. Only eight percent stated that they had not wanted to be present for the procedure (it was the expectation of the medical settings used for observation that all children be accompanied by parents), and an unspecified "vast majority" of parents felt that their presence had been of help to their children.

CARE-BY-PARENT UNITS

In recent years, increased attention has been given to care-by-parent units. In such units, parents adopt a more active, formalized role than is typical during rooming-in, being admitted to the hospital with their children and trained to provide a portion of their children's care. Functions performed by parents vary from routine caretaking and assessment of vital signs to more involved medical procedures that they will be required to continue at home. With greater responsibility given to parents, the need for hospital staff is correspondingly reduced. As a consequence, patient fees in care-by-parent units are typically lower. A recent analysis by Evans and Robinson (1983) confirms the economic advantages of this form of care. Average costs per episode were found to be 33 percent lower for general pediatric cases, 13.5 percent lower for tonsillectomy and adenoidectomy surgery, and 29 percent lower for other types of surgery when treatment was provided in a care-by-parent unit rather than a standard pediatric ward.

The literature available on care-by-parent units primarily describes their operation and the distribution of patients served, rather than evaluating the effects of this mode of care on children and their families (e.g., see James & Wheeler, 1969; Hardgrove & Dawson, 1975; Vermilion, Ballantine, & Grosfeld, 1979). However, limited attempts at evaluation have appeared.

Lerner, Haley, Hall, and McVarish (1972) conducted a series of studies to address three topic areas: 1) physician-parent communication in a care-by-parent unit, 2) the impact of hospitalization in a care-by-parent unit on the family, and 3) medical students' assessment of the unit. In none of the three studies were statistical analyses or control groups used.

Parents and physicians of 54 patients, hospitalized in a care-by-parent unit, participated in the first two studies. Interviews with parents were held after admission to the unit and upon discharge, with a subset of the parents also being contacted after return home. Physicians were interviewed following children's discharge. The authors had expected that communication between doctors and parents on the unit would be quite good, since parents were directly involved in their children's care and were frequently required to learn techniques to be continued at home. However, the results of the first study identified numerous discrepancies between the parents' and physicians' understanding of the child's diagnosis, prognosis, and care after leaving the hospital. The majority of parents were said to have a less than complete understanding of the procedures required for children's home care. The second study, conducted to assess the impact of hospitalization on the family unit, indicated that admission of a parent and child to a care-by-parent unit resulted in minimal family strain.

The sample for the third portion of the Lerner, et al. study consisted of sixty third-year medical students who had served clerkships on a care-by-parent unit, as well as a traditional pediatric ward. The medical students expressed a preference for the care-by-parent unit over a traditional ward, both as a setting for their own training and as a facility for providing patient care.

Caldwell and Lockert (1981) also present informal data concerning parent satisfaction with hospitalization in a care-by-parent unit. Parent responses to questionnaire items concerning their own reactions and those of their children were generally positive. Eighty-three percent of the parents whose children were currently hospitalized in a care-by-parent unit, but had previously been admitted to a traditional pediatric ward, favored hospitalization in the care-by-parent unit.

PARENT VOICE RECORDINGS

Tape recordings of parents' voices, sometimes accompanied by pictures of the absent parents, have been used in hospital settings as a means of reducing children's distress associated with separation. Three studies (Hennessey, 1974, 1976; Dart, 1980; McCain, 1982) have addressed the use of this intervention.

Hennessey (1974, 1976) investigated the responses of ten hospitalized children, seventeen to thirty months of age, while listening to audio recordings of their mothers' voices during brief separations. Mothers were asked to make a recording of themselves reading a story selected by the investigator, which emphasized themes of separation and mother-child relationships. Each mother was instructed to read the story as if her child were present, making modifications and comments as she deemed appropriate. Recordings were played daily for children for up to four consecutive days, yielding a total of 28 listening sessions. The book from which the story was read was available to children while the tape played. As children listened to the story, a nurse observer made notations of children's verbal and nonverbal responses.

Modifications of the story as read by the mother were frequent and included analogies and questions directed toward the child. Of the eighteen modifications on the theme of separation made by mothers, eleven concerned hope. All children indicated a recognition of their mother's voice when the recording was started. Most remained attentive during the listening session, frequently following the story in the book, though subjects fell asleep or showed signs of drowsiness upon completion of fifteen of the 28 sessions. Behaviors indicating pleasure occurred nearly twice as often as signs of displeasure.

Dart (1980) employed an experimental design to assess the effectiveness of mothers' voice recordings in altering children's responses to hospitalization. Forty-eight children, three to four years of age, hospitalized for tonsillectomy-adenoidectomy surgery, were randomly assigned to one of three conditions. During their 48-hour hospitalization, children in each condition had access to a toy television set, which displayed a picture and played a recorded tape. The television of subjects in the *mother group* depicted the child's mother and played a recording of her voice reading the child's favorite stories and rhymes. Subjects in the *stranger group* had a toy television that displayed an unfamiliar female face and played a recording of the child's favorite stories and rhymes as recited by a stranger. The television of *control group* subjects displayed a landscape and played classical music. Ratings of children's behavior were made at specified stress points. In addition, three observations of the frequency of selected behaviors were made while children were on the ward, and parents completed the Posthospital Behavior Questionnaire after discharge.

The *mother group* was found to manifest more positive behaviors at the stress points than the *stranger* or *control* groups. Moreover, behavioral observations on the ward indicated that the mother group displayed more frequent play behavior, curiosity and positive affect, and less frequent dependency, aggression, withdrawal, self-orientation, and negative affect than did children in the other groups. According to parent posthospital ratings, mother group subjects showed less regressive behavior than did other subjects after discharge, though, surprisingly, no difference was found among groups on the PHBQ separation anxiety factor.

McCain (1982) also asked parents of fifteen hospitalized children (four to eight years of age) to produce voice recordings. Among the formats for these tapes suggested by the investigator were a talking letter from family members, a tour of their house, and the reading of favorite stories. Completed recordings were played for children twice per day, for at least three days, at times when parents were not likely to be present. Analysis of the content of the recordings revealed that parents generally followed the format suggestions provided by the investigator.

Parents producing the tapes were asked to complete a brief questionnaire concerning their reactions to the process. As might be expected, all parents were supportive of the production of tapes for children, especially when separation is likely. When asked to describe the effect of the tape, a majority of the parents said that their children had "enjoyed it." However, only six of the fifteen parents surveyed cited an additional, beneficial effect of the recording.

Informal observations of children's behavior while listening to the tapes were also reported. All children were said to have listened intently to the recording each time it was played, with most asking to hear it again at times other than those designated for the study. No child was visibly upset by the experience of listening to the tape.

AVAILABILITY AND ADEQUACY OF SERVICES PROVIDED FOR PARENTS

Whether parents actually accompany their children to the hospital depends not only on the existence of policies permitting their presence, but also on the efforts of hospitals to encourage parent participation. Several surveys have been conducted in recent years to determine the prevalence and adequacy of services provided for parents (Hardgrove, 1975; Hardgrove & Kermoian, 1978; Alcock, 1977; Fagin & Nusbaum, 1978; Post, 1979; Thornes, 1983). Results of a portion of these surveys will be briefly summarized.

Hardgrove (1975) contacted 2,718 hospitals in the United States concerning the facilities they provide for parents. Respondents were asked whether beds were supplied for parents, if their facilities were considered adequate in quantity and quality, and whether parents were systematically informed of the services available. Finally, respondents were asked to rate the predominant staff attitude toward parent rooming-in. Responses were received from 1,498 general hospitals and 53 children's hospitals.

A greater percentage of children's hospitals were found to provide parent-oriented services than did general hospitals. For example, 83 percent of the children's hospitals provided some form of rooming-in, as compared to 54 percent of the general hospitals. Only 48 percent of the responding general hospitals contacted parents prior to admission to inform them of the availability of services, while 76 percent of the children's hospitals did so. Differences in staff attitudes toward rooming-in were similarly evident. Of the general hospitals surveyed, 41 percent encouraged, 39 percent tolerated, and 23 percent discouraged parental rooming-in. Corresponding proportions for children's hospitals were 59 percent encouraging, 33 percent tolerating, and 16 percent discouraging participation.

In a follow-up study, Hardgrove and Kermoian (1978) contacted 84 of the hospitals that had indicated in the previous survey that they: 1) supplied beds for parents, 2) considered their facilities adequate, 3) systematically informed parents of rooming-in, and 4) rated their staff as encouraging parent participation. Respondents were asked to describe their rooming-in program, indicating who was responsible for the program, how families were encouraged, and whether guidelines existed for promoting the effectiveness of staff and parent interaction with the patient. A response rate of eighty percent was obtained.

After reviewing the types of services provided by the responding institutions, Hardgrove and Kermoian concluded that:

> Institutional support for parental presence, for the most part, is limited to providing beds. Accommodations that would make parents more comfortable and relaxed—reserved bathing, kitchen, and meeting areas—were uncommon (p. 849).

Other supports, such as the presence of parent advocates, parent meetings, volunteers to provide relief for parents, and child care for well siblings, were each provided by fewer than 25 percent of the hospitals.

Fagin and Nusbaum (1978) sent questionnaires to 1,154 hospitals in the United States concerning visiting privileges in their pediatric units. Responses were returned by 636 institutions. Sixty-two percent of the responding hospitals permitted 24-hour visitation. Hospitals permitting unlimited visitation were not found to differ from other institutions in characteristics such as size of the unit, proportion of beds filled, age range served, most common patient diagnoses, or modal length of hospitalization.

It appeared that a small percentage of parents take advantage of rooming-in, even in facilities where it is permitted. Fagin and Nusbaum report that in 56 percent of the hospitals permitting 24-hour visitation, fewer than twenty percent of the parents actually roomed-in. Regional differences in the proportion of hospitals permitting 24-hour visitation were also noted. The highest percentage of hospitals providing unlimited visitation were in southern states (a finding also noted by Hardgrove, 1975), with the lowest proportion found in the northeast.

Finally, a recent survey on the availability of parent services in British hospitals indicates that the adoption of policies in that country to encourage parent participation has been slow, despite the passing of 24 years since the Platt Committee recommended liberalization of parent access to children. Thornes (1983) reports that, although 89 percent of the responding wards provided some form of overnight accommodation for parents, only 49 percent permitted totally unrestricted parent visitation. Limitations on parent visiting were especially prevalent in specialized ear, nose, and throat units. On the day of children's surgery, eighteen percent of these units restricted visitation, while another 24 percent completely prohibited it.

Chapter 6

PARENT AND SIBLING RESPONSES TO HOSPITALIZATION

Research reviewed in the preceding chapters has primarily addressed children's responses to hospitalization or other forms of health care, identifying factors such as separation that may contribute to their distress, as well as specific types of intervention that may reduce the upset associated with these experiences. The focus of the present chapter shifts from the reactions of children entering the hospital to those of other, nonhospitalized family members. Although the partitioning of research studies in this manner (alternately considering the response of hospitalized children and that of their parents and siblings) is conceptually convenient, this division should not obscure the interrelatedness of child and family reactions to hospitalization.

The studies reviewed in this chapter suggest that a substantial portion of parents are anxious or distressed during their children's hospitalization. Furthermore, the degree of anxiety manifested by parents in health care settings has frequently been associated with the amount of upset displayed by their children. There has been a tendency in the literature to assume that the direction of this relationship runs from parent to child, with the anxious parent fostering anxiety in the child. While this may, at times, be the case, the correlational nature of much of the research bearing upon this issue does not permit unqualified acceptance of this position. It may be equally true that greater upset among children, for whatever reason, causes the vigilant parent to become increasingly anxious. Or perhaps the relationship between parent-child anxiety is bidirectional and reciprocal, with anxiety displayed by either parent or child contributing to that experienced by the other party.

The research on parent responses further indicates that information given to parents by hospital personnel is beneficial in reducing the anxiety of parents and children alike. Yet, it appears that the likelihood of parents obtaining a maximum amount of information or otherwise actively participating in their children's hospitalization, by rooming-in, visiting, or freely approaching members of the medical staff is dependent on family demands and social characteristics, as well as personal qualities of the parents. Each of these factors that potentially inhibit parent involvement, and interventions designed to minimize the impediments, are considered in the present chapter.

Finally, research pertinent to siblings of hospitalized children is reviewed. Though it has been suggested that siblings are affected by the redirection of family resources toward the hospitalized child, nonhospitalized children, until recently, have been virtually ignored in the research literature. A limited number of studies have now appeared concerning the responses and participation of siblings during a child's hospitalization.

PARENTAL RESPONSES

Prevalence of Parent Anxiety

The prevalence of anxiety among parents of hospitalized children was assessed in one study appearing prior to 1965. Gofman, Buckman, and Schade (1957) reported the incidence and degree of parent anxiety to be great. All of the 100 parents surveyed expressed at least some anxiety about the hospitalization, with 57 percent considering this anxiety to be "overwhelming."

Several additional studies published since 1965 have considered the incidence of parent anxiety or fear associated with children's hospitalization, noting much the same results as those reported by Gofman, et al. For example, Skipper (1966) obtained parent self-ratings of distress before, during and after the tonsillectomy surgery of their children. "Intense" fear or anxiety was reported by 57.4 percent of the parents questioned, both the day before surgery and during the operation. The number of parents reporting intense fear two hours after the operation fell to 17.0 percent.

Skipper, Leonard, and Rhymes (1968) similarly report that more than sixty percent of a group of mothers, who responded to a questionnaire after the hospitalization of their children for tonsillectomy surgery, rated their anxiety as intense the day before surgery. The anxiety of mothers was also found to be high during children's surgery, though mothers who had received an experimental intervention (interaction with a specially trained nurse upon admission) reported lower anxiety during the operation than did those in the control condition. As in the Skipper (1966) study, anxiety among parents in both treatment conditions was considerably lower two hours after surgery.

Kessler (1969) interviewed mothers of young children with an acute illness, hospitalized for the first time and found eighty percent to be moderately or severely stressed by the situation. Maternal anxiety was found to vary with social class, with middle class mothers being more anxious than either upper or lower class mothers.

Frieberg (1972) surveyed 25 mothers of hospitalized children (15 months to 9 years of age) concerning their reactions to the hospital experience. Though presentation of data is unsystematic and the methodology used to obtain responses is not clearly delineated, Frieberg's results are consistent with those reported above. All mothers indicated that they felt "some degree of uneasiness, fear, or anxiety while their child was hospitalized, even if a specific frightening event had not occurred" (p. 1272). Among the factors most commonly cited by mothers as contributing to their anxiety were lack of information about diagnoses and procedures, and fears about treatments, procedures, and children's medical condition. Limited understanding of children's treatment was indeed apparent. Frieberg's questioning of mothers revealed that 15 of the 25 parents were lacking in knowledge of, or were misinformed about, important areas of care.

The Relationship Between Parent and Child Anxiety

The apparently high degree of distress experienced by parents during the hospitalization of their children has been of concern to investigators, not only because of its direct effect on parents, but also because of the possibility that parental anxiety may be conveyed to children, thereby contributing to their upset. Investigations of this so-called "emotional contagion hypothesis" were first conducted prior to 1965. For example, Levy (1960) failed to document a contagion effect, finding no relationship between mothers' reactions or their handling of their infants, on the one hand, and the incidence of crying noted among the infants during an injection. Campbell (1957), however, found that a higher percentage of mothers who had received fear-arousing instructions prior to the injection of their infants became tense during the procedure than those receiving neutral or informative instructions. Furthermore, significantly more infants in the "fear-arousing" group cried during the injection than did children in the neutral/informative condition. Other writers have suggested that a relationship exists between parental upset and children's posthospital adjustment (Woodward, 1959) and that supportive interventions directed toward mothers may reduce their upset, with this reduction, in turn, being reflected in decreases in children's emotional distress (Woodward and Jackson, 1961; Weinick, 1958).

Much of the more recent research examining the relationship between maternal anxiety and children's psychological upset has been conducted in dental clinics. For example, mothers' anxiety has been significantly associated with children's behavioral upset during a dental extraction (Johnson and Baldwin, 1968) or a routine dental examination (Johnson & Baldwin, 1969; Wright & Alpern, 1971). However, in his extensive review of the literature on children's fearful behavior in dental settings, Winer (1982) concludes that the purported relationship between mother anxiety and child behavior is "fragile." The relationship appears to be more evident in studies considering younger children (Wright & Alpern, 1971), rather than older subjects (Klorman, et al., 1979). Furthermore, although the association between parent and child anxiety has been recorded on initial visits, there is evidence that it diminishes as patients become more experienced in the dental setting (Koenigsberg & Johnson, 1972). Finally, interventions directed either toward children (Machen & Johnson, 1974) or mothers (Wright, Alpern, & Leake, 1973) have been shown to disrupt the relationship.

Research conducted in medical settings also suggests an association between maternal anxiety and the responses of children. Heffernan and Azarnoff (1971), for example, examined the anxiety of mothers and children in an outpatient medical clinic. Mothers participating in this study were questioned concerning their reactions to visiting *their own* physician. Responses were classified as indicating that maternal anxiety under those circumstances was either present or not. Children were separated from their mothers in the clinic waiting area, and their anxiety was assessed using a combination of the thematic apperception test and an adjective checklist. A Chi square test indicated that children with high anxiety in the outpatient clinic were more likely to have mothers who experienced anxiety when visiting their own doctor.

Significant correlations between mother and child anxiety have been reported in the prehospital period (Vardaro, 1978), as well as during hospitalization itself (Landes, 1973; Sides, 1977; Goslin, 1979). Vardaro (1978) examined the anxiety responses of eighteen children (36 to 66 months of age, scheduled for hernia repair) and their mothers prior to admission to the hospital. Anxiety of mothers and children was assessed by measuring excretion of 17-hydroxycorticosteroid (17-OHCS; a metabolite of cortisol, a hormone secreted by the adrenal cortex during periods of stress). Mothers collected 24-hour urine samples for themselves and their children in their homes before entering the hospital, also completing the State-Trait Anxiety Inventory (STAI; Spielberger, et al., 1970) and an assessment of children's prehospital behavior.

Strong, positive correlations between the two measures of maternal anxiety (17-OHCS and the STAI) were found. Presumably, the state and trait portions of the STAI were combined for this analysis, though this was not specified by the investigator. Both measures of maternal anxiety were strongly correlated with children's 17-OHCS level, but not with the prehospital behavior rating. The author's conclusion that "the mother has a significant effect on the emotional response of the child" (p. 14), is not defensible on the basis of this correlational study alone. Nevertheless, her suggestion that anxiety of children may be lowered through preadmission teaching directed toward parents is worthy of further investigation.

Three studies report data on the relationship between parent and child anxiety during the period of hospitalization (Sides,

1977; Goslin, 1979; Landes, 1973). Sides (1977) included measures of mothers' trait anxiety and their state anxiety during hospitalization as possible predictors of children's behavioral upset two weeks after discharge from the hospital. Zero-order correlations revealed a significant relationship between mothers' state (but not trait) anxiety and children's posthospital behavior. Goslin (1979) reports a significant relationship between parents' situational anxiety and the inhospital physiological arousal of their children, who had been admitted to the hospital under emergency circumstances for gastroenteritis.

Landes (1973) correlated two measures of mothers' anxiety (a self-report rating and a nurse's rating) with several child anxiety measures collected at admission, prior to surgery, and after surgery (including a nurse's rating, as well as data on pulse, temperature, and systolic blood pressure). Significant relationships between the nurse's ratings of mother and child anxiety were found during the admission and presurgical periods. The lack of independence between these observations (which were presumably made by the same nurse) undoubtedly contributed to the significance of these associations. Nevertheless, nurse ratings of parent anxiety in the pre- and postsurgical period were, respectively, correlated with children's presurgical temperature and their postsurgical pulse and temperature. Mothers' self-reported anxiety yielded only one significant association with a concurrent measure of children's upset. The self-reported presurgical anxiety of mothers was significantly related to children's presurgical pulse rates.

The Impact of Communication on Parent Anxiety

Indirect evidence of a relationship between parent and child anxiety is found in a series of studies considering the effects on the parent-child dyad of information and emotional support directed toward mothers (Mahaffy, 1965; Skipper, 1966; Skipper, Leonard, & Rhymes, 1968; Skipper & Leonard, 1968; Landes, 1973). The general finding of these studies is that increased communication between parents and hospital personnel results in reduced levels of upset among mothers (Skipper, 1966; Skipper, et al., 1968) and their children (Mahaffy, 1965; Skipper & Leonard, 1968). An exception to this pattern was noted by Landes (1973) who found that participation in a parent group was associated with *increases* in mothers' anxiety, and decreases in that of their children.

Skipper (1966) examined the association between the amount of information mothers had received and their feelings of distress during their children's hospitalization. Forty-seven mothers of three- to nine-year-old-children, hospitalized for tonsillectomy surgery, completed a questionnaire in which they rated their perceptions of the amount of information they had been given by physicians about the hospitalization and surgery. The parents were also asked to note their level of distress before, during, and after hospitalization. Self-ratings of anxiety for mothers who indicated that they had received "a great deal" of advance information were compared with those of mothers who had received "little or none."

Mothers who reportedly received greater information about the medical events had significantly lower levels of stress the day before, and during, the operation. Differences in the postsurgical period were not statistically significant. Skipper further notes that parents receiving more information about the hospitalization expressed significantly less desire for additional information and greater satisfaction with the hospital experience than those given limited explanations.

Since the Skipper (1966) study is nonexperimental in design and relies on parent report both for level of information and response variables, interpretation of the results should be made with caution. Nevertheless, the major implication of this study, that increased information results in lower anxiety among parents and possibly their children, is corroborated by other, more methodologically rigorous studies. For example, Mahaffy (1965) examined the effects of systematically providing mothers with emotional support and information beyond that normally provided in the research setting. Subjects for this study were 43 children (between two and ten years of age, hospitalized for tonsillectomy and adenoidectomy) and their mothers, who were randomly assigned to an experimental or control condition. Upon admission of their children to the hospital, mothers in the experimental condition were contacted by a nurse who answered their questions, assessed their needs, and supplied information accordingly. This contact was repeated at several specified times throughout the hospitalization. Control group mothers received routine hospital care. Presumably, the care received by children in the two groups did not differ, although those in the experimental group were undoubtedly aware of the research nurse's repeated presence.

No assessment of mothers' responses were made. However, the mean temperature, systolic blood pressure, and pulse rates of experimental group children were significantly lower than those of control group children preoperatively, postoperatively, and at discharge. Total volume and reported ease of fluid intake following surgery were also greater among children in the experimental group, and their incidence of vomiting was lower than that of control group children. Posthospital parent reports indicated that experimental group children had fewer medical problems after discharge and recovered from surgery more quickly than their control group counterparts.

In a study comparable to that of Mahaffy (1965), Skipper and colleagues (Skipper & Leonard, 1968; Skipper, Leonard, & Rhymes, 1968) examined the effects of providing information and emotional support to mothers of children ages three to nine years, admitted to the hospital for tonsillectomies. The study was conducted in two phases, varying only in the extent of experimental intervention to which mothers were exposed. In Experiment I, experimental-group mothers (N = 24) were met by a nurse upon admission who attempted to create a relaxed atmosphere, encouraged verbalization of mothers' feelings, and provided accurate information about hospital routines and procedures. The nurse also briefly contacted mothers at several times during the hospitalization when "anxiety-provoking events" were occurring. During Experiment II, nursing contact with experimental-group mothers (N = 16) was limited to interaction upon admission. Equal numbers of control group mothers were given routine hospital care, which was characterized by limited interaction with staff members and fragmented communication of information. No direct intervention with children in either the experimental or control conditions was given.

Results pertaining to mother responses are reported by Skipper, Leonard, and Rhymes (1968). Chi square analyses comparing experimental and control-group mothers' self-ratings of anxiety before, during, and after the operation failed to reach statistically significant levels, although the percentage of control group mothers indicating that their anxiety was "intense" during and after the operation was higher than that of the experimental group in both phases of the study. Ratings of mothers' anxiety and their adaptation to hospitalization were also made by nursing staff members who were unaware of the mothers' treatment condition. According to these ratings, anxiety of control-group mothers was significantly greater than that of experimental-group mothers during both portions of the study. Differences in ratings of mothers' adaptation were in the expected direction, though not significant.

Further analyses of mothers' posthospital self-reports revealed that the experimental condition in Experiment I was associated with less desire for additional information, less difficulty in feeling helpful, greater trust and confidence in the medical staff, and greater satisfaction with the hospital experience. In the corresponding analyses for Experiment II, the only result significant at the .05 level was that pertaining to desire for additional information.

Data from this study concerning children's responses, reported by Skipper and Leonard (1968), also support the effectiveness of the experimental condition, with the benefits being most pronounced for Experiment I (repeated nursing contact with experimental-group mothers). According to the results of this first phase, experimental-group children displayed consistently lower systolic blood pressure, pulse rates, and temperature, than control group children. Moreover, in the postoperative recovery period, they exhibited lower incidence of emesis, higher volume of fluid intake, and voided significantly earlier than their control-group counterparts. Nurses' blind ratings of the behavior of children in Experiment I indicate that experimental-group subjects adapted better to hospitalization than those in the control group. Fewer experimental-group mothers called their physicians following discharge, and more reported that their children had recovered within one week's time.

Children's responses during Experiment II are less consistently significant, though the smaller sample size, as well as the reduced amount of nursing contact with mothers, may account for this difference. Experimental-group children had lower pulse rates at discharge, lower temperature pre- and postoperatively, and greater fluid intake following surgery than control-group children. Post-hospital reports by mothers also indicate that more experimental than control-group children were fully recovered within one week of discharge.

In a study conducted by Landes (1973), one of the treatment conditions consisted of information and emotional support provided to parents in a preadmission group setting, rather than individually upon admission as in the previously discussed studies. Parents of 114 children (3 to 10 years of age) were assigned to one of four conditions. Those in the *Parents' Group* condition received explanations about their children's impending hospitalization from staff members and were encouraged to express their feelings about the event. In addition, parents were urged to discuss the hospitalization with their children. Parents in the *Puppet Play* condition attended a puppet show with their children, which depicted events to be encountered during hospitalization. Following the show, children were allowed to play with the puppets and medical equipment. A third group received both the Parent Group and Puppet Play interventions, while a control group received neither. Children's anxiety during hospitalization was measured by systolic blood pressure, pulse, temperature, and nurses' ratings, with each measure taken at admission, and pre- and post-operatively. Mothers' anxiety was assessed through a self-report rating and nurses' observation.

On the basis of correlations with other child and parent dependent variables, Landes selected systolic blood pressure as "the most stable indicator of child's anxiety" (p. 48) and, therefore, reports child outcomes using this measure only. Children whose parents were assigned to the *Parents' Group* condition had lower blood pressure at all three times of assessment than did children in other conditions. However, according to self-report measures, *parents* assigned to this condition were more anxious at admission than Puppet Play or Control Group mothers. Nurses ratings of parents in the *Puppet Play* condition, on the other hand, indicate that they were less anxious than those in the other conditions at the presurgical and postsurgical periods.

Landes summarizes these findings as indicating that the Parents' Group intervention increased parent anxiety, possibly by placing the burden of preparation on their shoulders, while lowering the anxiety of their children. Conversely, the Puppet Play condition reduced parent anxiety while increasing that of the children. It is suggested that this pattern occurs because parents attending a puppet presentation feel relieved of the responsibility of preparing their children, who, therefore, may be less adequately prepared.

Landes' interpretation of the data may, however, be unwarranted. In addition to the dubious, post hoc method of selecting a single dependent measure for consideration, the significant results reported are based on data from *all* families invited to participate in the preadmission experimental conditions, whether they actually did so or not. When only actual participants are included in the analysis (51% of those invited), it appears that differences are no longer significant. Data on these analyses are not presented.

Despite the methodological problems evident in a portion of the studies addressing the effects of communication and emotional support on mothers and children, the results obtained are reasonably consistent. Systematic communication provided to mothers by members of the hospital staff appears to be capable of reducing the anxiety of mothers (the possible exception being the case of Landes, where contact was made with parents in groups prior to admission), as well as that of their children.

Factors Influencing Parent Participation during Hospitalization

The literature on childhood hospitalization provides considerable evidence of the beneficial effects of parental visitation, rooming-in, participation in children's care, and acquisition of information. Nevertheless, parents frequently fail to avail themselves of these opportunities. The research presented in the following sections considers a combination of familial, social, and personal factors that have been associated with differing levels of parent participation in these activities.

Parent Rooming-in and Visitation. In 1959, the Platt Committee on the Welfare of Children in Hospital made a number of recommendations concerning the care of hospitalized children in Great Britain, including provision for unrestricted parent visitation and rooming-in. Although the Platt Committee recommendations were accepted by the Ministry of Health, movement toward implementation of its guidelines has been difficult (e.g., see Thornes, 1983).

A comprehensive examination of factors impeding implementation of the Platt Committee recommendations was undertaken and subsequently published by Stacey, Dearden, Pill, and Robinson (1970). In a portion of this investigation, Robinson (1970) reports that not all of the reluctance to accept liberalization of services rests with the institutions providing care. Familial factors, as well as parents' understanding of the necessity for involvement are implicated as well. Among the most important elements in the decision to either room-in or visit extensively were parents' commitments to other children at home. Based on interviews with parents concerning the possibility of rooming-in with their hospitalized children, Robinson reports that, "as family size increased so expressed readiness to live in decreased" (p. 41). When asked who would help out at home if they would room in, mothers were reported to cite a "restricted" range of possible helpers. For example, only two percent of the respondents mentioned that friends or neighbors might assist with the children remaining at home. If grandparents were unavailable, mothers reported that they would likely turn to other members of their household, who would then be forced to take time off of work or school to help.

In addition to problems of arranging for home care, reluctance to room in could also be attributed to parents' limited knowledge of the potential problems of parent-child separation. Robinson reports that mothers had little understanding of the reasons for rooming-in. For example, none of a group of rooming-in mothers who were interviewed for the study mentioned reduction of posthospital upset as a reason for remaining with her child.

Failure to participate in children's care may also be associated with parents' discomfort in the hospital environment. The relationship between mothers' visiting patterns and fears concerning their own potential hospitalization was also explored by Robinson (1968). On the basis of responses to four brief questions, mothers were classified according to the degree of fear they expressed about being hospitalized. The distribution of responses to questions regarding visitation suggests that greater fear in mothers is associated with an increased *desire* for unlimited visitation privileges. However, when actual visitation patterns were observed, there appeared to be an *inverse* relationship between mothers' fear and their tendency to visit children the maximum allowable time. Statistical tests of these relationships are not reported.

Factors influencing parental visitation of a special category of children, hospitalized newborn infants, were examined by Lampe, Trause, and Kennell (1977). It was the investigators' belief that attachment between parents and infants is more likely to be fostered in the intimacy of the family's home rather than in the hospital, and that a visible malformation of the infant would impede the attachment process. To assess these beliefs, the visiting patterns of parents in an infant unit were observed by members of the hospital staff who were unaware of the hypotheses. Frequency and duration of parental visitation, as well as their degree of involvement with the hospitalized infants, were used as indicators of attachment. Parents who had had their infants at home for two or more weeks prior to hospitalization visited significantly more often, stayed longer, and were more involved with their infants than those having their children home less than two weeks. Visitation patterns were not significantly affected by the presence of visible malformations in the infant.

It has also been suggested that socioeconomic factors effect visitation patterns, with inner-city parents, for example, spending a relatively small amount of time visiting their hospitalized children. Blitzer, Zuckerman, Pozen, and Blitzer (1983) investigated the visitation patterns of inner-city mothers and found that the time mothers spent with their children exceeded the expectations of the staff in the research setting. Members of the pediatric medical and nursing staff of a Boston municipal hospital were questioned concerning their perceptions of the length of mothers' visits. The majority responded that only twenty percent of the mothers would visit four or more hours per day, citing factors such as other children at home, work, and mothers' feelings of discomfort in the hospital for the limited visitation. Subsequently, mothers (who were unaware of the exact nature of the study) were asked to record the amount of time they spent with their children. These records were verified by intermittent staff observation.

Median length of visitation on the second day of children's hospitalization (selected because this day was considered to be representative and yielded the most complete data set) was six hours. Twenty-nine percent of the eighty participating mothers roomed-in with their children at least once during the hospitalization. Blitzer, et al. report that longer visits were associated with factors such as mothers' perceptions that visitation helped their child cope with hospitalization, history of breastfeeding, and mothers' rating of children's temperament as "easy." Interestingly, parents who reported that they felt unwelcome at the hospital had a significantly *greater* mean length of visitation on the second day of hospitalization than those not expressing this concern. Neither employment nor the presence of other children at home affected the length of maternal visits.

Earthrowl and Stacey (1977) report that, if parents from lower social classes fail to participate as actively in the care of their hospitalized children as do parents in other social classes, that failure is likely due to cultural and economic factors rather than differences in parents' appreciation of the child's situation. A survey of more than a thousand children discharged from hospitals in Wales in 1972 identified few significant class-related differences in parents' attitudes toward the importance of visiting their children or giving them explanations about the hospital. Though a somewhat higher percentage of upper class parents (92%) than lower class parents (77%) visited their children daily during hospitalization, the authors attribute this difference to economic factors, such as the cost of transportation to the hospital for lower class families.

According to Roskies, Mongeon, and Gagnon-Lefebvre (1978), the duration and timing of parental visits of hospitalized children, as well as parent behavior during those visits, are subject to modification through a preadmission intervention. Subjects consisted of mothers of children, one to five years of age, scheduled for elective surgery. During the control phase of the study, each mother was visited in her home and asked to complete a parent participation attitude scale and a detailed questionnaire concerning her child's daily habits.

After the hospitalization of 24 control group children, the experimental intervention was instituted, which consisted of extending the preadmission home visit by one-half hour to provide mothers with information about their children's hospitalization and how they might participate. Mothers were advised to visit daily for as long as possible. During the experimental phase, members of the nursing staff were invited to participate in weekly meetings with the investigators to discuss the emotional needs of hospitalized children and their parents.

Information on frequency and duration of mothers' visits were recorded by the nursing staff during control and experimental phases. In addition, periodic observation of parent, child, and staff interactions were made using a standardized observation schedule. Experimental group mothers were found to spend significantly more time with their children than did those in the control group. Roskies, et al. note that this difference is largely attributable to greater length of each visit rather than more total visits by experimental group mothers, since parents in both groups visited nearly daily.

Mothers in both treatment conditions were observed to spend almost all of their time at the hospital in direct involvement with their children. The nature of the activities undertaken by parents differed, however, with experimental group mothers spending significantly more time actively involved in their child's care.

Of further interest is the finding that the experimental intervention appeared to influence fathers' behavior, despite the fact that intervention efforts were directed solely toward mothers. Fathers in the experimental group were found to visit more often and for longer periods than those in the control group.

Parent Participation in the Acquisition of Information. Research reviewed earlier in this chapter indicates that acquisition of information helps to reduce the anxiety of parents and their hospitalized children. However, information (and the emotional support accompanying it) will be maximally effective, only if parents choose to cooperate in the process of dissemination. The greater the effort required of parents to obtain information, the less likely parents will be to participate in individual or group sessions designed to orient them to the hospital experience. Although acceptance rates are infrequently reported for the parent information studies cited above, it appears that when information is brought to the parent, either in the hospital or at home, the percentage of participation is quite good. For example, Skipper and Leonard (1968; also reported in Skipper, Leonard, & Rhymes, 1968) had one hundred percent acceptance of their inhospital intervention. Roskies, et al. (1978) also imply that parents readily agreed to a home visit, though supporting figures are not presented.

However, many of the interventions currently used by hospitals to provide information to parents and their children, such as inhospital, preadmission programs, require the active participation of the family. Reported levels of attendance at programs of this sort have been considerably below maximum possible participation. Meng (1980) reports a 41 percent attendance rate, and Landes (1973) a 51 percent rate, at experimental preadmission programs. Similarly, Schmeltz and White (1982) found attendance at preadmission meetings for parents of children scheduled for cardiac catheterization and surgery to average 45 percent of those invited, despite the fact that meetings were held in the evening to minimize conflicts with work schedules.

Several studies (which are considered in more detail in Chapter 10) have investigated the factors possibly influencing family participation in preadmission programming. Schmeltz and White (1982) found that parents were more likely to attend group meetings prior to hospitalization if their child were an infant or preschooler instead of schoolaged or adolescent, if they were of middle income rather than high or low, and if their child's diagnosis were classified as "mild" or "moderate," instead of "severe." As might be expected, distance from the hospital affected participation, with parents living more than two hours from the hospital being less likely to attend.

Among other distinguishing characteristics, group attenders were more likely to live in households with other relatives, were more willing to discuss feelings with psychosocial professionals, and had experienced fewer "upsets," such as deaths, miscarriages, separations, or divorce, than had non-attenders. Parents not attending the meetings were more likely to prepare their children for hospitalization close to the time of admission than were group attenders. Of those parents preparing their children two to four weeks prior to hospitalization, 75 percent had attended parent groups. In a final finding of note, the method of invitation to the group appeared to affect participation. Schmeltz and White observed that, although all parents received letters notifying them of the session, 85 percent of those who, in addition, were directly informed of the group by their child's cardiologist attended the meeting.

Schrier and Kaplan (1983) report on small samples of parents and children who had or had not attended a preadmission program offered by a hospital in South Africa. Families participating in the session of their own accord were of higher social class than nonattenders; mothers in these families were less likely to be employed outside of the home. All children of parents who attended the session without special invitation were either eldest or only children, while none of the nonattenders fit this description.

Meng (1980) found parents' familiarity with hospitalization to be an important factor in determining family participation in preadmission programming. Parents who chose to attend preadmission sessions had greater previous experience with hospitalization than did other parents and frequently cited their knowledge of the hospital as their reason for nonattendance. It appears from Meng's data that nonattending parents in this sample made use of their familiarity with hospitalization, discussing the impending admission with their children with a frequency equal to that of parents who had attended the preadmission sessions. Moreover, the range of hospital topics discussed by nonattenders with their children exceeded that of attending parents.

Once in the hospital (and in the absence of special interventions to provide parents with information) acquisition of information, other than that routinely given, depends on the parents' own efforts. However, not all parents are equally capable of initiating the interactions with hospital personnel necessary to obtain information. For example, Robinson (1968) reports a relationship between mothers' fears of their own hospitalization and their tendency to avoid hospital personnel. Mothers with higher levels of fear were found to be less likely to speak to the doctor in charge of their child's care, or to express complaints they might have about their child's hospitalization to staff members.

In a related study, Robinson (1972) examined the association between parents' attitudes toward authority and their "illness behavior" during children's hospitalization. A four-cell system of categorizing parents was used, based on parent responses to questions assessing two personality dimensions: 1) readiness to accept hospital authority, and 2) authoritarianism (a term not directly defined by Robinson, though discussion in the text suggests reference to persons who accept the power of authority, whether they dominate or are the ones dominated). The dimensions are believed to be independent. Thus, parents were classified as high or low on each, yielding the four separate groupings.

Although a number of parental behaviors and attitudes regarding hospitalization were surveyed and associated with parents in each of the four categories, those most relevant to the present discussion concern willingness to approach the hospital staff and to receive information. Parents who were rated as high on willingness to accept hospital authority, and also on the authoritarian dimension, were termed "submissive authoritarians." As a group, these parents were reported to have the least complaints about the care of their children and to be most satisfied with the information they received. However, they were also less likely to ask for information when needed, to express a complaint when one arose, or to speak to the doctor in charge of their child's case than were parents in two of the other three groups. Moreover, parents in the submissive authoritarian group were least likely to know the name of their child's surgeon and most frequently said it was unnecessary to speak to the doctor in charge of their child's care.

Parent Participation in Children's Care. When asked what role they would like to play in the care of their hospitalized children, parents have expressed a willingness to perform a variety of tasks. For example, Hill (1978) interviewed eighteen mothers of hospitalized one to four year olds concerning their desire to participate in their children's care by performing comfort measures, activities of daily living, and therapeutic functions, either alone or with assistance. The reported percentages of parents willing to perform the various activities indicates a nearly unanimous desire to engage in comfort measures and in simple daily living activities. The expressed willingness to participate in activities of daily living was somewhat lower if the child in question were in an oxygen tent or had an IV or other tubing. The majority of parents were also willing to perform therapeutic functions such as giving oral medications, monitoring IV rates, recording intake and output levels, and taking vital signs.

Beck (1973) surveyed 38 parents of children who had been previously hospitalized for cardiac conditions, concerning their attitudes toward participation in children's medical care. As in the Hill study, parents were most favorable toward providing emotional support for their children and performing caretaking tasks such as bathing and feeding. More uncertainty was expressed about performance of medical procedures such as taking temperatures, changing bandages, and measuring urine output. However, parent responses were most negative to items suggesting that nurses, rather than parents, perform specific tasks for children, such as administering simple medications and providing explanations of forthcoming procedures.

Jackson, Bradham, and Burwell (1978) report that the activities parents actually performed during their children's hospitalization corresponded to their previously expressed wishes for involvement. The responding subjects were 31 parents who planned to room-in during their children's hospitalization. Within 24 hours of admission, parents completed a questionnaire indicating which of eleven activities they were willing to perform (e.g., feeding, bathing, taking temperatures, etc.). On the third day of hospitalization, the questionnaire was readministered to see if their attitudes had changed. In addition, parents were asked to indicate whether they were, in fact, performing the functions as desired. According to Jackson, et al., most parents wanted to engage in nurturing activities, such as feeding and bathing, with a lesser number willing to perform more medically oriented tasks. Preferences reportedly remained virtually unchanged over the three-day period. Moreover, on the third day the activities preferred and those actually performed were found to closely coincide. Descriptive statistics and tests of significance are not presented.

Despite the apparent willingness of parents to actively participate in the care of their children, several factors have been identified as possibly impeding parental involvement. Among these factors are nurses' attitudes concerning parent participation and parents' uncertainty about their role in the care of their children. Concerning the first of these factors, two studies suggest that a discrepancy exists between the activities nurses believe mothers are willing to perform and mothers' actual stated preferences. Merrow and Johnson (1968) surveyed fifty mothers of hospitalized children and fifty pediatric nurses. Each was asked to classify thirty activities according to those a mother would prefer to do alone, would prefer to do with supervision, or would rather not perform. Statistically significant differences were found between nurses' and mothers' ratings of nine of the thirty items, with mothers typically being more willing to accept responsibility than nurses had predicted.

MacDonald (1969) surveyed 76 parents of pediatric patients and the nurses who cared for their children concerning activities that parents could perform. Though only a limited amount of the data are presented, MacDonald notes that discrepancies between nurses' and parents' perceptions were common, with 97.8 percent of the disagreements occurring with parents of children two or more years of age. Parents were reportedly more willing to engage in activities such as suctioning, changing dressings, taking vital signs, and restraining children during painful procedures than nurses had believed them to be.

The question of discrepancy between parents' and nurses' attitudes toward children's hospitalization was addressed in a somewhat different manner by Gohsman (1977). A semantic differential technique was used to assess nurses' and parents' attitudes toward twelve separate concepts (e.g., nurse, parents, doctor, nurse aid, shot). Differences in the responses of the 44 parents and 35 staff members questioned were relatively small and nonsignificant, though the greatest discrepancy was registered for the concept "parents." Nursing staff members considered "parents" to be less powerful (i.e., on the potency dimension of the semantic differential) than did parents.

Nonsignificant differences between nurses' and parents' attitudes toward another topic, a proposed bill of rights for children in pediatric settings, are reported by Suran and Lavigne (1977). However, a group of attending physicians, also surveyed in this research, expressed a significantly lower level of agreement with the bill than did parents. Differences between nurses' and attending physicians' assessments of the proposed bill were not significant.

The previously discussed study by Roskies, et al. (1978; in which a preadmission session with parents altered their visitation patterns, as well as the nature of their participation in child care) also indicates that staff attitudes concerning parent participation are modifiable through intervention. Nurses were asked to complete the Parent Participation Attitude Scale (Seidl & Pillitteri, 1967) at the beginning and upon conclusion of the experimental period, during which optional weekly meetings for staff members were held to discuss the needs of parents in the hospital.

Scores on the participation scale increased significantly from the pre- to post-test period, with greatest gains found among staff members who participated most actively in the meetings. Roskies, et al. also note that considerable increases were evident among staff members who were relatively young and inexperienced at the beginning of the experimental period. Less change was observed among older, more experienced, better educated staff members, since the attitudes of this group were generally favorable toward parent participation throughout the course of the study.

This finding corresponds to that of two other studies examining the relationship between the status of nursing personnel and their attitudes toward parent participation. Seidl (1969) found that nursing personnel of higher social position in the hospital, and those having higher levels of education, were more accepting of parent involvement in the care of children than were other staff members. Porter (1979) also found that nurses with higher educational levels were more receptive to family-centered care during a child's hospitalization than were their less educated counterparts.

The data presented by Roskies, et al. (1978) indicate that a change in *attitude* toward parent participation does not necessarily result in corresponding changes of behavior exhibited by nursing personnel. Despite the increase in positive attitudes regarding parent involvement noted among nurses over the course of the study, the experimental intervention did little to noticeably alter selected areas of behavior. Although observations indicate that nurses in the experimental period provided somewhat more play and emotional support than was offered to children under the control condition, only in the area of psychological preparation of patients was the amount of increase significant.

According to Roy (1967, 1968) a major hindrance to effective parent participation in the hospitalization of children is their own feeling of discomfort, which is fostered by the lack of a clearly defined parental role in the hospital environment. If so motivated, the nursing staff can improve the quality of parent involvement, Roy argues, by helping parents recognize their role in the care of their children through the introduction of "role cues." Three categories of cues are identified: 1) *congruent orientation cues* (in which the focus of the nurse's attention is adjusted, physically as well as verbally, to correspond to that of the mother), 2) *involvement cues* (the nurse communicates with the mother concerning the child's condition, treatment, activities, or behavior), and 3) *role reference cues* (the nurse directly tells the mother what she might do for her child). A measure of mothers' level of role adequacy, defined as the percentage of times a mother initiates an appropriate action in response to her child's "manifestation of sustenance or socialization needs," (1967, p. 179), was used to measure the effectiveness of the intervention.

The role adequacy of thirty mothers was assessed over a three-day period. The first day, in each case, was devoted to determining mothers' baseline level of adequacy, with no role cues being presented. During observation periods on each of the remaining two days, a portion of the mothers were exposed to cues presented by a staff nurse. Introduction of role cues was found to significantly increase the level of mothers' role adequacy.

A Note on Father Participation

The research reviewed in this and the preceding chapter frequently refers to "parent" actions, responses, or attitudes. In actuality, the parent referred to, with few exceptions, is the mother. The preponderance of research on mothers may be attributed to research traditions, societal beliefs, and the practicalities of conducting research. Medical psychology has, until recently, been dominated by Freudian theory, which places particular emphasis on the importance of the mother-child relationship. Early studies on the effects of separation on the hospitalized child, such as those cited by Vernon, et al. (1965), are rooted in this tradition and, therefore, almost universally attribute the negative responses of children to separation from *mother*, rather than other possible attachment figures. As hospitals have increasingly encouraged parent participation, society's traditional view of parenting roles, supported by the medical community's belief in the primacy of the mother-child relationship, has resulted in a greater number of mothers than fathers rooming-in and involving themselves in their children's care.

An indication that this situation is changing is offered by Lord and Schowalter (1979, 1982), who report an increase in fathers' involvement with their hospitalized adolescents in recent years (see Chapter 7). Moreover, as reported above, Roskies, et al. (1978) found that the level of father participation can be increased, even through the rather indirect means of an intervention targeted for mothers. Nevertheless, hospital-based researchers have typically found fathers to be less available for participation in studies and, for the most part, have eliminated them from consideration. In many cases where an attempt has been made to collect data from both parents, a substantially larger response has been obtained from mothers, with the imbalance being great enough to preclude examination of mother-father differences.

An example of the difficulty of getting father participation in hospital-based research is offered by Azarnoff, et al. (1975). Upon admission to the hospital, parents escorting their children were asked to complete a questionnaire on their children's behavior. With 128 patients in the study, questionnaires were completed by 116 mothers and only 68 fathers. A follow-up questionnaire was mailed to parents one week after discharge. Of the parents completing the first form, all but two mothers returned the second. However, ten of the 68 fathers who had completed the prehospital questionnaire failed to return the posthospital form. Since more mothers completed both questionnaires than fathers, the mothers' data were used for primary analysis.

Despite the low response rate of fathers, Azarnoff, et al. report limited analyses using this data. For example, there was some evidence that fathers' and mothers' perceptions of the hospital experience differed on the day of admission, following participation in one of three treatment conditions to which families were assigned—a tour of the pediatric unit. Parents were asked to rate their own understanding of the reasons for hospitalization, as well as their perceptions of their children's understanding. Fathers in the tour group tended to assess their own understanding as high, but that of their children as low. The opposite relationship was true for mothers, who rated their own understanding as low, while that of their children was rated high. However, when data were considered together from subjects in all three treatment conditions (the tour group, a *booklet group,* which was read a preparation pamphlet upon arrival at the hospital, and a control group), fathers were found to have a lower assessment of their own understanding than mothers, *if* their child were a girl.

Zabin and Melamed (1980) attempted to assess the possible relationship between the disciplinary practices of fathers, as well as mothers, and children's inhospital and posthospital anxiety reactions. A questionnaire assessing parents' styles of interacting with their children was sent to families within a year following children' hospitalization. This information was then correlated with data on children's reactions to hospitalization gathered in conjunction with an earlier study (Melamed & Siegel, 1975). Little difference was reported in the response rate to the questionnaire by fathers (54%) and mothers (60%).

The results indicated that fathers' use of punishment (characterized by instructing the child that failure to engage in a feared behavior would result in unpleasant consequences) and their reinforcement of children's dependency behaviors were directly associated with several measures of children's anxiety. Fathers' modeling of desirable behavior and their providing of reassurance were inversely related to a measure of preoperative anxiety. Direct associations were also found between the level of children's anxiety behaviors and mothers' use of force or their reinforcement of children's dependency, whereas positive reinforcement by mothers was inversely related to child anxiety.

Apart from the few findings discussed in this section, little documentation exists concerning the behavior, attitudes, or responses of fathers during the course of a child's hospitalization. A similar gap exists in knowledge of children's responses to fathers' involvement in their care, or of child reactions to separation from this parent.

SIBLING RESPONSES TO HOSPITALIZATION

The research concerning sibling responses to, and participation in, the hospitalization of children is nearly as scarce as that pertaining specifically to fathers. However, in recent years an encouraging trend toward greater investigation of the impact of hospitalization on nonhospitalized children has been evident.

An early indication that hospitalization may affect nonhospitalized siblings appears as an incidental finding in a study by Sipowicz and Vernon (1965). The authors, in this instance, note that previous studies on hospitalized children had been deficient due to their failure to include adequate control groups of nonhospitalized subjects. They argue that, because of this deficiency, attribution of the psychological upset reported among hospitalized children to the experience of hospitalization itself is unwarranted. In an attempt to compensate for this problem, Sipowicz and Vernon conducted an investigation comparing the behavior of twins, one of whom in each pair was hospitalized.

Twins were selected as subjects since it was assumed that: 1) each pair was roughly similar in behavior before hospitalization, 2) mothers would be able to compare accurately their children's behavior after hospitalization, and 3) "the hospitalization of one twin did not constitute stress for his co-twin" (p. 229), an assumption which the data subsequently proved to be faulty. Mothers of 24 sets of twins were asked to compare the behavior of their children through use of a modified form of the Posthospital Behavior Questionnaire (Vernon, et al., 1966), which was mailed to their homes six days after the hospitalized twin's discharge.

In sixteen of the 24 pairs, the hospitalized twin, as expected, was judged to be more upset than the home twin. In three cases, no overall difference was apparent. However, for five of the pairs, the home twin was found to be significantly more upset than the child experiencing hospitalization. Data obtained from parents on changes in behavior of the home twin while the sibling was in the hospital were examined. Sipowicz and Vernon report that:

> Changes were noted in 13 of the 24 pairs of twins. In ten of these the absence of the hospital twin, or the absence of the mother visiting the hospital twin, was apparently upsetting to the home twin (p. 230).

The authors further note that those home twins who did *not* exhibit negative affect in response to their sibling's hospitalization were considerably younger (mean age of 2.04 years) than those displaying upset (4.45 years).

Despite this evidence that hospitalization might be upsetting for nonhospitalized siblings (at least in the exceptional case of twins), virtually no additional research on the impact of hospitalization on siblings appeared for more than a decade. Responses of healthy siblings have, however, been reported in studies assessing family adjustment to the chronic illness of a child member. Research has considered the adjustment of siblings of children with asthma (Taylor, 1980), congenital heart disease (Aply, Barbour, & Westmacott, 1967; Taylor, 1980), leukemia (Binger, Ablin, Feuerstein, Kushner, Zoger, & Mikkelsen, 1969), myelomeningocele (Hunt, 1973), spina bifida (Tew & Lawrence, 1973), and cystic fibrosis (Burton, 1975; Harder & Bowditch, 1982; Taylor, 1980).

At least two studies, the results of which are conflicting, have directly compared behavioral responses of siblings of children with differing types of medical conditions. Gath (1972) contrasted behavioral ratings of schoolage siblings of children with Down's syndrome or with surgically repaired cleft palates, finding no difference in the adjustment of these groups when compared to each other or to their respective control groups. Lavigne and Ryan (1979) compared the behavioral adjustment of siblings (age 3 to 13 years) of pediatric hematology, cardiology, and plastic surgery patients with a control group of siblings of healthy children. Siblings in the combined illness groups were found to be more withdrawn than the control group children. Moreover, comparison of illness groups showed that siblings of children with a visible condition (i.e., plastic surgery patients) were rated higher on social withdrawal than siblings of patients with "invisible" conditions (hematology and cardiology). Among younger children (3 to

6 years of age), siblings of plastic surgery patients were also rated as higher on a general psychopathology scale than siblings of children in other illness categories.

Descriptions of the adjustments made by nonhospitalized siblings and their families during the brief hospitalization of schoolage children are provided by Knafl (1982) and Knafl and Dixon (1983). Data for these reports were gathered through two intensive interviews with parents, the first being conducted within 24 hours of admission to the hospital, with the second interview occurring four to six weeks after discharge.

The role of nonhospitalized siblings during the period of hospitalization was classified as either *active* (siblings assuming additional tasks or responsibilities) or *passive* (siblings expected to accept changes in routine). Of the 59 participating families, Knafl (1982) reports that sibling involvement was active in 21 cases. Among families with active sibling participation, eight reported instances of one sibling providing care for others at home. In the other 13 active cases, siblings assumed responsibility for at least a portion of their own care. Families classified as having *passive* sibling participation (N = 38) were further subdivided according to the degree of change in routines nonhospitalized siblings were asked to accept. Subcategories included *high change* (siblings with substitute caregivers outside of their own homes; N = 12), *moderate change* (substitute caregiving in the home; N = 14), or *low change* (no change in caregiver or location; N = 12).

Parent perceptions of sibling responses to the hospitalization were also obtained and classified as being *negative* (e.g., atypical behavior, emotions, or complaints), *concerned* (curiosity expressed about the hospitalized child's condition, with no overt change in behavior), or as demonstrating *no response.* Only thirteen of the 59 families reported negative responses, with but two of these considered severe. Non-severe negative behaviors disappeared either upon the hospitalized child's return home or within a week's time. The authors report that negative responses were found to cluster in siblings of the high-change subgroup (Knafl, 1982), and among children 4 to 11 years of age (Knafl & Dixon, 1983).

Knafl and Dixon (1983) also provide information on the contact maintained by siblings during a child's hospitalization. Of the 104 nonhospitalized children under eighteen years of age in the families considered, 69 percent maintained direct contact via telephone or visitation, with forty percent of the siblings visiting the hospitalized child. The percentage of sibling visitation was found to increase with age, a reflection of policy in the hospitals studied, which prohibited visiting by children younger than twelve years. Despite this official prohibition, seventeen of the fifty siblings four to eleven years of age, and two of 27 younger than four years, were permitted to visit. Instances of negative sibling responses appeared to be unrelated to the method of contact maintained by siblings.

The impact of sibling visitation has also been examined in two specialized cases concerning infants. Schwab, Tolbert, Bagnato, and Maisels (1983) assessed sibling visitation in a neonatal intensive care unit, while Trause, Voos, Rudd, Klaus, Kennell, and Boslett (1981) considered the effects of visiting both mother and newborn infants following childbirth.

Schwab, et al. randomly assigned sixteen siblings (3.8 to 7.25 years of age) of thirteen infants, hospitalized for two or more weeks in a neonatal intensive care unit (NICU), to a visiting or nonvisiting condition. Approximately a week after the infant's birth, each sibling was brought to the hospital. Those in the visiting group spent fifteen to thirty minutes in the NICU. Sibling interactions with infants varied from touching to holding and feeding them. An observer was present during each visit to note the sibling's reactions. Following this period, siblings in both groups were interviewed. Parent ratings of sibling behavior were also obtained at three points: 1) upon admission, 2) prior to the hospital visitation, and 3) one week after the visitation.

No significant changes were found in the behavior of siblings in either group over time, nor were differences in the behavior of visiting and nonvisiting siblings significant. Though five of the sixteen subjects failed to respond to an investigator's questions following the visitation period, those responses obtained suggest greater acceptance of the hospital by siblings in the visiting group. Four of the six nonvisiting siblings responding to the interview gave negative or fearful descriptions of the hospital, while all five of the visiting siblings who completed the interview were said to be positive or noncommittal in their descriptions. Observations indicated that visits were neither disruptive of patient care nor upsetting to the visiting sibling.

Trause, et al. (1981) examined the reactions of 31 firstborn children (1 to 3.5 years of age) to the birth of a sibling. Subjects were randomly assigned to a visiting condition (N = 17) or a nonvisiting condition (N = 14), with children in the visiting group allowed to spend one hour per day with their mothers. Home visits were made two to four weeks before mothers' hospitalizations, and one to two weeks following discharge. During the home sessions, an investigator observed the behavior of mother-child dyads and asked each mother to complete a form on her child's behavior. Observations were also made of children's behavior when brought to the hospital to be reunited with their mothers upon discharge.

Visitation was found to be unrelated to alteration in children's behavior in the posthospital period, with both groups of siblings displaying heightened disturbance. Increases in sleeping problems, temper tantrums, and excessive activity were noted among visiting and nonvisiting children alike. Observation revealed that mothers in both groups issued more angry and stern commands following hospitalization, and that their children stayed near them significantly more than in the prehospital period. Hospital visitation, however, was associated with differences in children's behavior with mothers at discharge. Those in the nonvisiting group more often ignored or avoided their mothers when they entered the waiting room, ignored or refused mothers' requests for a hug or kiss, and ignored or responded negatively to their parents' questions of whether they liked the new baby than did children participating in daily visitation.

An objection frequently raised in opposition to sibling visitation is that the introduction of siblings to patient care areas will increase the risk of infection. Schwab, et al. (1983) and Trause, et al. (1981) each considered this factor when conducting their visitation studies. In neither case was an increased incidence of infection associated with sibling visitation. These findings are in agreement with those of Umphenour (1980) who found no increase in bacterial colonization in a well-baby nursery following sibling visits.

The published studies addressing the question of sibling visitation and infection have focused on visitation in infant units. To determine whether evidence exists concerning sibling visitation in other pediatric units, and whether legal barriers prevent such visitation, Shuler and Reich (1982) conducted a series of three informal surveys. In the first of these, 52 state health departments were contacted and asked 1) whether their state regulations prohibited sibling visitation, 2) whether they could provide documentation that visitation is associated with increased risk of infection, and 3) whether the state makes specific recommendations regarding health screening in facilities allowing visitation.

Of the 25 departments responding to the survey, one reported that its state limited visitation to children fourteen years of age or older. Another five states restricted the visits of children less than twelve years of age. Two of the states restricting visitation were said to permit sibling visits in "family-centered" maternity units. None could provide evidence of increased infection when sibling visitation was allowed in maternity wards. Twenty-three of the responding states reported that health screening was left to the discretion of the individual hospital; the remaining two states provided guidelines.

Subjects of the subsequent two surveys conducted by Shuler and Reich (1982) were, respectively, pediatric hospitals and selected physicians. The majority of the responding hospitals permitted visitation by young children and reported positive attitudes among health care personnel toward this practice. None of the institutions had formally studied the effects of visitation or infection rates, though five reported no noticeable increase in infection following implementation of sibling visitation.

The limited number of physicians contacted in the final survey were reported to be generally positive toward some form of sibling visitation. As was true of the other surveys, the physicians could cite no empirical data pertaining to the association between increased infection rates and sibling visitation.

Chapter 7

ADOLESCENT HOSPITALIZATION, HEALTH CARE, AND ILLNESS

The research literature on hospitalized adolescents differs considerably from that pertaining to younger children, both in total volume of research available and in the nature of the studies that have been conducted. Of the studies reviewed in this text concerning reactions to health care experiences, some twenty percent include subjects thirteen years of age or older. However, only a few of these exclusively consider adolescents (Green, 1976; Kaplan, et al., 1981; Mahon, 1980). The remaining studies in this category that include adolescents typically examine subjects of a wide age range, with this range averaging nearly twelve years. In these instances, young adolescents merely serve as the upper boundary of the sample, with their characteristic responses to health care seldom isolated for consideration.

Of the limited number of studies solely devoted to adolescent hospitalization and illness (27 studies in all), the majority are surveys assessing adolescents' general attitudes and opinions about their health care or their responses to specific aspects of their experience while hospitalized. The research methodology of these studies is frequently presented in a cursory manner. Systems used for classifying responses and the reliability of such systems, are seldom reported.

Aside from research using survey techniques, there has been little attempt to assess directly the immediate or posthospital effects of hospitalization on adolescents. Only a single observational study exclusively considering the activities of hospitalized adolescents was identified (Kaplan, Rosenstein, Skomorowsky, Shenker, & Ramsey, 1981). The stated purpose of this research was instrument development, rather than hypothesis testing. Clough (1978) included young adolescents in his observational study of orthopedic patients, who ranged in age from nine to fifteen years. However, the primary function of this research was to investigate the comparability of observations of subjects made by three independent groups of observers. Age-related responses were not at issue.

Use of self-report measures to evaluate levels of psychological upset among hospitalized adolescents is equally rare. The only study discussing development of a self-report scale designed to assess the anxiety of adolescents in the hospital (Parker & Gibson, 1977) was conducted with a group of nonhospitalized subjects. No evidence of this instrument's subsequent use with a population of hospitalized adolescents was discovered.

Virtually no application of experimental research designs is found in the literature on adolescent hospitalization. Despite the profusion of research assessing the merits of preoperative preparation for children and adults, fewer than ten percent of the preparation studies considered in Chapter 10 of this text include subjects thirteen years of age or older. None of the identified studies has specifically evaluated adolescent preparation. Neither have other interventions, implemented in hopes of minimizing the emotional distress of hospitalized adolescents (e.g., the institution of adolescent units, recreational programs, or group meetings), been subjected to systematic evaluation.

Topics addressed by the existing research, presented in this chapter, include assessments of adolescent's conceptions of health and illness, as well as surveys of their perceptions of health care problems and delivery systems. Studies documenting the distribution of diagnoses among hospitalized adolescents are examined to underscore the differences between general pediatric and adolescent populations. Following this review, the limited number of studies assessing adolescent responses to hospitalization are presented, as is the research sampling adolescent opinions concerning visitation patterns and information providers. Other areas considered are parent reactions to children's illness and hospitalization, and studies pertaining to the institution of adolescent units. Finally, the results of two studies are presented on the knowledge and attitudes of hospital personnel about adolescents.

ADOLESCENT HEALTH CARE CONCEPTS AND ATTITUDES

Conceptions of Health and Illness

Of the numerous studies reviewed in Chapter 3 on children's conceptions of health care and illness, Only Millstein, et al. (1981) focused on the period of adolescence, with the attention of this study being limited to subjects eleven to fifteen years of age. Seventy-seven nonhospitalized junior high school students were asked to explain how they know when they are sick. Multiple responses were accepted, and all were coded using a system developed by Campbell (1975) consisting of eleven theme categories, the most sophisticated of which refer to covert symptoms, specific diagnoses, and psychosocial states, rather than more apparent external symptoms. The frequency of adolescent responses in the higher categories (characterized by Campbell as "adult-favored") was recorded for comparison with the responses of Campbell's sample of children and adults.

Although the responses most frequently given by adolescents referred to simple, external symptoms (cited by 90% of the subjects), 35.5 percent of the Millstein, et al. sample mentioned psychosocial states in their responses. Frequency of use of adult-favored themes by adolescents fell between that of the children and adults interviewed by Campbell, though closer to the level of children than adults. The researchers had anticipated that *within* the adolescent group the total number of themes mentioned, as well as the frequency of adult-favored themes, would increase with age. However, the hypothesized patterns were not found.

If, as Millstein, et al. suggest, young adolescents' concepts of health and illness are closer to those of children than adults, exploration of further development in later periods of adolescence is warranted. Research to date, operating primarily from a Piagetian framework that allows for no qualitative change in cognition from adolescence through adulthood, has neglected this area of investigation.

Health Concerns of Adolescents

More frequently examined than concepts of health and illness have been adolescents' perceptions of the health care problems existing among their peers. Three surveys addressing this topic (Brunswick, 1969; Sternlieb & Munan, 1972; Parcel, Nader, & Meyer, 1977) differ in geographic location of data collection and in the age and socioeconomic status of the respondents—differences that likely account for some the variability in the reported results. Nevertheless, despite the regional and socioeconomic differences, several common themes emerge from this research. Problems related to drugs, sex, school, and families are typically cited, reflecting the pervasiveness of anxiety associated with these issues.

In the earliest of these studies, Brunswick (1969) interviewed 122 adolescents (12 to 17 years of age) in a predominately lower-middle and working class section of New York City. Among other questions, respondents were asked to identify "the biggest health and medical problems for young people living around here" (p. 1734). Subjects were allowed to cite multiple problems.

The most frequently mentioned problems (with the percentage of adolescents identifying each response given in parentheses) were: cigarette smoking (44%), drugs (34%), drinking (32%), and air pollution (18%). When asked to rate their own current health status, 83 percent said it was "good" or "very good." Fewer felt that their dental condition was as favorable, with only two-thirds rating it as "good" or better.

Sternlieb and Munan (1972) sought a sample representative of the general population of "youth" (defined as 15 to 21 years of age) living in Sherbrooke, Quebec. Some 1400 subjects completed a health care questionnaire in their school or place of employment. Though data on socioeconomic status are not reported, it may be assumed that the sample is somewhat more diverse than that contacted by Brunswick. Subjects were presented with lists of "health problems" and "personal problems" and were asked to select those which were currently of concern to them. As in the Brunswick study, multiple responses were permitted.

The most commonly cited health problems were nervousness (29.2%), dental problems (27.2%), menstrual problems (22.4% of the female respondents), and acne (18.3%). Most common personal problems were attributed to school (30.1%), family (20.9%), sex (16.5%), and religion (16.2%). Two of the health problems frequently cited by the Brunswick (1969) adolescents, drugs and drinking, were classified by Sternlieb and Munan as personal problems. Both were cited by fewer than seven percent of the Canadian youths. In what may be another reflection of cultural differences, the remaining two problems most frequently noted by Brunswick's New York City adolescents, cigarette smoking and air pollution, do not appear in the lists of either personal or health problems submitted to respondents by Sternlieb and Munan.

Parcel, et al. (1977) obtained questionnaire responses from 3,255 students in two high schools in Galveston, Texas, representing upper to lower class families, but with nearly half of the respondents from lower-middle or lower class families. Students were presented with lists from which they were to identify "health concerns" (i.e., areas associated with adolescent health about which respondents might have questions or worries), and "health problems" (matters with which students might wish to receive help). Commonly cited health concerns involved school (44.0%), drugs (39.3%), sex (38.2%), and parents or family (35.2%), while most frequently expressed health problems were related to acne (30.0%), sex (29.2%), depression or sadness (23.3%), and obesity (22.8%).

Despite the different systems of categorization used by Parcel, et al. (1977) and Sternlieb and Munan (1972), a number of the expressed concerns were shared by respondents to both surveys (i.e., problems with school, family, sex, and acne). As was also true of the Sternlieb and Munan survey, Parcel, et al. did not include cigarette smoking (the most frequently cited problem in the Brunswick study) in their list of health problems or concerns.

Attitudes Toward Adolescent Health Clinics

The highly personal nature of several of the health issues identified as being of concern to adolescents makes attention to them through traditional health care channels less than satisfactory. For example, use of the family physician for information on sex or contraception, or for assistance with a problem of drug abuse, may be unacceptable. Alternate sources of help may be either unavailable, too expensive, or unknown to adolescents who may, as a consequence, avoid professional help, thereby compounding the problem.

One suggested means of providing alternative care is through community-based adolescent clinics. Typically sponsored by an existing hospital or health care agency, adolescent clinics are designed to provide sensitive, low-cost, confidential care. Two of the studies previously reviewed were, in fact, conducted to assist in planning such services (Sternlieb & Munan, 1972; Parcel, et al., 1977). Each included questions specifically pertaining to this type of health care facility. A third study (Resnick, Blum, & Hedin, 1980) also considered adolescents' evaluation of this type of service.

Adolescents responding to the Sternlieb and Munan (1972) survey were asked to specify factors that inhibit their visits to doctors. One-third of the subjects responded that they were never sick. However, 27 percent of the sample cited cost of care as an impediment. Fear of the physician was the third most frequently cited limiting factor, although this was mentioned by only 5.2 percent of the respondents.

Sternlieb and Munan, as well as Parcel, et al. (1977), questioned subjects concerning the type of information they felt adolescent clinics should supply. The results of both surveys are in essential agreement, despite minor variations in the order and percentage of subjects responding to each item. The Sternlieb and Munan Canadian sample most frequently mentioned sex education (65.2%), drugs (63.5%), venereal disease (43.2%), alcoholism (42.0%), and family planning (38.4%). The comparable list for the Parcel, et al. sample of Texas adolescents included drugs (66.8%), sex education (58.0%), venereal disease (57.3%), birth control (52.5%), and alcohol (50.0%).

When asked with whom they would like to discuss their health problems in an adolescent clinic, the Sternlieb and Munan sample most frequently mentioned general practitioners (47.9%), followed by friends (39.2%), parents (35.3%) and psychologists (26.6%). Interestingly, the most frequently mentioned means of obtaining information at clinics was *not* through personal contact, but rather through films (mentioned by 59.2% of the subjects).

Parcel, et al. used a different format for identifying adolescent preferences for information providers. Respondents were presented with a series of seven situations concerning "a friend" and were asked to whom the individual should go in each case. Parents, physicians, and community agencies were cited most frequently, with the precise order of preference depending on the problem under consideration. For example, parents were the preferred source of assistance for personal situations such as contemplation of suicide or running away from home. Physicians were recommended for consultation concerning venereal disease or stomach aches, while community agencies were suggested for questions on alcoholism, contraception, and pregnancy.

Sternlieb and Munan (1972) further asked respondents to identify characteristics they felt were important in physicians staffing adolescent clinics. Qualities most frequently mentioned were the physician's understanding (92.6%), friendliness (84.1%), personality (81.4%), and informal manner (65.3%). The age, sex, and dress of physicians were each mentioned by fewer than thirty-five percent of the sampled adolescents. Finally, when asked whether they would use an adolescent clinic if the need arose, 94.0 percent of the sample responded affirmatively.

General reactions of groups of adolescents in Minnesota to adolescent health services are reported by Resnick, Blum, and Hedin (1980). Participants were more than 800 high school students from over twenty schools and organizations who met in discussion groups of five to seven members. Each discussion group designated a leader who read questions and recorded comments. Responses obtained from the 170 discussion groups are reported using "qualitative techniques of content analysis" (p. 138), which were said to identify recurrent themes. However, percentages of groups or individuals raising specific issues are not reported.

According to Resnick, et al. the quality and style of the personnel staffing adolescent clinics were highly regarded by participants. Clinic staff members were viewed as technically competent, compassionate, and direct. The environment of such clinics was noted as being comfortable and age-appropriate, with the absence of small children and parents considered to be an important element. Affordability and confidentiality of clinic services were also commended.

Negative responses were most frequently registered by rural respondents. Among the concerns they expressed were the potentially high cost of adolescent clinics to the community and the possibility that the availability of adolescent health services would cause dissension in families or encourage irresponsible behavior. Moreover, concern was raised that clinic confidentiality might limit parents' knowledge of potentially serious conditions.

THE HOSPITALIZED ADOLESCENT

Diagnoses of Hospitalized Adolescents

The distribution of diagnoses among hospitalized adolescents has been documented in two studies (Tonkin, Ng, & Sheps, 1981; Oelberg & Finkelstein, 1981). Percentages of patients in the designated categories vary between studies due to differences in the types of hospitals examined and in the systems used for classifying patients. Nevertheless, the data indicate that conditions necessitating hospitalization of adolescents frequently differ from those of younger children. In particular, pregnancy, accidents, and, to a lesser extent, psychosis account for a substantial portion of adolescent admissions.

Tonkin, et al. (1981) examined the adolescent populations of two major pediatric referral and tertiary care facilities that were to be combined to form a single children's hospital in Vancouver, British Columbia. Information was obtained on all patients eleven to nineteen years of age discharged from the two hospitals between 1971 and 1978. Patients were categorized on the basis of the length of their hospitalization and severity of their diagnosis. Percentages of total patients, as well as percentages of total bed days, accounted for by each category are presented.

In absolute numbers of patients, adolescents admitted for short-term stays (1 to 3 days) and having no significant secondary diagnoses were most common, accounting for 43.9 percent of all discharges. However, over the eight years for which records were examined, the percentage of total adolescent bed days accounted for by this group was far lower, ranging from 9.8 to 11.7 percent. Patients admitted for long-term stays (15 or more days) or with significant secondary diagnoses, on the other hand, constituted only 16.3 percent of the total adolescent discharges, but 56.9 percent of total adolescent bed days. Violence-related conditions (including suicide or homicide attempts or accidents) accounted for 20.9 percent of adolescent bed days during a one-year period (1977) selected for detailed examination. Pregnancy accounted for 16.9 percent of all adolescent discharges in the hospitals studied.

Oelberg and Finkelstein (1981) reviewed the records of all adolescents, twelve to eighteen years of age, admitted to the University of Texas Medical Center in 1977. More than two-thirds of the 2,208 patients considered were females. This disproportionate distribution was attributed to the prevalence of obstetrics/gynecology admissions, which constituted 48 percent of all adolescent admissions to this facility. Ninety-five percent of this group was admitted to obstetrics. Adolescent admissions to other hospital services included surgery (29% of the admissions), pediatrics or internal medicine (13%), psychiatry (10%), and dermatology or radiology (less than 1%).

In addition to compiling this information, Oelberg and Finkelstein conducted a detailed examination of the charts of 325 adolescents admitted during 1977 to assess the adequacy of the baseline information contained in the patients' records. They report that information on diet, substance use or abuse, immunization status, perinatal events, social history, and menstrual history (excluding obstetrics records) were infrequently recorded in adolescents' charts.

Adolescent Responses to Hospitalization

In recent years, several reviews of the theoretical and clinical literature on the effects of hospitalization on adolescents have appeared (e.g., see Conway, 1971; Jackson, 1973; Lincoln, 1978; Schowalter, 1977). This material suggests that hospitalization and illness negatively affect adolescents' body image and self-esteem. Moreover, fears of death associated with illness are reported to be prevalent, as are concerns over the loss of independence that hospitalization or illness may entail. Specific elements of hospital life, such as the intrusions on privacy, or the existence of regulations limiting adolescents' choices or impeding their access to peers, are identified as contributing to the upset experienced by this group during hospitalization. Unfortunately, the theoretical guidance and clinical insights evident in this literature have not been translated into a program of rigorous investigation. Few systematic studies have appeared that assess the nature and prevalence of inhospital or posthospital reactions of adolescents, nor has their been sufficient effort to determine the individual or environmental elements that contribute to adolescent responses.

Symptomatic of the lack of concerted investigation on the reactions of adolescents to hospitalization is the virtual absence of instruments to assess variations in adolescents' anxiety or behavior. Noting the lack of such investigative measures, Parker and Gibson (1977) began development of their own instrument, the Hospitalized Adolescent Anxiety Tool (HAAT). Through a review of the literature on adolescent hospitalization, and examination of instruments designed to measure anxiety in other populations, Parker and Gibson compiled a series of 28 statements pertaining to seven developmental and situational categories: body image concerns, independence/dependence concerns, perceptions of peer interaction, identity formation, situation-specific phenomena, manifestations of the properties of anxiety, and adolescent activities/frame of reference. Adolescents completing this instrument were asked to designate the degree to which they felt each item accurately described themselves, with responses on a four-point scale ranging from "not at all" to "very much so" (e.g., "I am content with how I look," or "I feel that things have interfered with my plans").

Unfortunately, the only reported piloting of this instrument by Parker and Gibson was conducted with nonhospitalized adolescents. Analysis of the internal consistency of the instrument, performed on the pilot data, indicated that four items should be deleted from the scale. No assessment of validity of the scale was reported. Nor is there evidence in the identified literature of the subsequent use of this measure with hospitalized subjects.

Adolescent anxiety over the integrity and acceptability of their bodies, another of the concerns frequently cited in reviews of the clinical and theoretical literature, has been investigated by Green (1976). Eight adolescent males, fourteen to seventeen years of age, were interviewed and observed for five days following emergency appendectomies. Expressions about their body experiences were recorded and analyzed for content, frequency, and change in pattern over the period of recovery from surgery.

Subjects' attention to their bodies was described as intense and continuing, with the number of body-related expressions reaching a maximum level on the second day of hospitalization, gradually declining thereafter. Three-fifths of the expressions pertained to body *function*, and more than one-third to body *sensations*. Few expressions were related to *appearance*.

The expressions of the adolescent males were further categorized according to the types of concerns they expressed about body *integrity* (i.e., capability, endurance, or intactness) or body *condition* (impairment, improvement, or uncertainty). Nearly half of the concerns about integrity related to capability, while more than half of the expressed concerns about body condition referred to impairment. However, an increase in the body expressions of *improvement* was noted over time.

Mahon (1980) examined the relationship between selected presurgical characteristics of fifty scoliosis patients, 11 to 23 years of age, and their recovery from surgery. Presurgical assessments, conducted in the hospital approximately a week before surgery, measured adolescents' trait anxiety, active-independent orientation, emotional poise, and level of cognitive development. It was predicted that subjects low in trait anxiety, and high in the other assessed presurgical characteristics, would fare better during the postsurgical period. To test this hypothesis, two separate canonical correlations were computed, the first relating the presurgical measures to assessments of state anxiety and depression made in the hospital approximately one week after surgery, and the second relating the same presurgical measures to the amount of pain medication required by patients and the number of days they spent in the hospital prior to discharge.

The first of these analyses proved significant. Examination of zero-order correlations between presurgical characteristics and postsurgical indices revealed that the significance of the correlation is largely due to the strong relationship between trait anxiety and both postsurgical measures of psychological state. The second canonical correlation, using medications and days in the hospital as outcome measures, instead of the anxiety and depression ratings, was nonsignificant. Mahon contends that this was due to an artificial restriction in the variability of time spent in the hospital after surgery—a period kept relatively constant for all patients. The second canonical correlation was, therefore, recomputed substituting another measure, presence or absence of urinary and/or bowel elimination difficulties, for postsurgical days.

The reanalysis yielded significant results. Zero-order correlations again suggested that the significance of this analysis is primarily due the association between trait anxiety and one of the outcome measures—in this case, elimination difficulties. Thus, although Mahon contends that the assessed presurgical characteristics are predictive of postsurgical adjustment, it appears that a single characteristic, trait anxiety, makes the strongest contribution to this relationship.

The only structured observational study of adolescent activities while in the hospital was reported by Kaplan, et al. (1981), who developed the Hospitalized Adolescent Interaction Scale, a thirty-item checklist for documenting adolescents' activities while alone or interacting with staff members, visitors, or other patients. Observations using this instrument are made at predetermined intervals for ten seconds, with the observer recording all items occurring in that period, as well as the location of the observation.

Pilot-testing of this instrument consisted of observations of activities on two separate adolescent units, one of which offered patients significant autonomy and had an active program of adolescent activities, with the other being more restrictive. Although the data reported were not intended to be a comparison of the differing approaches to patient care, the authors found remarkable similarity in the interactions of adolescents in the two settings. Examination of combined categories of activities revealed that more than half of adolescents' time in both settings was spent in solitary pursuits or inactivity. Interaction with other patients occurred infrequently. When interaction *was* observed, it was more likely to be with adults than with fellow patients. The four most frequently occurring checklist items, which appeared in the same order of frequency at both hospitals, were: 1) television on, 2) visitor in room, 3) patient watching television, and 4) visitor and patient talking.

Aside from these few studies, little systematically obtained information exists on adolescent reactions to, or activities during, hospitalization. Moreover, the limitations of the data presented by the studies reviewed are several. For example, two of the studies limited their samples to a single, relatively narrow group, with Green (1976) considering young, male adolescents recovering from appendectomies and Mahon (1980) investigating scoliosis patients. None of the studies addressed adolescent reactions during the posthospital period. The need for further research on the inhospital and posthospital reactions and behaviors of adolescent patients, hospitalized for a range of medical and surgical conditions, is apparent.

Adolescent Visitation Patterns

Information on the frequency and identity of the visitors of hospitalized adolescents is presented by Lord and Schowalter (1979). Visitation patterns for two hundred patients admitted to an adolescent unit were determined through interviews. An equal number of male and female patients, younger and older than fourteen years of age were included in the sample. Subjects reported averaging slightly more than four visitors per day, although the total number of visitors received varied with patients' age. Patients younger than fourteen years had one-third fewer visitors than the older adolescents. Parents accounted for half of the younger group's visitors, but only a third of those received by older subjects. The percentage of visitors who were siblings or other relatives was comparable for both groups, representing approximately one-third of each group's total. Older adolescents received more visits from friends than did younger subjects.

In addition to patient age, the severity of the adolescent's illness affected visitation patterns. Subjects rated as having a "mild" illness averaged one more visitor per day than adolescents with more serious conditions. Severe illness was associated with longer periods of visitation, especially when the patient was male.

On a given day, 93 percent of the mothers and 67 percent of the fathers of the adolescents were said to have visited. Average length of parental visit was nearly three hours, though mothers' visits averaged an hour longer than those of fathers.

Adolescents' evaluations of the visitation patterns were also obtained. When questioned about the total number of visitors they had received, 52 percent of the adolescents said they were satisfied, and 43 percent wanted more, while 5 percent would have preferred fewer visitors. Seventy-two percent of the subjects found the length of individual visits to be satisfactory, although 32 of the two hundred adolescents noted that at least one visitor had stayed too long. When asked whom they preferred to have visit them, 26 percent identified parents as their first choice. An additional 19 percent specifically identified their mothers as the most preferred visitor, while only three individuals so designated their fathers. Age differences were apparent in patient preferences for visitors, with older adolescents preferring friends over parents.

Adolescent Preferences for Information Providers

The preferences of adolescents for information providers and for the type of information received are reported in studies by Craft (1981), who sampled a general population of hospitalized adolescents, and by Levenson and colleagues, who surveyed a group of adolescent cancer patients (Levenson, Pfefferbaum, Silberberg, & Copeland, 1981; Levenson, Pfefferbaum, Copeland, & Silberberg, 1982; Pfefferbaum & Levenson, 1982; Levenson, Pfefferbaum, & Overall, 1983). Craft obtained questionnaire responses from forty subjects, twelve to seventeen years of age. Subjects were presented with a series of topics (identified through earlier meetings with adolescents as commonly arising during hospitalization) and were asked to designate the preferred source of information for each: parents only, health professionals only, parents and health professionals together, or another source. Of the 560 total responses to individual items, health professionals only was designated most often (255 responses), followed by both parents and professionals (201 responses), parents only (101 responses), and other sources (3 responses).

Preference for health professionals was strongest when the topic in question required technical expertise, such as questions concerning medications, examinations, and length of hospitalization. Age was also a factor in the selection of information providers, with older adolescents more likely to prefer health care professionals over parents. A separate survey of parents of adolescents revealed a preference that information be given by both parents and professionals.

Results reported in the series of studies conducted by Levenson and colleagues are quite similar to those of Craft, despite Levenson's use of a more selective group of adolescents—those receiving treatment for cancer. Respondents in this research included 63 adolescent patients (11 to 20 years of age), 60 parents, and 53 physicians. When asked who currently provides information about the patient's illness, adolescents, parents, and physicians agreed that the physician was the primary source of information (Levenson, et al., 1981). Substantial agreement was also apparent on questions of the preferred means of providing adolescents with information concerning their illness, with 59 percent of the patients, 60 percent of the parents, and 68 percent of the physicians citing private discussions with a health professional as most preferable. More than 65 percent of the respondents in each category said that the health professional providing the information should be the physician. Less agreement was apparent concerning the inclusion of parents in these discussions. While a majority of adolescents (68%) and parents (75%) favored parent inclusion, only seventeen percent of the physicians wanted the parents present.

Although there was general agreement that physicians should be the primary source of information for adolescent cancer patients, Pfefferbaum and Levenson (1982) report a discrepancy between adolescents' opinions of the information that is important to them and physicians' perceptions of adolescents' views. Adolescents and physicians were asked to rank a series of thirty questions about illness in order of importance, with physicians told to adopt the patient's perspective when making this rating. Patient and physician rankings differed significantly on fifteen of the thirty items. Questions for which no conclusive answers exist (e.g., "what causes cancer?" "how can cancer be prevented?") tended to receive high rankings from patients. Physicians, on the other hand, gave such questions lower rankings, with higher ratings being given to questions concerning adolescent socialization issues (e.g., participation in care, appearance, relationships).

Patient rankings of the types of information desired were

not significantly related to characteristics such as subjects' sex, diagnosis, time elapsing since their diagnosis, or disease status. However, after performing a factor analysis on subjects' responses, Levenson, Pfefferbaum, and Overall (1983) found a limited number of intuitively reasonable relationships between the eleven information factors identified through the analysis and selected patient variables. For example, they note that patient diagnosis was related to the factor labelled "physical appearance," with those adolescents having a type of cancer likely to result in physical impairment or disfigurement ranking questions in this category as high in importance. Age was related to the factor termed "teenage identification," which included questions on payment of bills, the effects of alcohol, smoking, and drugs on the illness, and means of utilizing the experience of other cancer patients in solving problems. Patients younger than sixteen years of age ranked questions in this category as significantly less important than did older adolescents.

Parent Responses to the Illness and Hospitalization of Adolescents

The relationship between parents and their adolescent children during the adolescent's illness was investigated by Peterson (1972). Data for this study, which consist entirely of adolescent perceptions of the relationship, were obtained through questionnaires completed by 6,725 adolescents in high schools throughout the United States. Participants responded to questions concerning parental *control* over adolescents' activities (defined as attempts to modify or direct children's behavior in accordance with predetermined standards of conduct) and *interest* in their activities (the degree of concern or regard parents have for their children's pursuits) under conditions of illness and health. For purposes of analysis, respondents were categorized on the basis of their current and past health status.

No direct relationship was found between parents' general interest in, or control over, their children's activities and adolescents' current health status. However, adolescents with a history of health problems *did* perceive changes in relationships with other family members during periods of illness. For example, adolescents classified as chronically ill, especially chronically ill females, reported changes in parents behavior when they (the adolescents) were ill.

Parents were said to display more attention and affection during these periods, with only a minority of the reported parental changes (2.4%) classified as negative. Moreover, adolescents with a history of illness (apparently including those with past hospitalization or serious illness, as well as those chronically ill) perceived parents as exercising more control and having more interest in their activities during illness than did adolescents with no such history.

Adolescents with a history of illness also perceived alterations in the behavior of their siblings during periods of illness. Under such circumstances, siblings were reported to be more kind and more interested in the ill adolescent. As in the case of parent changes during illness, only a small percentage of the changes in siblings' behavior were seen to be negative.

Parent responses during adolescent hospitalization have been documented by Lord and Schowalter (1979, 1982; Schowalter & Lord, 1969). This series of studies is of particular interest since it represents one of the few successful attempts in the literature on hospitalized children to gather data on fathers' reactions. Furthermore, this research suggests that a dramatic shift in the involvement of fathers with their hospitalized adolescents has occurred over a ten-year period.

Fifty mothers and fifty fathers of children ten to eighteen years of age, admitted to an adolescent unit, were interviewed in 1970 (reported by Lord & Schowalter, 1979). More than half of the children of the interviewed parents were reported to be severely ill. Although methods used for assessing and categorizing responses are not presented, Lord and Schowalter report that 82 percent of the parents of both sexes manifested symptoms of anxiety or depression.

Parent motivation for visiting the hospitalized adolescent was also discussed. Eighty-six percent of the mothers were said to visit out of "genuine concern for their children" (p. 8), with the remainder motivated by duty or guilt. Slightly more than half of the fathers interviewed were said to be motivated to visit by affection and concern for their children. Other fathers were characterized as being outspoken in their dislike of visiting, doing so mainly out of moral obligation.

Ten years later, a follow-up study was conducted with parents of adolescents hospitalized in the same unit (Lord & Schowalter, 1982). Forty-five couples (parents of moderately to severely ill patients ten to twenty years of age, hospitalized for at least one week) were selected for the study. Each parent was interviewed separately. Data on this sample of parents were compared with that portion of the 1970 sample who, like subjects in the follow-up study, were interviewed at least one week after their child's admission. The resulting subset of the 1970 sample consisted of nineteen mothers and nineteen fathers.

As in the earlier study, details of methodology are not presented, nor were statistical tests used to compare differences between the 1970 and 1980 samples. Nevertheless, the distribution of fathers' responses suggest that change had occurred in the intervening period. For example, as compared to the 1970 sample, a smaller proportion of the 1980 fathers expressed dislike of the hospital (1970: 32%; 1980: 13%), expressed anger toward the patient (1970: 32%; 1980: 11%), or used denial as a means of detaching themselves from the situation (1970: 53%; 1980: 11%). Fathers in the later sample were also reported to spend more time on the ward, and to attend parent meetings with greater frequency, than was true in 1970.

Further changes were noted in the motivation for visiting expressed by both parents. Declines were reported in the percentages of fathers and mothers motivated to visit by duty (Fathers—1970: 32%, 1980: 13%; Mothers—1970: 5%, 1980: 0%). In fact, a higher percentage of the fathers than mothers in the 1980 sample were said to visit primarily out of interest and concern for their children (Fathers: 80%; Mothers: 73%).

A limited amount of information on parent attitudes and reactions to adolescent hospitalization is provided by Schowalter and Lord (1969). Interviews with one hundred parents of hospitalized adolescents were conducted, during which parents registered their opinions concerning preparation of adolescents for hospitalization and expressed concerns about their children's admission. Ninety-six percent of the parents felt that adolescents should be forewarned about hospitalization, with 44 percent stating that prospective patients should be prepared as early as possible. These responses were contrasted with opinions expressed in separate interviews by children of the responding parents. Eighty-seven percent of the adolescents favored some form of preparation, although 62 percent of these said that it should occur no more than one week prior to admission. Schowalter and Lord report that many adolescents felt that they had been informed of the hospitalization too early.

Parents were also asked for their perceptions of their children's greatest worry upon entering the hospital. These responses were compared with those listed by the adolescents themselves, which included medical procedures (mentioned by 31% of the patients), separation (17%), the hospital atmosphere (9%), and physical disability (8%). Parents were found to underestimate their children's fears of procedures and separation, though figures detailing parents' responses are not presented. Forty-six percent of the parents said that nothing worried their children, while only 35 percent of the adolescents actually gave this response. When asked to identify their own principal worries upon admission, more than half of the parents (52%) mentioned concern over their child's diagnosis or condition.

Adolescent Units

The establishment of separate adolescent units has been frequently advocated by health care professionals (Hofmann, Becker, & Gabriel, 1976; Lindheim, Glaser, & Coffin, 1972). These settings are believed to provide adolescents with autonomy, independence, and support of peers that is typically unavailable to them in either pediatric or adult wards. Though expressed support for adolescent units is common, little systematic research has been conducted on the effectiveness of these units, or the specialized programs they provide, in reducing the upset of adolescent patients. As in other areas of adolescent study, the majority of the research on adolescent units consists of surveys of patient or staff attitudes. Moreover, with a single exception (Rigg & Fisher, 1971) the existing studies have made no attempt to compare the attitudes of respondents exposed to differing types of settings. Thus, the inferences that may be drawn from this body of research are limited.

An early investigation the prevalence of adolescent units, and the types of services they provide, was conducted by Rigg and

Fisher (1970). Surveys were sent to 53 hospitals in the United States and Canada that were characterized as having an interest in adolescent medicine. Responding hospitals having adolescent units or outpatient clinics were asked to provide information on the services they offered.

Of the 49 hospitals responding to the survey, 24 had adolescent units. The physical location of these units within the hospital, room arrangements, and criteria for admission are discussed. In addition to the adolescent units, thirty adolescent clinics (defined as either a separate physical area, or a separate time within a clinic reserved for adolescents) were identified. Information was gathered on clinic staffing, the numbers of adolescents served, and the types of diagnoses most frequently encountered. The list of adolescent units and clinics identified though the survey was not considered to be exhaustive.

In a subsequent study, Rigg and Fisher (1971) attempted to compare staff and patient attitudes in hospitals with or without adolescent units. Twelve hospitals identified in the 1970 study as having both an adolescent unit and clinic were compared with a second group of eight hospitals, each having an adolescent clinic, but no separate inpatient unit. Questionnaires were sent to the clinic directors and to either the head nurse of the adolescent unit or, in the case of the comparison group of hospitals, to the nurse in charge of the unit where most adolescents were admitted.

Characteristics of the two groups of hospitals were compared. Results are presented descriptively, with no statistical tests of significance performed. Hospitals having adolescent units were said to offer patients greater privileges than other hospitals, including visitation by friends, permission to smoke, opportunities for socializing, and use of kitchen facilities. Clinic directors in hospitals with adolescent units felt that the presence of a separate unit facilitated continuity of care from outpatient to inpatient settings. Furthermore, concentration of adolescents in a single unit was seen as advantageous to the training of physicians and nurses since it permitted observation of patients with similar and contrasting conditions. Clinic directors in hospitals without adolescent units commented on the disadvantage of their settings for the continuity of care and for the training of health care professionals. Comments from nurses concerning their evaluation of adolescent units were similarly favorable. Although some head nurses of adolescent units noted problems of discipline in their settings, all respondents from both categories of hospitals felt that a separate unit was desirable for adolescents.

In addition to surveys of clinic directors and nurses, groups of patients from the two types of hospitals, plus a third group of patients from hospitals with neither an adolescent unit nor clinic, were interviewed by Rigg and Fisher (1971). Again, comparisons are presented without use of statistical analyses. No group differences were noted in adolescents' perceptions of the ways in which hospital staff members managed the wards or interacted with patients. The majority of respondents in all three types of settings rated staff members as being age-appropriate in approach, as providing clear explanations of disease and follow-up care, and as being honest.

More surprising were patients' opinions of the preparation they received for admission. A higher proportion of subjects hospitalized in adolescent units than in other settings rated their preparation as only "adequate" as opposed to "good." However, subjects in adolescent units rated their recreational facilities more favorably than did other patients. Finally, Rigg and Fisher report that the "vast majority" of all subjects interviewed expressed preference for hospitalization in a ward exclusively devoted to adolescents.

The remaining surveys of attitudes concerning adolescent care confined their samples to subjects admitted either to an adolescent unit (Schowalter & Lord, 1969; Schowalter & Anyan, 1973) or to a general pediatric unit (Louis & Lovejoy, 1975). The results are not unexpected. Subjects admitted to adolescent units viewed this system of care favorably, while those hospitalized in other settings were more critical of the care they received. However, the lack of comparison groups within these studies limits the usefulness of their results.

Schowalter and Lord (1969) conducted semi-structured interviews with 100 parents and 100 patients admitted to an adolescent unit. Ninety-five percent of the parents expressed unconditional approval of the unit. Of the five remaining parents, two were said to be indifferent and three were concerned about the housing of male and female adolescents on the same floor. Eighty percent of the patients approved of the adolescent unit. Schowalter and Lord report that all patients expressing disapproval were thirteen years of age or younger and were also disturbed by the admission of both sexes to the unit. The interviews further indicate that parent and patient knowledge of diagnoses was good. All parents and 90 percent of the adolescents either knew the patient's diagnosis or knew that it had not yet been determined.

Similarly favorable data are presented by Schowalter and Anyan (1973). A Ward Atmosphere Scale, consisting of sixteen true/false statements about experiences on an adolescent unit, was completed by 112 adolescents, twelve to seventeen years of age. Other than three items indicating dissatisfaction with their doctors for unpredictable schedules, inadequate explanations, and lack of time spent with patients, and an additional item indicating that nurses failed to spend enough time talking with patients, the majority of the responses to each remaining item were positive. Hospital staff members were said to be interested in the feelings of the patients, to treat them as individuals, and to foster contacts among patients. Relationships with peers and opportunities for activities were also rated positively.

In contrast to these findings are the data gathered by Louis and Lovejoy (1975). Eighty-seven adolescent patients hospitalized in a large pediatric facility with no separate adolescent unit were interviewed after the second day of their hospitalization. In addition, parents were interviewed at admission and asked to complete a questionnaire assessing their reactions to the adequacy of services provided for them and their children. Sixty-six percent of the patients were reported to be dissatisfied with the hospital atmosphere and rules. Complaints of sharing one's room with younger children, and of the absence of lounges or reading areas, were common. Relationships between adolescents' attitudes and their age or duration of admission were generally nonsignificant. However, patients classified as seriously ill were significantly less satisfied with the psychological atmosphere of the hospital.

Of the parents questioned, 76 percent felt that more privacy was needed during discussions with professionals. Thirty percent expressed complaints about facilities for parent visitation, and 28 percent were critical of admission procedures. However, despite these criticisms, 84 percent of the parents thought that "the hospital's physical and psychological facilities were conducive to optimal adolescent adjustment and early discharge" (p. 1047).

Staff Members' Knowledge and Perceptions of Adolescents

Studies have been conducted to evaluate hospital staff members' knowledge of normal adolescent development (Lavigne, 1977) and their opinions of the behavior of adolescents differing in racial-ethnic background (Finkelstein, Medina, & Vegehla, 1981). In each case, considerable discrepancy was noted between staff members' responses and standards of comparison derived from other research.

Lavigne (1977) contends that most pediatric hospital staff members receive little training in adolescent growth and development. Moreover, the training that they do receive is likely to be influenced by psychoanalytic theory, an approach that "promotes the notion of adolescence as a time of turmoil, stress, and personality problems" (p. 98). Recent research cited by Lavigne suggests that psychoanalytic theory inaccurately characterizes normal adolescence, exaggerating the frequency of symptomatic behavior. For example, although an increase in depressive affect is observed in adolescence, psychiatric symptoms and severe parent-child alienation are atypical. Inadequate understanding of normative adolescent behavior, Lavigne argues, may cause hospital staff members to ignore or misinterpret true indications of psychopathology.

In conjunction with an inservice training program on adolescent development, Lavigne administered a questionnaire to three groups of hospital personnel: pediatric residents (N = 13), staff nurses (N = 20), and adjunct personnel, including chaplains, recreational therapists, child care workers, respiratory therapists, speech pathologists, and ombudsman staff members (N = 12). The questionnaire consisted of nine true/false statements, each epitomizing a popular notion about adolescence that had recently been addressed by longitudinal studies or surveys. Correct responses were based on results of these studies.

Only three of the nine items were correctly answered by a majority of the subjects in all three groups. Of the remaining six items, fifty percent or more of at least one group disagreed with the correct response. Analysis of the individual groups indicates that adjunct personnel fared best, with at least fifty percent of this group responding correctly to seven of the nine total items. The majority of pediatric residents responded correctly to four items, with the majority of staff nurses correctly answering only three items.

Finkelstein, et al. (1981) surveyed 290 employees of a medical school and its hospital concerning the characteristics and behaviors of adolescents. Each respondent was given a questionnaire containing a list of 36 attributes. Subjects were initially asked to rate the degree to which each of the characteristics accurately described the general population of adolescents. After completing this portion of the survey, respondents were asked to review the list of items, this time giving their perceptions of the likelihood that adolescents in each of four racial-ethnic groups (caucasian, Black, Mexican-American, and oriental) would exhibit each characteristic.

Although subjects had little trouble completing the first portion of the questionnaire, considerable reluctance to complete the second half was evident. Fifty-three subjects failed to answer the latter portion of the questionnaire. Responses of the remaining subjects were frequently incomplete. However, of those responses obtained, Finkelstein, et al. report that "respondents were of the opinion that white and oriental adolescents are more likely to have positive or neutral behaviors and black adolescents negative behaviors" (pp. 3–4). Subjects' ratings were compared with the results of other published surveys in which adolescents of the racial-ethnic groups in question rated their own behavior. Correspondence between the two ratings was poor. Finkelstein, et al. conclude that the data reveal "significant stereotyping of adolescents in general and of various racial-ethnic groups" (p. 6).

Chapter 8

THE HOSPITAL MILIEU

The unfamiliarity of the hospital setting has been identified as a factor contributing to the psychological upset of pediatric inpatients (Vernon, Foley, Sipowicz, & Schulman, 1965). A portion of this unfamiliarity is a product of the medical procedures and equipment children encounter while hospitalized. However, it may also be attributed to more subtle sources such as changes in children's daily routines and the sudden, often unpredictable demand for periods of intense interaction with relative strangers, alternating with periods of inactivity and social isolation. The research reviewed in the present chapter considers these elements of the hospital milieu, which distinguish the medical environment from that to which children are accustomed. Children's everyday activities in the hospital, including their television viewing habits and their contact and communication with others, are documented. In addition, the impact of a frequently distracting and intrusive environment on the sleep patterns of children is examined.

THE ACTIVITIES OF HOSPITALIZED CHILDREN

Though researchers have repeatedly documented the behaviors and responses of children indicative of emotional distress, both during the period of hospitalization and following discharge, few attempts have been made to record the more mundane activities of hospitalized children. The exceptions include Kaplan, et al. (1981), who conducted a time-sample study of patient activities in an adolescent ward, and Cataldo, et al. (1979), who observed the behavior of children in a pediatric intensive care unit.

Kaplan, et al. found adolescents to spend much of their time alone while in the hospital. Moreover, they note that on those occasions when adolescents were observed interacting with others, it was more likely to be with adults rather than other patients (see Chapter 7). Cataldo, et al. report that children hospitalized in an intensive care unit were either awake, or awake and alert, during fewer than half of the periods of observation. Among children who were rated as awake and alert, verbalizations were noted in only eighteen percent of the observation periods. This same group was seen to engage in activities (e.g., playing alone or with others, or watching television) 36 percent of the time (see Chapter 4).

In a third study, not previously discussed, Schulman, Kaspar, and Child (1970) videotaped the activities of nineteen children (2 to 7 years of age, hospitalized for elective herniorrhaphies) while in their hospital room. Each subject was admitted to a six-bed ward equipped with a one-way mirror through which the videotape recordings were made. The equipment was programmed to record twenty-second samples every five minutes from 9:00 am to 6:00 pm for each of the three days the child was hospitalized. Subsequent analysis of the tapes indicate that children spent the majority of their time *outside* of the room, except on the day of surgery. A small portion of their daytime hours was spent sleeping, again with the exception of the day of their operation. In only two percent of the observations on the day of admission, and ten percent of those on children's discharge day, was sleep noted. This compares with recordings of sleep in 23 percent of the preoperative and 41 percent of the postoperative observations on the day of surgery.

Television Viewing Habits

Television viewing is a common activity of hospitalized children. In their observational study of adolescents, Kaplan, et al. (1981) found that two of the three most frequently occurring events, from their checklist of thirty items, were "television on," and "patient watching television." Cataldo, et al. (1979) found that 13 percent of the children who were awake and alert in a pediatric intensive care unit were watching television.

A more detailed consideration of the television viewing habits of hospitalized children is found in the studies conducted by Guttentag, Albritton, and Kettner (1981, 1983). This research, which was conducted in a hospital equipped with television sets in each patient room, reports high levels of television viewing among children of all ages throughout the daytime hours.

In their initial study, Guttentag, et al. (1981) observed the behavior of 845 patients ranging in age from newborns to seventeen years. Each child was observed at half-hour intervals between 9:00 am and 5:00 pm, with observers recording whether the child was present in his or her room and whether the television was on or off. If on, the observer further noted the type of programming viewed, whether other persons were present, and whether the child was engaged in other activities.

Television viewing was found to be lowest in the morning, with 21 percent of the patients watching television at 9:00 am. The peak viewing time for the morning was 11:30 am, when 61 percent of the patients were watching. Early afternoon viewing levels remained moderately high (with 45 to 60% watching television during this interval), peaking for the day at 4:00 pm, when 75 percent of all children were viewing television programming. The total amount of time children spent watching television during daytime hours (an eight-hour period) was found to exceed the level reported by a separate source for nonhospitalized children during a 24-hour period.

To a great extent, viewing patterns were indiscriminate. Channels were reported to remain unchanged over most of the periods of observation. Although children frequently did something else while watching television (e.g., playing, reading, eating), an average of forty percent of the viewers across all observation periods engaged in no other activity while viewing programming.

Factors potentially influencing television viewing patterns were also examined by Guttentag, et al. (1981). Time spent watching television was found to decline with increasing length of hospitalization. In addition, children in isolation viewed more television than did nonisolated children, and patients with same-aged roommates watched less television than those with roommates more than two years different in age.

After the introduction of a closed-circuit television channel, which broadcast programming appropriate for hospitalized children, Guttentag, et al. (1983) reexamined patient television viewing habits. The daily pattern of viewing was similar to that found in the initial study, with viewing levels lowest early in the morning, peaking temporarily at noon, then rising to a late afternoon high for the day. The total amount of time children spent viewing television was found to increase after introduction of the channel.

Despite limited changes in the quantity and pattern of children's television viewing, the content of the programs watched was affected by the introduction of closed-circuit children's programming. The presence of the new children's channel, which presented prerecorded programming, as well as a live, one-hour daily broadcast, dramatically increased the percentage of viewers watching programs intended for children. Although morning viewing patterns were little affected by the introduction of the hospital channel, a shift in viewing habits toward the closed-circuit channel was observed in late afternoon, a period when commercial stations broadcast virtually no children's programming. Overall, 45 percent of children's television-viewing time was devoted to the alternative hospital programming.

Factors affecting television viewing were reexamined after the introduction of the hospital channel. As in the earlier study, isolation and roommates' ages were found to influence viewing habits. In addition, a positive relationship between number of roommates and viewing time was found. Other significant relationships were noted for age (with older children viewing more television) and sex (with boys viewing more than girls). However, in contrast to the 1981 study, length of hospitalization was unrelated to amount of time patients spent watching television.

CHILDREN'S INTERACTIONS WITH OTHERS IN THE HOSPITAL

Amount of Contact with Others

The amount or frequency of contact hospitalized children have with others has been examined by Schulman, et al. (1970) and by Grant (1983). In the first of these studies, Schulman, et al. reviewed videotape recordings of children's activities in their hospital rooms to document the amount of time they spent with other people. As mentioned above, the elective surgical patients spent the majority of their daytime hours outside of their rooms, except on the day of surgery. Nevertheless, when subjects were in their rooms and awake, they were alone approximately half of the periods of observation. Depending on the day in question, parents were present 16 to 39 percent of the time. Nurses were present 9 to 16 percent of the time. Physicians, on the other hand, were not observed with children other than on the day of discharge—a finding that the authors note may be misleading, since surgical rounds typically occurred earlier than 9:00 am, which marked the beginning of the research observation period.

Schulman, et al. also rated children's mood during each observation period, noting differences in affect depending on who was present with the child. Children's mood was described as, "best when the parent is present, a little worse . . . when the child is alone, and again worse when the nurse is present" (p. 730–731).

Although Schulman, et al. found children to be alone during approximately half of the observation periods when in their rooms, this finding does not necessarily indicate that children encountered extended periods of uninterrupted isolation. In fact, a quite different situation may exist, with children subjected to exceedingly brief, but repeated exposure to others. Grant (1983) documented the frequency with which people entered a six-bed unit of a children's hospital in New Zealand. On five separate days, from 6:00 am to 6:00 pm, an observer recorded the number of people entering a child's room, the identity of each person, and the length of their stay. An average of 327 separate entrances, made by 106 *different* people, were recorded per twelve-hour observation day. Members of the nursing staff accounted for the greatest number of both entrances and different individuals entering the unit, followed by visitors, and doctors. The majority of all visits were less than one minute in length.

The Nature of Children's Contacts with Nurses

Nurses are among the most common contacts of hospitalized children, certainly in terms of frequency of contacts (Grant, 1983), if not duration. The nature of the interactions occurring between children and nurses has received the attention of several investigators. Among the topics addressed by these studies are the frequency and duration of nurse-child interactions (Cleary, 1977, 1979; Smith, 1976), the influence of parents' presence on nurse-child contacts (Schulman, et al., 1970; Smith, 1976), and the designated functions of these encounters (Smith, 1976; Cleary, 1977, 1979). The data suggest that nurse-child interactions are brief in duration and are primarily initiated for performing nursing functions rather than for providing children with emotional support or social stimulation.

The distribution of nursing attention in a 22-bed open pediatric ward was documented by Cleary (1977, 1979). Observations were made three times per hour for sixteen hours per day over three separate weeks. When a nurse was present in the ward during the period of observation, a *sighting* was recorded. If, in addition, the nurse were doing something with a child, a *contact* was recorded. Cleary reports that during more than forty percent of the observation periods, no nurse was present in the ward. The greatest number of sightings occurred at lunchtime, breakfast, and during midafternoon. Of the total number of sightings recorded over the three weeks of observation, only 44.4 percent involved contact with the patient.

Smith (1976) reports that when contacts occur, they are typically brief in duration. In this case, fifteen nonacutely ill children (18 months to 5 years) were observed for unspecified periods of time. The average duration of the 168 contacts observed was less than 1.5 minutes. Only three contacts lasted more than ten minutes, the purpose of which, in each case, was to bathe a child.

The brevity of the nursing contacts observed by Smith is consistent with the previously mentioned findings of Grant (1983). Although Grant did not provide a breakdown of length of contacts by each category of visitor, it was reported that entrances to the unit studied were made most frequently by nurses, and that the majority of all visits lasted less than one minute.

Two of the studies cited have investigated the assertion that members of the nursing staff tend to avoid contact with children when parents are present. The data of Schulman, et al. (1970) confirm this pattern of avoidance. Nurses were significantly more likely to be observed with children in parents' absence than when parents were visiting in their children's rooms. Smith (1976), on the other hand, detected no avoidance of children when parents were present. Moreover, the length of individual nursing contacts, though brief, was virtually identical whether parents were present or not.

According to Smith (1976) a majority of the observed contacts occurring between nurses and hospitalized children were initiated for performance of nursing functions, rather than to provide social interaction. Similar data are reported by Cleary (1977, 1979). The percentage of nurse sightings classified as involving social contact with children varied from 24 percent to 29 percent, depending on the week examined. Cleary suggests that the task assignment system of nursing practiced in the hospital where observations occurred (i.e., each nurse providing a specific service to multiple children) contributed to the lack of social interaction recorded.

Interpersonal Communications

Documentation of Communication Patterns. Little information exists on the nature of children's communications with others in the hospital environment. The only comprehensive study of children's verbalizations to adults was conducted by Pidgeon (1974a, 1974b), the purpose of which was to examine the function and content of verbal contacts initiated with adults by hospitalized children. The sample consisted of 24 moderately ill preschool children, half of whom were from families receiving welfare (termed "disadvantaged" children). The remaining half were from families considered to be economically and socially advantaged.

Subjects' verbal interactions with others were observed in the absence of parents in structured and unstructured settings. Each verbal contact was classified according to its *function* (being either *expressive* or *evocative* of wants, feelings, or cognitions) and its *referent* (*objects* or *persons* either in the hospital or elsewhere).

More than sixty percent of children's verbal contacts were either expressive or evocative of cognitions, with cognitions defined as items of factual, reasoned, or imagined information (e.g., facts, generalizations, or judgments). The majority of these were *expressive* in nature and referred to persons and objects in the hospital environment. In more than one-third of the expressed cognitions, children themselves were identified as the referent. Contacts with adults to express *wants* were less common, accounting for 21.1 percent of all children's verbal contacts. Expressions of *feelings* were exceedingly rare, occurring in only 1.7 percent of the cases. Evocative verbal contacts (i.e., those eliciting the cognitions, wants, or feelings of an adult) accounted for only 15.3 percent of children's verbalizations.

The total number of verbal contacts initiated with adults by advantaged and disadvantaged children did not differ. However, group differences were found in the content of their verbalizations. For example, advantaged children expressed more wants for services, while disadvantaged subjects more frequently expressed wants for attention. Moreover, disadvantaged children were found to verbalize less about their parents, than did advantaged subjects.

Pidgeon's study is limited to *children's* contribution to adult-child communications in the hospital. No documentation of the contribution of adults, as well as children, to interactions occurring in inpatient settings was found, though Klinzing, Klinzing, and Schindler (1977) published a preliminary report on a possible method for assessing such interactions. The observational scale described by the authors consists of eleven items. Coding of an interaction begins when a staff member and child come in contact with each other and continues for 7.5 minutes or until the contact ends. The precise method of recording observations is not specified.

Pilot work with this instrument was conducted in a pediatric hospital over a four-week period and included more than two thousand episodes of interaction. The most frequently coded scale item during this period was "silence," accounting for approximately forty percent of all codings. The authors recommend further modification of the scale to distinguish among three types of silence, termed positive, negative, and neutral. Other frequently coded items included "staff to staff or staff to parent talk" and "staff member gives facts or opinion." "Patient talks" ranked fourth in order of frequency during each week of observation.

Two studies conducted in outpatient settings have documented the patterns of doctor, parent, and child communications (Freemon, Negrete, Davis, & Korsch, 1971; Pantell, Stewart, Dias, Wells, & Ross, 1982). Freemon, et al. (1971) reviewed tape recordings of interviews conducted during 285 patient visits to a pediatric walk-in clinic. Communications between the parent or child and the physician were examined and coded for content and affect. The great majority of the recorded communications occurred between parents and physicians, with 48.8 percent being from doctor to mother, and 38.6 percent from mother to doctor. The physicians' statements to children represented 10.5 percent of all communications. In only 2.1 percent of the communications did children speak directly to physicians.

The majority of mothers' communications to doctors related to medical history. Doctors' statements to mothers also frequently pertained to medical history (34.1% of all doctor to mother statements), as well as to children's treatment (30.1%). Discussion of the *cause* or *prognosis* of children's illness by the physician was rare, with each accounting for less than four percent of the doctors' total statements to mothers. Less affect was noted in doctors' communications than in those of mothers. Relatively few of the physicians' statements to mothers communicated friendliness or reassurance, although nearly half (46.0%) of the doctors' utterances to children did so.

Quite a different pattern of communication among parent, child and physician is reported by Pantell, et al. (1983). The sample for this study consisted of 115 children (4 to 14 years of age) accompanied to an outpatient clinic by an adult. Videotapes of physicians' interviews with the children and adults were coded for 1) the direction of the communication, 2) the type of transaction occurring (statement, response, or interruption), and 3) content (with 10 categories used).

In contrast to the Freemon, et al. findings that communication between doctor and child occurred less than thirteen percent of the time, Pantell, et al. found that doctor-child interactions accounted for 45.5 percent of all communication. More information on children's current condition was directly obtained from patients than from their parents, though more explanation of the problem was given to parents. A positive relationship was found between children's age and the amount of substantive communication occurring between doctors and children. Pantell, et al. suggest that the discrepancies between their findings and those of Freemon, et al.

may be due to differences in the settings of the studies, socioeconomic status of the samples, and the greater psychosocial sophistication of the staff in the latter research.

The Effects of Interpersonal Communication. In addition to describing the patterns of communication with medical personnel, one may also consider the influence such communications exert on patients and parents. Though this topic has received little direct attention in inpatient settings, the previously discussed research on communicational interventions directed toward parents (Mahaffy, 1965; Skipper, Leonard, & Rhymes, 1968; Roy, 1967, 1968; see Chapter 6) and children (Fernald & Corry, 1981; see Chapter 4) suggests that verbal interactions are capable of altering subjects' behaviors and reducing their emotional distress.

Three studies, each conducted in an outpatient setting, have examined the relationship between physicians' style of communication and selected responses of parents and children (Korsch, Gozzi, & Francis, 1968; Francis, Korsch, & Morris, 1969; Hyson, Snyder, & Andujar, 1982). Two of these studies (Korsch, et al., 1968; Francis, et al., 1969) are based on data from the same sample of eight hundred outpatient visits to a pediatric clinic (a subset of which also formed the sample for the Freemon, et al. study discussed above). Parents of children receiving care at the clinic were interviewed by researchers two weeks after the clinic visit to determine their perceptions of the visit and how it had affected their subsequent behavior.

Korsch, et al. (1968) found 76 percent of the parents to express high or moderate satisfaction with the clinic visit. Characteristics of the visit possibly contributing to parent satisfaction were investigated. Satisfaction was found to be unrelated to either the amount of time the physician spent with the patient or to the patient's diagnosis. However, parents' perceptions of the physicians' interpersonal communication style were related to their satisfaction levels. A greater proportion of parents who described the physician as friendly, or commended the physician's communication skills, expressed satisfaction with the visit than did others. The fulfillment of parent expectations concerning their visit was also associated with parent satisfaction. Displeasure was expressed by parents who had expected to be given a cause or diagnosis of their child's condition, yet were given none. Moreover, the majority of parents whose children did not receive shots, tests, x-rays, or medicine when such treatment was anticipated were dissatisfied with the clinic visit.

Francis, et al. (1969) found that parent compliance with medical advice (including use of medicine, adherence to treatment and diet, and the return to the clinic for follow-up care) was also related to perceived characteristics of doctor-parent communication. Noncompliance was found to be greater among parents who described the physician as business-like rather than friendly, and among parents who said the physician did not understand their concerns. In another finding analogous to the Korsch, et al. (1968) study, Francis, et al. found that reduced compliance rates were associated with the failure of physicians to meet parents' expectations that a diagnosis or cause of children's illness would be provided.

The only study to directly examine the relationship between the physician's style of interaction and children's behavior in an outpatient medical setting is that of Hyson, Snyder, and Andujar (1982). Forty-eight children, two to seven years of age, were observed during routine examination by one of six participating doctors. Three characteristics of the doctors' interactions during the examinations were assessed: 1) *warmth* (physical proximity to the child, and expressions of empathy), 2) *child involvement* (extent to which the physician talked with the child and let the child handle medical instruments), and 3) *mother involvement* (extent of the doctor's conversation with the mother and his encouragement that she hold the child on her lap during the examination). Children's responses were rated as positive, negative, or neutral. The methods used for scoring doctor and child behaviors are not fully described.

The authors report that doctors' warmth and, to a lesser degree, their child involvement behaviors were associated with positive reactions by children. Neutral, passive behavior exhibited by children was associated with a style of interaction characterized by low warmth and limited child involvement. Occurrence of negative behaviors was unrelated to physicians' characteristics, but rather was associated with children's age. Data supporting these findings are not included in the research report.

Research in the dental literature also indicates that one's manner of communicating with children during treatment is capable of affecting patients' behavioral and subjective responses to care. Melamed, Bennett, et al. (1983) randomly assigned 42 dental patients (4 to 12 years of age) to one of four conditions signifying the type of reinforcement dentists would provide during restorative treatment. Children in the *positive reinforcement group* were verbally praised for compliance with instructions. Noncompliant behavior was ignored. Subjects in the *punishment condition* were criticized for instances of noncompliant behavior, but were given no praise for their cooperation. Other treatment conditions consisted of a combination of *positive reinforcement and punishment* and a *neutral* condition, in which behavior was neither praised nor criticized. Observational, subjective, and physiological measures were used to assess patient compliance and anxiety.

The punishment condition was associated with greater disruptiveness and noncompliance than were other treatment conditions. In fact, those children in the punishment condition who had initially rated their own fear level as low exhibited a significant *increase* in self-reported fear following treatment. However, use of criticism in combination with positive reinforcement was found to be as effective as other conditions in eliciting children's cooperative behavior. Fleece (1979), who also conducted an experimental evaluation of the effects of differing reinforcement strategies used by dentists, failed to detect significant group differences.

Results similar to those of Melamed, Bennett, et al. are provided by Weinstein, Getz, Ratener, and Domoto (1982a). Videotape recordings of 25 dental practitioners with preschool patients were coded and analyzed using lag sequential techniques, a method of analysis through which one can determine the probability that a target behavior will be followed by other types of behavior (see Sackett, 1978). It was found that behavior indicative of children's fear was reduced following dentists' use of directive commands or their reinforcement of children's behavior. Coercion or coaxing by the dentist was most likely to be followed by fear-related behavior.

The effects of dentists' empathic behaviors were also considered by Weinstein, et al. (1982a). The likelihood of occurrence of fear behavior was reduced after dentists questioned children about their pain or acknowledged its presence. Reassurance in response to children's expressions of pain appeared to be less effective, while the ignoring or ridiculing of these expressions was associated with a high probability of subsequent fear-related behavior.

The data were re-examined by Weinstein, et al. (1982b) to determine whether dentists adjusted *their* behaviors in response to children's manifestations of fear. Following instances of children's fear-related behavior, dentists were less likely to use either direction or reinforcement—the techniques that the preceding study had suggested were most effective in minimizing children's fear. Instead, children's fearful behavior was more often followed by relatively ineffective or counterproductive actions by dentists, including statement of rules, coercion, coaxing, reassurances, and ridicule. Direction and reinforcement by dentists were found to occur with higher probability following nonfearful behavior.

Research on the effects of staff members' communications on the psychological responses of children in inpatient settings is quite limited. Vernon, et al. (1967; also reported in Schulman, et al., 1967) found that children's reactions to anesthesia induction varied with the anesthetist conducting the procedure. The researchers speculate that this difference may have been associated with variations in the amount of time individual anesthetists spent trying to establish rapport with the children before beginning the procedure. Other inpatient studies indicate that increased attention and emotional support from staff members are effective in reducing children's psychological upset (Minde & Maler, 1968; Fassler, 1980; Schwartz, et al., 1983; see Chapter 10).

THE SLEEP PATTERNS OF HOSPITALIZED CHILDREN

Given the unfamiliarity of the hospital environment, the disruptions of daily routines, and the intense, yet sporadic interactions with others that children experience, health care professionals have expressed concern that children's sleep patterns will be altered as well, and this at a time when the need for rest is great. Two studies have considered the sleep of hospitalized children, examining factors that either promote or disturb it. Beardslee (1974, 1976) documented the sleep of children during afternoon nap time, while Hagemann (1978, 1981a, 1981b) considered children's night sleep.

Subjects in the Beardslee study were 24 children, two to five years of age, hospitalized for medical or surgical problems. Each child was observed on a minimum of four days, with each observation lasting from lunch to the end of scheduled nap time, a period of approximately two hours. A total of 125 separate observations were conducted, with notations made of children's care prior to nap time, environmental phenomena occurring in their proximity, and their behavior during the scheduled sleep period. Findings were presented in terms of children's *wakefulness* (failure to fall asleep during nap time), *sleep,* and *sleep disruption* (arousal from sleep during nap time).

Children's *wakefulness* was clearly related to disturbances in the environment. Greater incidence of wakefulness was noted among subjects in rooms near service areas. Moreover, a positive relationship existed between the amount of time staff members spent in a child's unit and the duration of his or her wakefulness. Wakeful periods also tended to last longer on days when on-going ward activities were moderate or high, and were more common among children who had experienced two or more stressful experiences (e.g., restraining of children's movements, or transferring children to another location when parents were absent).

Given the factors affecting wakefulness, and the restricted period of observation, it is not surprising that an increase in ward activities and the location of a child's room near a service area also affected the duration of children's sleep. However, in the majority of occasions when a staff member was observed in the room of a sleeping child, the child's sleep was not disturbed. Beardslee explains that few of the entrances by staff members involved physical contact with the child. When such contact did occur, it nearly always affected the child's sleep. In addition to direct contact with the patient, sleep disruption generally occurred in response to on-going ward activities (e.g., cleaning of floors) and other stimuli such as telephone rings or public address announcements. Disruptions were noted on forty percent of the observation days when children fell asleep. Forty-three percent of those experiencing sleep disruptions were able to fall asleep again.

Hagemann (1978, 1981a, 1981b) reports on the night sleep of 34 children, three to eight years of age. Observations of children were made for fifteen to thirty seconds, every five minutes, from 8:00 pm to 8:30 am, with the observer noting whether the child was asleep or awake, as well as the causes of any arousals. Duration of children's sleep (which ranged from 4 to 10.5 hours, with a mean of 7.8 hours) was determined by 1) the time of sleep onset, 2) the time of sleep termination, and 3) the amount of sleep disruption. Delays in onset of sleep were usually attributed to distractions in the ward, involvement in activities initiated by others, physical discomfort, or self-initiated resistance to sleep. Termination of sleep occurred spontaneously in less than twenty percent of the children. In most cases, children were awakened by nursing staff, laboratory technicians, or by noise and light in their vicinity.

Sleep disruptions were classified as *internal* (e.g., physiological needs, or discomfort) or *external* (environmental stimuli or caretaking functions). Nearly two-thirds of the sleep disruptions were the result of external causes, with the majority of these occurring for caretaking measures, typically the obtaining of vital signs. Half of the arousals from internal causes were due to discomfort, with nearly all of this experienced by children admitted to the hospital with medical diagnoses. Hagemann (1981b) reports that disruptions, "occurred with such frequency and distribution that very few children were able to sleep uninterruptedly through more than half of the sleep period" (p. 139).

Chapter 9

PLAY AND THE HOSPITALIZED CHILD

The literature on the relationship between children's play and stressful circumstances (whether health care experiences or other potentially stressful events) contains two seemingly contradictory strains. One body of research suggests that play behavior is not immediately necessary for survival and that when critical, stressful environmental factors intervene, play behavior declines (Schultz, 1979). Reductions in play behavior in response to transitory or prolonged stressors have been noted in children (Barker, Dembo, & Lewin, 1941; Hetherington, Cox, & Cox, 1979) and in laboratory animals (Mason, 1965).

A parallel body of research postulates a relationship between play and stress operating in the opposite direction. That is, play is believed to be used by children as a means of reducing anxiety produced by stressful conditions. Though this function of play is primarily espoused by writers adopting a psychoanalytic orientation, others have drawn upon this theory to posit a compensatory role of play. Piaget (1962), for example, describes his daughter's play as she pretends to hold her newborn cousin after being warned not to touch the baby. Such play, according to Piaget, "enables the child to relive his past experiences and makes for the satisfaction of the ego rather than for its subordination to reality" (p. 167). In other words, play enables the child to distort possibly upsetting aspects of reality into more agreeable patterns. Expanding upon this view, Singer (1977) states that "imaginative play can be viewed as a major resource by which children can cope immediately with the cognitive, affective, and social demands of growing up. It is more than a reactive behavior, however, for it provides a practice ground for organizing new schema and for transforming and storing material for more effective later expression in plans, actions or verbalizations" (p. 10).

Of course, the most comprehensive expression of the therapeutic value of play is found in the psychoanalytic literature. For example, Erikson (1963) describes the actions of children apparently using play to minimize the emotional impact of disturbing circumstances. He contends that by, "utilizing his mastery over objects, the child can arrange them in such a way that they permit him to imagine that he is master of his life predicament as well" (p. 217). Play is also thought to benefit children by allowing them to symbolically repeat disagreeable circumstances, reducing their aversiveness in the process. Wälder (1933) describes this activity as "a method of constantly working over and, as it were, assimilating piecemeal an experience which was too large to be assimilated instantly at a swoop" (p. 217).

Play is finally thought to be beneficial to children by permitting "catharsis," or the discharge of negative affect. An aggressive impulse spurred, for example, by the departure of a parent may be suppressed in "real life," but released in the safety of the play setting. The implication is that failure to discharge negative feelings in an appropriate manner results in socially unacceptable means of discharge and in the emotional upset of the child.

Though the literature on the play behavior of hospitalized children presented in this chapter is not extensive, it includes evidence pertinent to both of the postulated relationships between play behavior and stress. In particular, documentation of reductions or alterations in children's play during hospitalization exists. In addition, there is evidence that, under certain circumstances, children spontaneously use play to aid their adjustment to the hospital setting. The research further suggests that intervening variables, such as the degree of anxiety or defensiveness manifested by children, may determine whether they use play materials in a manner that could be considered therapeutic. After presenting the research pertaining to these relationships, the literature concerning the effectiveness of play interventions in reducing children's upset is discussed. The chapter concludes with a brief overview of research concerning the characteristics of hospital-based play programs in the United States and Canada.

THE EFFECTS OF HOSPITALIZATION ON CHILDREN'S PLAY

Disruption of Play

Tisza, Hurwitz, and Angoff (1970) provide evidence that circumstances of hospitalization may indeed result in reductions of children's play activities, especially among preschool children. The original goal of this research project was to study systematically the content and character of children's free play activities in a hospital playroom. It was hypothesized that play activity would result in a decrease of children's anxiety, which would in turn lessen the amount of regression noted in children during and after hospitalization. However, when the researchers observed that little play occurred among young children when not supported by their mothers or a mother substitute (such as the playroom supervisor), the focus of the project shifted to, "the examination of the child's feelings, needs, and emerging relationships which eventually could lead to development of the ability to play" (p. 517). Thus a study of the changes in children's play behavior over a three-day period was initiated.

Children in three age groups were included in the study (three to four year olds, four to six year olds, and six to eight year olds), with eight children in each group. Observations were made twice daily by child psychiatrists observing either individually or simultaneously. Notes recorded during daily observation periods were used to complete checklists on children's behavior. Categories of behavior examined were said to include indices of the grief and recovery processes, use of toys, and interactions with adults and children. The precise behaviors observed and criteria for their categorization are not presented. Moreover, the results are primarily descriptive, with little reference to the frequency of occurrence of behaviors.

Descriptions provided by Tisza, et al. suggest that a disruption in the behavior and activities of children in all three age groups occurred on the first day in the playroom. For example, evidence of "neuromuscular regression" (i.e., awkwardness in movements and grasping) was reported initially for each age group, yet gradually diminished over the three days of observation. Constriction of children's play behavior on the first day was most pronounced in the youngest age group. Three- to four-year-old children were described as immobile, generally remaining in the spot where they were initially located throughout the period of observation. Few attempts at interaction were made by this group, and their use of toys was restricted, though it increased over successive days of observation. Children in the older age groups displayed more mobility, a wider range of affect, and greater use of toys on the initial day of observation than did three to four year olds. Nevertheless, the play activities of the older children also became more differentiated and complex with time.

The amount of this apparent play disruption that is attributable to hospitalization is indeterminate, Since Tisza, et al. did not compare the inhospital play of children with either their own play before and after hospitalization, or with the play of a comparable group of nonhospitalized subjects. Also unspecified are the situational factors possibly responsible for disruption in children's play. For example, it is unclear whether parents were present with their children during any or all of the observations. Therefore, the alterations in play activities noted may solely represent a reaction to separation rather than to other elements of the hospital experience. Despite these ambiguities, the increasing complexity of play behavior noted over three days suggests that something about the hospital environment may, at least temporarily, have altered the pattern of children's play.

Further indication of the disruption of play during hospitalization is provided by Burstein and Meichenbaum (1979), who studied the relationships existing among children's play, anxiety, and their level of defensiveness. Children, four to nine years of age, were observed while playing with selected sets of toys prior to, during, and after hospitalization for minor surgery. The amount of time spent playing with materials was recorded for each play session. A significantly greater amount of play disruption (i.e., time spent *not* playing with available toys) was noted *during* hospitalization than either before or after. The authors observe that the, "play disruption behavior appeared to be due to a disposition not to play rather than merely because of a distraction to novel stimuli of the hospital environment" (p. 125). The play patterns of hospitalized children were contrasted with those of a control group of nonhospitalized subjects, who were also observed at three separate times. The total amount of play exhibited by the latter group did not significantly differ across sessions.

The activities of children in a pediatric intensive care unit, who were awake, alert, and judged as being capable of engaging in play, were recorded in separate studies conducted by Cataldo, et al. (1979) and Pearson, et al. (1980). In each case, little interaction with toys was observed prior to an intervention consisting of directed play. Though the number of children who had access to materials before the intervention was not reported by Cataldo, et al., the limited preintervention play activity was not necessarily a product of the unavailability of toys. Pearson, et al. observed low preintervention levels of play, despite the presence of toys or play activities for all subjects.

Aggression in Play

In addition to the disruption of play activities, it has been suggested that another alteration in the play of children may occur during hospitalization—an increase in the aggressiveness of their play behavior. Vredevoe, Kim, Dambacher, and Call (1969) contend that aggressive behavior is manifested by children in response to frustration. Working on the assumption that hospitalization for surgery represents a frustrating experience, the researchers hypothesized that the postoperative play of surgical patients would be more aggressive than that of nonsurgical patients or of nonhospitalized children. The play of four- and five-year-old children in each of these groups was, therefore, examined.

Play sessions of all children were fifteen minutes in length. Each child was provided with a standard set of materials including blocks, a family of dolls, a telephone, and a dump truck. Surgical patients (N = 14) were observed in play sessions before and after surgery. Nonsurgical patients (N = 7) and nonhospitalized children (N = 20) were also observed during two play periods held 24 to 48 hours apart. Videotapes of the play sessions were coded for 22 separate behaviors, seven of which were considered to be aggressive responses. No significant differences were noted among groups during either play session. Moreover, few behavioral changes within groups were noted between the first and second play sessions. Of those changes found, none indicate an increase in aggressive play associated with either hospitalization or surgery.

THE USE OF PLAY BY HOSPITALIZED CHILDREN

The data of Tisza, et al. (1970), Burstein and Meichenbaum (1979), Cataldo, et al. (1979), and Pearson, et al. (1980) suggest that some disruption in the play of children occurs during hospitalization. Despite these indications of disturbance, the literature also provides evidence that, when children do engage in play, they use this activity to facilitate their adjustment to the hospital. For example, research indicates that play activities are used by children to establish supportive relationships with adults and peers and to gain a sense of mastery (Tisza, et al., 1970). Furthermore, there may be an increased tendency for hospitalized children to select play materials relevant to their condition, which would be consistent with the psychoanalytic view that play is used to assimilate and master stressful circumstances (Gilmore, 1966). However, children with extreme levels of anxiety or defensiveness may avoid play materials relevant to their condition, thereby denying themselves the potential benefits that play may provide (Gilmore, 1966; Burstein & Meichenbaum, 1979).

Spontaneous Therapeutic Activities. As mentioned above, Tisza, et al. (1970) report that the play behavior of hospitalized children changed over a period of three days. The alterations varied among subjects in different age groups, though children at each age level demonstrated an increasing amount of interaction with others and a tendency to use play in a manner that might be considered therapeutic. For example, three- to four-year-old children, who made little use of toys on the first day of observation, frequently used play materials on the second day to establish adult relationships, either offering objects to, or requesting them from, the adults. This use of toys continued on the third day, with children additionally imitating the activities of the playroom supervisor. Tisza, et al. also report that children of this age began to use toys "in the service of mastery" on the third day of the study.

Interactions with peers were found to emerge early in the hospitalization of four- to six-year-old children. Toys were also used by children of this age for activities ranging from simple manipulative behavior to dramatic play. The oldest group of children observed, the six- to eight-year-olds, initially used play materials to "orient themselves, establish familiarity, and maintain continuity" (p. 523). This form of activity was soon replaced by use of toys to attain "pleasure in the mastery of their function" (p. 523). Motor play was frequently observed, while dramatic play was relatively uncommon. When dramatic play was observed among children in the older two age groups, it reportedly depicted themes of denial of separation, smallness, and vulnerability. However, no child in the three days of observation used dramatic play to act out aspects of hospitalization relating to medical procedures.

Selection of Relevant Play Materials. The absence of spontaneous medical play reported by Tisza, et al. is surprising if one accepts the psychoanalytic position that children recreate troubling situations in order to assimilate and master them. However, another study, conducted under more controlled circumstances, provides results consistent with psychoanalytic thought. In this case, Gilmore (1966) focused on children's selection of play materials rather than the themes observed during free play. It was predicted that "when a child experiences strong affects he will play with objects relevant to the perceived source of his anxiety" (p. 399).

In an initial test of this hypothesis, the toy preferences of eighteen tonsillectomy patients (5 to 9 years of age) were compared with those of a matched group of nonhospitalized subjects. Each child was presented with three sets of toys, one set at a time, which consisted of hospital-relevant and irrelevant items. Preference was measured by the amount of time children spent playing with each toy during the six minutes allowed per set. As expected, the hospitalized children showed a greater preference for the hospital-relevant toys than did the control-group subjects.

Since the preference for hospital-relevant materials noted among pediatric inpatients may have been attributable to increased *interest* in medical procedures, rather than increased anxiety, Gilmore conducted a second experiment in a non-medical setting controlling for the factor of interest. In this case, school children, who had volunteered to join a "secret club" with the knowledge that part of the initiation might be painful, were randomly assigned to 1) a *visual fear* group, 2) an *auditory fear* group, or 3) a *control* group. All children were taken individually into an office where subjects in the fear groups viewed an apparatus they were told would be used to give them a brief, painful stimulus (either a bright light or a loud sound, depending on their group). Control group children did not see the apparatus, but were told about the initiation procedures. They were also informed that they would be permitted to join the club without submitting to the painful experience. Thus the procedures were of interest to these children, but not a personal threat to them.

After this introduction, and before the anticipated initiation, all children were allowed to play with materials relevant to the auditory or visual modality. Following this play period, children in the fear groups were informed that they would be allowed to join the club without the painful experience. Again, children in all three groups were permitted to play with the materials. The results indicate a significant "modality by trial by group interaction consistent with the hypothesis that, under conditions of anxiety, children prefer toys according to their relevance to that anxiety" (p. 408). This effect was most prominent among children in the auditory fear group, who showed a marked preference for auditory toys in the first session (when their anxiety was presumably high) and a sharp decrease in the second play session.

To check the replicability of this finding, Gilmore conducted a third experiment, similar to the second, yet dealing only with auditory stimuli. As in the second experiment, children's toy preference was significantly affected by their treatment condition. However, the direction of that effect was unexpected, with children in the auditory fear group significantly *avoiding* interaction with auditory toys in their first play session. An examination of children's anxiety levels (assessed by a set of standardized questions during each of the three experiments) indicated that children in both the experimental *and* control groups of the third experiment were significantly more anxious than children in the previous studies. Thus Gilmore suggests that:

> The presence of anxiety in a child has an important influence on a child's choice of toys for play. This influence takes the form of a markedly increased or a markedly decreased interest in toys relevant to the source of the anxiety. Which of these changes will occur depends upon as yet unspecified addition factors, but the most likely candidate would seem to be the absolute magnitude of the fear of anxiety (p. 416).

The previously mentioned Burstein and Meichenbaum (1979) study is based, in part, on the work of Gilmore. While Burstein and Meichenbaum agree that level of anxiety may influence children's selection of play materials when under stress, they suggest that another factor, children's defensiveness, may also be applicable. In support of this position, the authors cite Janis' (1958) work with adult surgical patients, which reports that a moderate level of anxiety prior to surgery was predictive of satisfactory postsurgical adjustment. Moderate anxiety is said to stimulate thoughts and images of impending events thus enabling prospective patients to develop mechanisms for coping with the events. Janis also reports that patients high in defensiveness tended to be low in presurgical anxiety and therefore did not engage in the "work of worrying." The postsurgical adjustment of such patients was consequently poorer. Applying the Janis model and the results of the Gilmore studies, Burstein and Meichenbaum predicted the existence of: 1) a curvilinear relationship between hospitalized children's stress level and their selection of hospital-relevant toys, and 2) an inverse relationship between defensiveness and relevant toy selection.

Twenty children, four to nine years of age were assessed in their homes one week prior to hospitalization for minor surgery, in the hospital the night before surgery, and at home again one week after surgery. Defensiveness was measured during the first session using a questionnaire developed by Wallach and Kogan (1965). Children's anxiety was assessed at each time period using Gilmore's (1966) scale. In addition, preference for play materials was determined by recording the amount of time each child spent playing with hospital-relevant or non-relevant toys before, during, and after hospitalization.

Correlations between concurrent measures of children's anxiety and time spent playing with hospital-relevant materials were nonsignificant. However, a significant relationship between children's *prehospital* play and *posthospital* anxiety was noted such that increased play with hospital-relevant toys prior to admission was associated with reduced anxiety following discharge. Furthermore, children's level of defensiveness was *negatively* related to their amount of play with hospital-relevant toys in the prehospital period and positively related to posthospital anxiety.

Burstein and Meichenbaum interpret their results as revealing two groups of children who demonstrate different response patterns when confronted with stress. Children in one group (which the authors describe as the "work of worriers") are low in defensiveness prior to hospitalization, actively play with relevant materials in the prehospital period, and display minimal anxiety following discharge. Subjects in the second group (termed "deniers") are high in defensiveness, avoid prehospital play with hospital-relevant toys, and report higher levels of anxiety following hospitalization.

To further understand the characteristics distinguishing these groups of children, a follow-up study was conducted seven months after discharge. At this time, four children considered representative of the "work of worriers" group and four "deniers" were interviewed, with subjects in these groups matched on age and sex. Children's responses indicate that "worriers" had developed a more articulated perception of hospital-related experiences and threats than did "deniers." Although the two groups did not differ on the total number of items recalled about hospitalization, significantly more of the events recalled by the "worriers" pertained to hospital or medical procedures. "Worriers" also recalled more preparatory statements given by parents before hospitalization—a result that is apparently not a product of differences in parents' approaches. Separate interviews with parents revealed no appreciable difference in the types of information provided to children in the two groups. On projective assessments, "worriers" identified significantly more specific threats, and offered more self-delivered reassurances concerning hospitalization and surgery than did "deniers."

The Burstein and Meichenbaum results are partially supported by the data of Tarnow and Gutstein (1983; also reported in Gutstein, 1980). Approximately three days prior to tonsillectomy surgery, 34 children (4 to 9 years of age) and their parents participated in a preparation program. At that time, the activities of children were videotaped during three separate five-minute periods. In the first, children were left alone to play freely with materials in two boxes, one of which contained hospital equipment, while the other held an assortment of age appropriate toys. Following this session, children were observed during medical play with an experimenter, who asked each subject to demonstrate what would happen in the hospital. Finally, parents rejoined their children and were asked to use the medical play materials to prepare their children for surgery.

Children's level of active preparatory behavior in each session was rated using a four-point scale ranging from 0 (total non-involvement) to 3 ("active involvement in an integrated fashion"). Self-report and observational assessments of children' distress were made during each of the three observation periods. In addition, parents completed forms concerning their children's behavior and fearfulness on the day of preparation and again one week after surgery. Relationships among levels of children's preparatory behavior across observation periods, as well as relationships between preparatory behavior and the other outcome measures, were assessed.

Ratings of children's preparatory play when alone were significantly associated with ratings made when with the experimenter and with parents, indicating some degree of consistency in their involvement in preparation across sessions. When children's preparatory behavior was related to observational and self-report measures of distress during preparation, only one significant relationship emerged, and that with only a portion of the sample. Observational ratings of distress for older subjects (6 to 9 years) were negatively associated with levels of preparatory play. However, in a finding comparable to that of Burstein and Meichenbaum (1979), Tarnow and Gutstein report significant relationships between children's play and their posthospital behavior and fearfulness. Specifically, higher levels of active preparatory play when alone or with the experimenter were associated with lesser posthospital behavioral disturbance. Moreover, active involvement when with parents was significantly correlated with reduced levels of fear after discharge.

The data reported above suggest that children respond to stressful events with differing styles, either openly approaching the threatening circumstances, initiating a constructive process of worrying, or defending themselves against contemplation of the events. The nature of children's play, or at least the materials chosen for play, is reflective of their coping style. Those children more willing to confront events, as demonstrated by their choice of relevant play materials, are also less likely to display upset following the event.

Another nonexperimental study examining the relationship between play and anxiety suggests that children's selection and current use of toys may be associated with anxiety displayed during a *previous* health care experience—in this case, dental treatment. McTigue and Pinkham (1978) considered children between 42 and 66 months of age who had previously undergone a dental restoration procedure, which included an injection of a local anesthetic. During the earlier treatment, children's behavior had been rated as definitely negative, negative, intermediate, or definitely positive.

Fifteen children from each category were included in the present study. Each child was allowed to play for five minutes with materials including a miniature dental chair, a doll patient, a dental handpiece, and toy dental instruments, as well as several non-dental toys. Children's toy selection, use of dental toys, and verbalizations were recorded at fifteen second intervals. Ratings of children's involvement with dental toys varied, depending on whether children looked at the toys (1 point), touched them (3 points), or actively manipulated them (6 points).

Univariate analyses of variance revealed group differences in the use of four dental items (significant at $p < .10$): the doll patient, a needle, mirror, and toothbrush. For each item, children in the "definitely positive" group displayed more active play than did children in the "definitely negative" group. Thus, while Burstein and Meichenbaum (1979) found play behavior to be related to subsequent anxiety, McTigue and Pinkham suggest that past manifestations of anxiety may be related to subsequent play.

Of considerable interest, though not discussed by the authors, was the play behavior of the *intermediate* group. For three of the four dental items for which significant group differences in play were found (doll, needle, and toothbrush), the highest mean play score was recorded *not* by the "positive" group, as the authors' discussion implies, but by the intermediate group. If past dental behavior may be viewed as indicative of children's level of anxiety concerning forthcoming dental encounters, the elevated amount of stress-relevant play among the intermediate group may be reconciled with the findings of both Janis (1958) and Gilmore (1966). Janis suggests that moderate anxiety is most effective in stimulating the "work of worrying." Thus, it is not unreasonable that the greatest amount of interaction with dental toys was noted among the group displaying a moderate amount of upset during past treatment. The McTigue and Pinkham results may also be seen as consistent with Gilmore's suggestion that children will select toys relevant to their stressful condition unless extremely anxious, in which case such materials will be significantly avoided.

In a subsequent study, Pinkham and Kerber (1979) attempted to replicate the McTigue and Pinkham results with a group of 27 schoolaged children. Ten children previously displaying negative behavior during dental treatment and seventeen children exhibiting "definitely positive" dental behavior were allowed to play with a set of toys including dental equipment, as well as non-relevant materials. A discriminant analysis of data on children's play (collected in a manner similar to that of the earlier study) accurately reclassified all children into their appropriate dental behavior groups. Subjects in the positive behavior group made greater use of the dental items than did those previously displaying negative dental behavior. However, when use of individual items by children in the two groups was directly compared, a significant difference in only one item was found, the dental mirror, with "positive" group children using it more extensively.

The preceding studies indicate that a relationship exists between children's play behavior and their responses to stressful medical and dental events, though the nature of that relationship is not fully understood. It appears that children who are neither highly anxious nor highly defensive will frequently select toys relevant to their condition for their play. The research further suggests that play with stress-relevant materials may be beneficial to children, possibly resulting in reduced disturbance in the period following health care. The small group of studies examining this proposition through experimental research will be considered in the following section.

THE EFFECTS OF PLAY INTERVENTIONS

Play Interventions and Children's Upset

Despite indications from clinical data and correlational studies that play may be beneficial in reducing upset, experimental evaluation of the effectiveness of play has seldom been conducted. Excluding research incorporating play as an adjunct to preparation (see Chapter 10), four of the identified studies have investigated the capacity of structured play to alter children's upset. The format of the play intervention in each of the identified studies is markedly different. Lockwood (1970) provided a single free play session with medical toys. Clatworthy (1978, 1981) offered daily, thirty-minute play sessions using a variety of toys, only a portion of which were directly relevant to the hospital setting. Schwartz, et al. (1983) used a play condition consisting of a single session with materials unrelated to hospitalization as a control for a preparation intervention. Finally, Clegg (1972) assessed the effectiveness of participation in child life programming (which included play and educational opportunities) on hospitalized children's anxiety.

Lockwood (1970) examined the impact of situational doll play on the responses of children, four to six years of age, hospitalized for elective surgery. Upon admission to the hospital, the twenty children participating in the study were given the Hospital Picture Test, a projective instrument developed by Barton (1964), which yields scores on anxiety-defense, dependency, aggression, and anxiety-fear dimensions, as well as indices of children's total stress and of the focus of their stress reactions. Following administration of the test, half of the children participated in a play session with a nurse. Children were given the option of playing doctor or nurse and were allowed to manipulate a variety of medical toys and items. For children in the experimental group, the projective test was readministered immediately after the play session. Control group children were tested a second time after an intervening period of one half-hour.

Though data analysis is not fully presented, Lockwood reports that the situational doll play did not significantly reduce children's total stress scores. However, the anxiety-defense scores of experimental group subjects were found to be significantly lower following play sessions. In addition, the stress reactions of children receiving the play intervention were increasingly focused on doctors and medical procedures. Lockwood summarizes these findings as indicating that:

> A situational doll play session on the day of admission to the hospital broke down the child's defense mechanisms or learned patterns of coping with crisis situations; and that the child's anxiety fears were focused upon a more clearly perceived and realistic object: the doctors and/or medical procedures (p. 118)

As noted above, Burstein and Meichenbaum (1979) suggest that children's level of defensiveness is indicative of their willingness to play with relevant materials, thereby initiating the "work of worrying" process. Children engaging in "worrying" are said to display more clearly articulated conceptions of threats and to experience less anxiety following hospitalization. The findings of Lockwood suggest that play may not only *reflect* children's willingness to approach threatening circumstances, but when provided in structured settings may also *facilitate* their approach by reducing children's defensiveness and anxiety.

Clatworthy (1981) conducted a series of three experiments involving daily, unstructured play sessions, finding play in each case to have a beneficial effect on the anxiety levels of children. Phase I of the study (results of which are also presented by Clatworthy, 1978) involved 23 children hospitalized for four days in a children's hospital. During Phase II, 26 children hospitalized in the same setting for two-day periods were considered. Phase III was conducted in a university hospital with 65 children, admitted for longer hospitalizations. The procedure for each phase was similar. Children five to twelve years of age were randomly assigned to either the experimental or control condition. The anxiety of all children was measured at admission using the Missouri Children's Picture Series (Sines, Pauker, & Sines, 1974), with this test readministered either at discharge or on the seventh day of hospitalization.

Experimental play sessions lasted thirty minutes each and were conducted by a nurse therapist who provided materials such as dolls, cars, paints, a punching bag, hospital equipment, and story books. Play sessions was said to be directed in part by the child, with the nurse therapist providing reflection and some interpretation of the feelings revealed by children during their play.

Results were consistent across all three phases, with control group children found to be more anxious at the final evaluation than children receiving the play treatment ($p < .10$). However, the play intervention did not appear to decrease children's anxiety over the course of their hospitalization. Rather, experimental group children maintained their initial anxiety levels, while significant *increases* in the anxiety of control group children were noted over time.

Schwartz, Albino, and Tedesco (1983) also provide limited evidence that nondirective play in the presence of an adult may be helpful in modifying children's upset during hospitalization, even when the play is unrelated to hospital experiences. The primary purpose of this study was to evaluate the effectiveness of a preparation protocol, which consisted of information about an impending surgical procedure presented through play techniques. Subjects were 45 children, three and four years of age, who were hospitalized for dental surgery. In addition to the experimental group of children who received relevant information and play (the so-called "related play therapy" group), two other conditions were used. A control group received no preoperative preparation, while an "unrelated play therapy" group was allowed to play with a toy barn and farm animals for twenty minutes under the supervision of the same child life specialist who conducted the "related play" sessions. Conversation during unrelated play sessions was limited to the farm toys, with no mention of the surgery. The therapist tried to create a pleasant atmosphere during the play sessions, conducive to gaining children's trust and confidence.

Children's manifest upset and cooperation were rated at a series of stress points using the scales developed by Wolfer and Visintainer (1975). Examination of group differences at individual stress points revealed that children in the "related play" group were consistently more cooperative and less upset than control group children. However, ratings of children in the related and unrelated play groups were significantly different at only one point, with related play children less upset during anesthesia induction than those in the unrelated group. Thus it appears that an opportunity to play under the supervision of a supportive adult is at least somewhat effective in altering children's upset behavior. This conclusion is further supported by Minde and Maler (1968; see Chapter 10), who found no difference in self-reported anxiety or length of hospitalization of children who received either an explanation of their illness, or an opportunity to play and talk with an adult, who made no reference to the child's condition.

An increasing amount of play for hospitalized children is provided by specially trained professionals, commonly known as child life specialists. The final study considered in this section, Clegg (1972), represents the only attempt to date to assess the effectiveness of a comprehensive child life program. Unfortunately, methodological problems severely limit the interpretation of Clegg's results.

The anxiety of forty children (6 to 10 years of age, hospitalized for major elective surgery) was assessed using the Palmar Sweat Index at admission, after surgery, and again after four hours of participation in a child life program. Child life activities occurring in the morning were said to include individualized schooling, group educational experiences, creative arts and crafts, and a communal lunch. Afternoon activities consisted of free play, arts, crafts, and recreation. The particular activities to which subjects were exposed during their four-hour experiences are not specified. Clegg reports a significant reduction in anxiety levels of children following participation in the child life program. However, since no control group was used for comparison, it is unclear whether the reduction in anxiety is attributable to the child life program or to other factors such as general adjustment to the hospital setting, improvement of physical condition following surgery, or anticipation of returning home.

Three of the intervention studies considered above indicate that supervised play sessions with materials, either related or unrelated to the medical setting, may be helpful in minimizing children's upset during hospitalization (Lockwood, 1970; Clatworthy, 1978,

1981; Schwartz, et al., 1983). However, the precise role of play in altering children's emotional distress remains ambiguous. None of the studies considered above used either an attention control group (i.e., interaction with an adult, but no play) or an unsupervised play condition (play opportunities, without adult support). One cannot, therefore, determine whether play itself is directly effective in altering anxiety and upset, or perhaps operates indirectly by providing a vehicle for the development of supportive relationships, which is, in turn, the operative factor in reducing children's distress.

Play Interventions and Children's Behaviors

Three studies have examined the effects of supervised play experiences on specific behaviors of children, rather than on the higher order construct of children's psychological upset. Two related studies have assessed the impact of a play intervention on children's affect, as well as their attention to and interaction with play materials, while in an intensive care unit (Cataldo, et al., 1979; Pearson, et al., 1980). In the third study, Williams and Powell (1980) examined alterations in designated positive and negative behaviors of children when supervised play was introduced to an outpatient waiting area. In each case, supervised play was found to dramatically alter the identified behaviors. Withdrawal of supervision, even when toys remained available, resulted in a return to the patterns of behavior exhibited prior to the intervention.

Cataldo, et al. (1979) selected for observation eleven ICU patients (1 to 21 years of age) who were judged to be awake and alert. Each participated in an intervention consisting of three five-minute segments. During the first segment, two groups of children were given no play materials (other than those already available to them), while the third received toys with no supervision. During the middle segment, children in all three groups were provided with play materials, plus the supervision of a child life specialist. In the final period, play materials were taken from children in one group, but were left with those in the other two. Subjects were observed during the fifteen-minute intervention, with their affect and their *attention to* and *interaction with* play materials recorded.

Also noted were instances of inappropriate behavior.

The introduction of play materials and supervision greatly increased children's attention to and manipulation of materials. In addition, subjects provided with toys, either before or after the period of supervision, displayed moderately high levels of attention and interaction, though not as great as during supervision. Withdrawal of toys following the supervision period resulted in marked reductions of these behaviors. Increases in positive affect and reductions of inappropriate behavior were reported for individual subjects during periods of play and supervision.

Pearson, et al. (1980) also examined the behavior of children in the ICU in response to a play intervention. The eleven children included in the sample ranged in age from two to fourteen years, were of stable physical condition, and were judged to be capable of manipulating play materials. Children's interactions with materials and their affect were recorded before, during and after a period of play intervention. In the preintervention period, subjects were provided with neither supervision nor play materials, though all eleven children had materials of their own available to them at that time. The play intervention phase consisted of a child life specialist approaching individual children with toys, engaging each in activities for a twenty-minute period. Upon conclusion of the intervention, play materials were left with the children. Unlike the Cataldo, et al. (1979) study (in which children were observed immediately after intervention, revealing moderately high levels of interaction when toys were left with them), Pearson, et al. delayed postintervention observation for 30 to 45 minutes after the conclusion of the play session.

Significant increases in children's positive affect and their interaction with materials were recorded when the intervention was instituted. Despite the fact that toys were left with children following the intervention, a significant reduction in manipulation of materials was noted when supervision was withdrawn. In fact, the amount of interaction in the postintervention period was significantly lower than during the preintervention phase.

Williams and Powell (1980) investigated the effectiveness of a structured, supervised play program in altering children's behavior in an outpatient waiting area. The study was conducted in two stages. In the first of these, observations were made during a control period (in which no play supervision and few toys were available) and an experimental period (consisting of supervision and an adequate supply of toys). Occurrences of negative behaviors were recorded, which included crying, screaming, nail-biting, aggressive play, and hostile parent-child interaction. In addition, positive parent-child interaction and constructive play behavior were noted. During the control period of the first phase, 421 positive and 641 negative behaviors were recorded. This compared with 879 positive and 144 negative behaviors noted during the experimental period.

To assess the contribution of supervision to the reduction of negative behaviors in the outpatient area, a second research phase was conducted. In this portion of the study, an experimental period, identical to that used in the first phase (i.e., supervision and toys), was contrasted with a modified control period, in which toys were available *without* supervision. Results were similar to those of the earlier phase. The control period yielded 566 positive and 1034 negative behaviors, versus 1078 positive and 144 negative behaviors under the supervised condition. Thus, the dramatic change in children's behavior was not solely a product of the introduction of play materials, but may be largely attributed to the presence of trained supervisory personnel.

The studies conducted by Cataldo, et al. (1979), Pearson, et al. (1980), and Williams and Powell (1980) indicate that the introduction of directed play experiences is capable of temporarily modifying children's behavior, increasing interaction with materials, altering affect, and reducing negative behaviors. However, the studies further suggest that providing play materials alone, without direct supervision, is less successful in altering the designated behaviors.

Infant Stimulation

Another form of play-related intervention receiving research attention in recent years is the stimulation of hospitalized infants. In the past, conventional medical practice discouraged the stimulation of premature or low-birth-weight infants, beyond that necessary for basic care, on the grounds that these children are too fragile to be treated in this manner. However, the wisdom of this practice has been questioned by a series of studies indicating that systematic stimulation may promote infants' physical growth, as well as their cognitive and social development (Scarr-Salapatek & Williams, 1973; White & Labarba, 1975; Rausch, 1981; Porter, 1972; Kramer, Chamorro, Green, & Knudtson, 1975).

In the most extensive of these interventions, Scarr-Salapatek and Williams (1973) alternately assigned thirty consecutively born low-birth-weight infants to an experimental or control condition. From birth onward, experimental group children were provided with visual, tactile, and kinesthetic stimulation, said to approximate good home care of infants. For example, objects were hung in the infants' isolettes where they could easily be seen by the children. When able to maintain their body temperature for thirty minutes, infants were removed from their isolettes for feeding and for play sessions, which consisted of rocking, patting, fondling, and verbal stimulation. In contrast, control group children were kept in the isolettes at most times, and were fed and changed with minimal disturbance.

Although control group infants weighed more than the experimental group infants at birth, and had higher scores on the Brazelton Newborn Scales administered at one week, these differences were reversed after four weeks of the stimulation program. Experimental group infants gained significantly more weight during this period than control group subjects.

After discharge from the hospital, experimental group infants and mothers were visited by a social worker to enable these subjects to continue their program of stimulation at home. Toys and activities appropriate to the child's developmental level were provided by the social worker, who instructed mothers in their use. After one year of this program, experimental infants were found to have a significantly higher developmental status than that of control subjects—a level nearly equal to the norms for one-year-old children.

Other interventions discussed in the research literature have been more restricted, both in time and in the scope of stimulation activities provided. Nevertheless, positive effects have been typically noted among infants receiving experimental treatment. White and Labarba (1975) randomly assigned twelve premature infants to an experimental or control condition, with experimental group children receiving four fifteen-minute periods of tactile and kinesthetic stimulation daily for ten days. Upon the conclusion of the intervention, experimental group subjects' weight and formula intake were significantly greater than that of control group infants. Group differences in number of feedings, frequency of voiding or stooling, body temperature, respiration and heart rate were nonsignificant.

Rausch (1981) provided twenty premature infants with a fifteen-minute period of of tactile and kinesthetic stimulation daily during the first ten days after birth. Responses of these children were compared with those of a group of infants, matched on weight, gestation, sex, race, and ability to breathe spontaneously, who received no experimental treatment. Though the weight gain of the experimental group exceeded that of control group infants over the ten-day period, this difference was not significant. However, over the latter half of the intervention period, significant group differences in feeding intake and frequency of stooling were recorded, with each difference in favor of the infants receiving systematic intervention.

Stimulation programs examined in two additional studies were limited to either the kinesthetic or tactile modality. Porter (1972) reports significant developmental differences between experimental and control group infants (4 to 40 weeks of age) in favor of those receiving kinesthetic stimulation—cycling motions of arms and legs, provided four times daily, six days per week for two months. Kramer, et al. (1975) provided an extra 48 minutes of tactile stimulation per day, for a minimum of two weeks, to an experimental group of eight premature infants. No significant difference was found when their rate of physical growth was compared with that of six premature infants who had received no stimulation. However, the rate of social development of infants in the tactile stimulation group was found to be greater than that of control group subjects.

Use of Music

Music has been used as an adjunct to hospital play programs, with children directly involved in musical play, or with music provided as a background for other activities. The effects of this use of music on hospitalized children's emotional status has not been addressed in the identified research. However, Ammon (1968) suggests that the playing of music may have a therapeutic effect on the medical condition of at least one group of patients—young children in respiratory distress. Subjects included twenty children, 2 to 24 months of age, whose condition necessitated placement in a high humidity environment. Children randomly assigned to the experimental condition were allowed to listen to a tape recording of classical music for one hour, while control group children heard no recording. Vital signs of experimental subjects were checked before and after the intervention. Those of control group children were recorded at a comparable interval, without the intervening music. A significantly greater reduction in respiratory rate of experimental than control group subjects was noted.

DEVELOPMENT OF HOSPITAL-BASED PLAY PROGRAMS

At least eight surveys assessing the prevalence and functioning of hospital-based play programs have been conducted since 1965. Two surveys of the general pediatric services provided by hospitals in portions of Canada include questions concerning the play opportunities available to children (Alcock, 1977; Post, 1979). The remaining surveys pertain specifically to the characteristics of child life programs, and the professionals staffing them, in the United States and Canada (Dombro, 1967a, 1967b; McCue, Wagner, Hansen, & Rigler, 1978; Rutkowski, 1978; Mather & Glasrud, 1981; Ricks & Faubert, 1981). The results of surveys in this group conducted prior to 1980 are summarized and discussed by Larsen (1980).

Despite the progress in establishing hospital-based play programs documented in these surveys, resistance to the institution of play programs remains. Hall (1977, 1978) reports on observations made in two children's wards in Great Britain before and after the introduction of trained play personnel. Physicians in these settings were said to be supportive of the therapeutic goals of play programming, but since they spent only limited time on the units, they exerted little influence on the practical operation of the programs. Nurses tended to use play leaders as "an extra pair of hands," having them deal with difficult children or those less seriously ill so that they (the nurses) could devote more time to patients with greater illness. Conflicts were also noted between playleaders and ancillary ward personnel. The latter typically encouraged sexually stereotyped play and were often disturbed by the disorder of play activities.

Chapter 10

PSYCHOLOGICAL PREPARATION FOR HOSPITALIZATION AND HEALTH CARE PROCEDURES

The preparation of children and parents for health care encounters has received more research attention in recent years than any of the other topics considered in the present text. Vernon, Foley, Sipowicz, and Schulman (1965) identified a mere six studies appearing prior to publication of their literature review pertaining to the psychological preparation of children for hospitalization (Cassell, 1963; Jackson, et al., 1953; Jessner, et al., 1952; Prugh et al., 1953; Vaughan, 1957; Weinick, 1958). Since 1965, more than ten times that number of research reports (65 in all) have appeared examining the use of preparation interventions with children and parents in medical or dental settings.

Of the studies considered in this chapter, 42 evaluate the effectiveness of interventions designed to reduce the upset of children and parents engendered by hospitalization. Thirty-one of these are experimental in nature, characterized by deliberate assignment of subjects to specified treatment or control conditions. Eleven are nonexperimental or correlational studies, examining the characteristics or responses of subjects differing in their preexisting levels of preparation for forthcoming events. An additional six studies, all of which use experimental designs, examine the effectiveness of preparation for specific, isolated medical events (e.g., injections, rectal temperatures, cast removal, and anesthesia induction).

Interventions outside of the medical setting have also been conducted. For example, the value of preparation for dental experiences has been addressed in thirteen experimental studies. Two additional studies examine the impact of classroom-based interventions on the attitudes toward hospitalization and health care procedures of healthy schoolaged children. The final two studies considered in this chapter are surveys of institutions concerning their implementation of preparation programs.

Despite the volume of material available on preparation, examination of individual studies reveals limitations in the research conducted to date. These limitations may be illustrated by closer examination of the 31 experimental studies on the preparation of children and parents for hospitalization. Figure 1 depicts the percentage of these 31 studies involving children of each age group. Since samples of broad age range are frequently used in this research, the numbers total well above one hundred percent. As may be seen, most research of this type includes late preschool and schoolaged children in their samples. Involvement of children in the older age groups is less frequent. Fewer than forty percent of the studies include twelve-year-old children. Moreover, only three of the 31 studies in this group consider subjects thirteen years of age or older. Thus, the value of preparation among older pediatric populations is yet to be established.

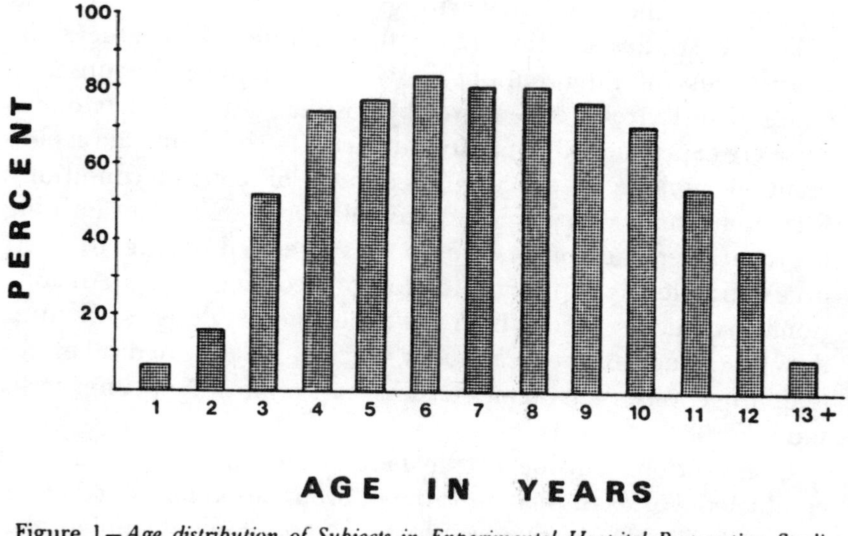

Figure 1—*Age distribution of Subjects in Experimental Hospital Preparation Studies.* The percentage of total studies (N = 31) including subjects of each age level.

Further problems in generalizing the results of existing preparation research become apparent when one examines the conditions for which participating children have been hospitalized. Some ninety percent of the 31 preparation studies under consideration involve children admitted for surgical or diagnostic procedures, while only three individual studies evaluate the effectiveness of inhospital explanations given to patients hospitalized with medical diagnoses. Of the 28 studies involving preparation for surgery, 26 include subjects variously described by the authors as minor, elective, or short-term surgical patients. Diagnoses in this category consist primarily of tonsillectomy and/or adenoidectomy surgery, though admission for hernia repair, myringotomies, and certain diagnostic procedures requiring brief hospitalization are also included in this group. In contrast, only a single experimental study is devoted exclusively to preparation for cardiac surgery (Hackett, 1976), though two preparation studies in the nonexperimental category also consider this condition (Gabriel & Danilowicz, 1978; Schmeltz & White, 1982).

The majority of the research has been limited to inhospital preparation interventions, rather than those occurring prior to hospitalization. More than eighty percent of the experimental, medical preparation studies involve interventions conducted *after* children have arrived at the hospital. In contrast, three studies examine interventions occurring in the home prior to admission (Roskies, et al., 1978; Ferguson, 1979; Wolfer & Visintainer, 1979). Moreover, despite the prevalence of preadmission programs as a means of preparing children for hospitalization (Azarnoff & Woody, 1981), only two experimental studies consider this form of preparation (Landes, 1973; Peterson, 1978), though six nonexperimental studies examine preadmission sessions, comparing the characteristics of subjects who attend such programs with those who do not.

The review of research in the present chapter begins with studies providing procedural information to subjects in a simple, didactic manner. Following this discussion, research varying the method of instruction or the type of information provided is considered. Basic presentations of information about the hospital, procedures, and equipment have been modified in several ways. One group of studies has incorporated *play activities* in the preparation process, allowing children to manipulate and familiarize themselves with the equipment to be used in their care (Cassell, 1965; Johnson & Stockdale, 1975; Williams, 1980; Schwartz, et al., 1983). The content of other preparation protocols has been modified to emphasize the sensations children experience while undergoing health care procedures (e.g., Johnson, Kirchhoff, & Endress, 1975; Siegel & Peterson, 1980, 1981). Child-oriented approaches to preparation also include the use of *filmed modeling* (Vernon, 1973, 1974; Melamed & Siegel, 1975) and the teaching of *coping skills* such as relaxation techniques or comforting self-talk (Peterson, 1978; Nocella & Kaplan, 1982).

Parents have also been frequently included in preparation activities, sometimes as the sole recipients of intervention efforts (Mahaffy, 1965; Skipper & Leonard, 1968; Roskies, et al., 1978). In other cases, parents are provided with preparatory information in conjunction with activities directed toward their children. One approach to preparing subjects, referred to as stress-point preparation, combines parent participation with other elements such as the providing of information, rehearsal for events, and consistent contact with a member of the nursing staff during designated periods of risk (Wolfer & Visintainer, 1975, 1979; Visintainer & Wolfer, 1979).

Many of the techniques used to prepare children and their families for health care encounters, including stress-point preparation, involve extended contact with a supportive person, in addition to whatever type of information may be provided. The question of the potential contribution of emotional support to the reduction of children's upset, therefore, arises. Studies addressing this question are also reviewed (c.f., Minde & Maler, 1968; Fassler, 1980).

After considering the experimental data on the various approaches to preparing children and parents for health care events, the nonexperimental research is considered. Studies in this category are of two principal types. In the first instance, an assessment is made of the adequacy of children's preparation (presumably given by parents at home) upon their arrival at the hospital, with this level of preparation being related to children's perceptions of stress (Menke, 1972, 1981) or to their behavioral responses while hospitalized (Milosavljević, et al., 1972). The remaining nonexperimental studies examine participation in preadmission programs, comparing attending and nonattending subjects on family characteristics or children's responses.

BASIC INFORMATIONAL APPROACHES

A primary means of preparing children and their parents for health care encounters is by providing accurate information about the impending events. In the literature reviewed by Vernon, et al. (1965) an accurate understanding of one's circumstances was said to be beneficial for two related reasons. First, threats of which one is aware are believed to be less upsetting than those that remain vague and ill-defined. Second, unexpected stress is held to be more disturbing than that which one anticipates.

Vernon, et al. also note that, in practice, preparation is typically not limited to mere presentation of information. Through the process of preparation, children are allowed to establish a trusting relationship with a member of the hospital staff. Furthermore, expressions of children's emotions are frequently elicited during the process. Either of these elements may contribute significantly to the psychological benefits of preparation.

However, rather than evaluating the relative contributions of information, emotional support, and the opportunity for expression of feelings, most preparation research has incorporated all three elements in experimental protocols, varying the method of presentation or the content of the information itself. (A notable exception to this rule is the research on filmed modeling, a process that requires neither the establishment of a relationship nor the elicitation of emotional expression.) The studies reviewed in this section concern the presentation of basic information to children about their condition or treatment, without elaboration of the content or incorporation of ancillary techniques such as play, filmed modeling, or instruction in relaxation skills. After considering the research of this sort pertaining to medical illness, surgery, and dental procedures, the question of the relationship between knowledge obtained through preparation and children's psychological upset is examined.

Information about Medical Conditions

Among the research providing subjects with basic information about their condition are three studies involving patients with medical diagnoses (Minde & Maler, 1968; Goslin, 1979; Rie, Boverman, Grossman, & Ozoa, 1968). In each case, children were given explanations of their condition after admission to the hospital, following commencement of their treatment. Thus, a portion of the information provided pertained to events that had already occurred, a situation that distinguishes these studies from the others to be considered.

Subjects in the Minde and Maler (1968) study included 108 children, five to twelve years of age, hospitalized for medical conditions. On the second and third days of their hospitalization, children in the experimental condition were visited by a child psychiatrist who spent 30 to 45 minutes per day with each subject discussing the child's illness and treatment, as well as fears commonly expressed by hospitalized children. Control group subjects received no such visits. Nurses' ratings of children's behavior and a self-report questionnaire were completed before and after the period of experimental intervention for subjects in both conditions.

A significant decline in the experimental group's self-ratings of anxiety was noted following the intervention, though nurses' ratings of children's behavior over the same period revealed no significant differences. Data on the duration of children's hospitalization indicate that subjects in the experimental group were hospitalized for a significantly shorter time than control group subjects, despite lack of group differences in type or severity of admitting diagnoses.

The value of an informational intervention in reducing the upset of children admitted to the hospital under emergency circumstances was assessed by Goslin (1979). The sample consisted of forty children, eighteen months to six years of age, with the admitting diagnosis of gastroenteritis. Children who were randomly assigned to the experimental condition were read a story about a child entering the hospital with that diagnosis, with the story addressing fears and misconceptions common among hospitalized preschool and schoolaged children. Control group children received no intervention. Subject's temperature, pulse, and respiration rates were measured before and after the intervention period. In addition, parents completed the Posthospital Behavior Questionnaire. Experimental group subjects were found to have significantly lower temperatures than control group children in the evening following the intervention. However, the groups did not differ in other physiological measures or in their posthospital behavior.

The impact of information provided to children hospitalized with rheumatic fever was considered by Rie, et al. (1968). Fifty-two children, eight to eleven years of age, were assigned to one of two treatment conditions, both of which consisted of a series of three small-group meetings. Children assigned to the *tutorial* group were taught about rheumatic fever's onset, treatment, and follow-up care. Those in the *psychotherapy* group explored the concerns and fantasies that hospitalized or ill children typically express, yet were given no information about rheumatic fever. The Children's Manifest Anxiety Scale (CMAS) and two other instruments specifically designed for this study to assess children's knowledge of, and concerns about, rheumatic fever were administered before treatment, within one day of completion of the group sessions, and again some nineteen months after children had been discharged. Data were also gathered on subjects exposed to neither treatment condition.

Immediately following their respective interventions, subjects in both treatment groups exhibited improvements in their knowledge scores, while the scores of control group children remained unchanged over a comparable period. However, the subsequent, follow-up assessments indicated that children in the psychotherapy group, but not the tutorial group, were able to maintain improvements in knowledge over an extended period. The authors suggest that failure to address the concerns and anxieties of tutorial group children about their condition may have interfered with the durability of the information they had acquired. Although a reduction in the CMAS scores of the tutorial group subjects was recorded in the immediate postintervention period, neither group showed a significant change in anxiety scores between admission and follow-up assessments.

Information about Hospitalization and Surgical Procedures

The preparation of children for hospitalization and surgical procedures through presentation of basic information has been evaluated in two additional studies (Thomson, 1972; Azarnoff, Bourque, Green, & Rakow, 1975). Thomson (1972) examined the effects of a preoperative explanation provided to children by an operating room nurse. Subjects ranged in age from six to ten years and were hospitalized for mild to moderate short-term surgical procedures. Following admission to the hospital in the afternoon prior to surgery, experimental group children (N = 10) were given explanations of the procedures they would experience. Though instructional outlines were prepared to guide the nurses conducting the sessions, each instructor was encouraged to adapt explanations to conform to the interests and attention span of individual children. Control group subjects (N = 10) received no visit or instruction from operating room personnel. Children's manifest anxiety was rated by nurses at five points prior to and following surgery. Children who had received preoperative instruction were found to be consistently less anxious than control group subjects.

Azarnoff, et al. (1975) compared two methods of providing information to children and their families upon arrival at the hospital—the reading of a preparation booklet and a hospital tour. In this case, the sample consisted of 128 children, four to eleven years of age, most of whom were admitted for elective surgery or diagnostic procedures. Upon admission, children were randomly assigned to one of three groups. Those in the *booklet* group were read a publication that explained hospital routines and activities and addressed topics such as separation from parents and possible misconceptions about treatments. The *tour* group visited hospital areas including the kitchen, nurses' station, a patient room, playroom, treatment room, and surgical waiting room, with an explanation provided for each area. *Control* group children received neither intervention. Assessments of children's stress levels were made upon admission and on the day of discharge using self-report and parent-report measures.

Examination of the characteristics of children in the three conditions revealed significant group differences in sex, ethnicity, number of previous hospitalizations, admitting diagnoses and length of hospital stay, thereby making interpretation of results difficult. No simple main effects for experimental condition were reported, though the authors discuss possible differential effects of the selected interventions for children varying in age, sex, and prior hospital experience.

Information about Dental Procedures

Although dental preparation studies have commonly incorporated specialized forms of intervention, such as the use of filmed modeling or instruction in coping skills rather than presentation of information alone, the latter approach was adopted by Herbertt and Innes (1979). The sample consisted of 422 children ranging in age from five to eleven years. Each subject was scheduled for two dental sessions, the first consisting of a basic examination and the second involving treatment.

Prior to each of the two visits, subjects were assigned to one of three conditions (control, preparatory information, or familiarization). The type of intervention provided on the initial visit was not necessarily the same as that received when children returned for treatment. The *control* condition consisted of a brief lesson in dental health, containing no information about specific dental procedures. The *preparatory information* condition included the dental health lesson given to control group subjects, as well as an explanation of the procedures to be performed that day. Children in the *familiarization* condition were also given the dental health lesson and were taken into the dental operatory, but were given no specific information about their treatment. Observations of children were made to assess their cooperation with procedures and their anxiety during each dental session.

Children's reactions during a given dental visit did not vary with the type of instruction received prior to their treatment. However, Herbertt and Innes created a ranking of the total amount of information received in the two preparation sessions, positing that the control condition would supply the least information and the preparatory information condition the most. Furthermore, since the outcome measure used for this analysis was children's behavior during the second (dental treatment) session, information provided immediately prior to that session was ranked higher than that given before the initial session. A trend analysis revealed a significant curvilinear relationship between the derived ranking of information received by children and their manifest anxiety during treatment, with a moderate amount of information resulting in the least upset.

The Value of Information

Several of the studies discussed above provide at least partial support for the value of providing children with information about their condition (Minde & Maler, 1968; Goslin, 1979; Rie, et al., 1968; Thomson, 1972), yet in none of this research is the relationship between information and children's upset clearly delineated. Herbertt and Innes (1979) suggest that either too much or too little information may result in elevated levels of anxiety. However, this conclusion may not be justified since the measure they used to quantify information was, in actuality, merely a subjective ranking of the amount of *opportunity* one has to acquire information in an organized fashion, rather than a direct assessment of the information *received* by children or their understanding of that information.

In their discussion of the limitations of the research literature they had reviewed, Vernon, et al. (1965) observe that the direct effects of interventions such as preparation are seldom measured. This criticism remains valid for most of the research conducted in subsequent years. Of the six studies reviewed in the preceding sections, only one incorporates a direct measure of children's knowledge (Rie, et al., 1968). In that case, both tutorial and psychotherapy interventions resulted in increased knowledge immediately following treatment, though this increase was maintained over a nineteen-month period by the psychotherapy group only. The Rie, et al. study does not, however, clarify the relationships among the type of instruction given, children's acquisition of knowledge, and their anxiety in response to health care. The psychotherapy group, it will be recalled, emphasized emotional concerns rather than presentation of information. The relationship between children's knowledge and their anxiety scores was not examined.

To directly demonstrate the effects of information on children's responses to health care, it would be necessary to document that: 1) preparatory instruction results in increased knowledge about one's condition, and that 2) increased knowledge is associated with reduced upset. Most of the limited number of studies addressing the relationship between information and upset examine no more than one of these propositions. For example, in an assessment of a slide-tape presentation given to nonhospitalized schoolaged children, Roberts, Wurtele, Boone, Ginther, and Elkins (1981) found that subjects viewing a program about the hospital had better knowledge of medical terms and procedures than did subjects viewing an unrelated program, thereby confirming the first proposition. Although reductions in anxiety were reported among children viewing the hospital slide-tape presentation, the relationship between knowledge and anxiety was not directly examined.

Other studies provide some support for the second proposition, indicating that increased knowledge, whether from preparation or other sources, results in reduced upset (Lende, 1971; Thompson, 1983). Lende (1971) found that children's responses to tonsillectomy and adenoidectomy surgery were unrelated to the method by which they had been prepared (book, discussion, play, or attention control condition). However, results of a questionnaire designed to assess children's *knowledge* about the surgical procedure were significantly related to children's behavior, such that high levels of upset were associated with low knowledge. Thompson (1983) found that children's ability to identify and describe the function of a series of medical instruments was inversely related to their upset levels during examination by a physician in an outpatient clinic.

The only study to examine both propositions, investigating the effects of preparation on children's knowledge, as well as the relationship between their knowledge and upset, was conducted by Melamed, Dearborn, and Hermecz (1983). The authors report that subjects who had viewed a hospital-relevant film had significantly greater knowledge of hospital procedures than did children who had viewed a control film. Previous hospital experience was also associated with increased knowledge. Moreover, when the relationship between children's knowledge and upset was examined, it was found that greater knowledge was associated with less intense reactions to the hospital, less reaction to anesthesia induction by mask, and fewer days spent in the hospital.

Although direct assessments of knowledge acquired through preparation are infrequently reported, the small amount of available data suggest that instruction in health care topics *does* result in increased knowledge. In addition, increased levels of knowledge, whether acquired through preparation interventions or other sources, have been associated with reductions in children's upset.

SENSORY INFORMATION

The content of explanations given to children in the research reviewed thus far has been primarily procedural, emphasizing routines and describing the occurrence of events. Other researchers have suggested that, rather than merely providing information on the mechanical aspects, of forthcoming procedures, one should also inform patients of the sensations that they will experience. According to Johnson, Kirchhoff, and Endress (1975) the intensity of one's emotional response to a threatening event may be a function of the discrepancy between that which a person expects and what is actually experienced during the event. By providing accurate sensory information, this discrepancy, and the upset it produces, may be reduced.

To test this proposition, Johnson, et al. (1975) randomly assigned 84 children (6 to 11 years of age, scheduled for removal of an orthopedic cast) to one of three groups. The *sensory information* group listened to a tape recorded message describing the sights, sounds, smells, and tactile sensations associated with the procedure, and including a few seconds of the noise of a cast saw. The *procedure information* group heard a taped message describing the mechanics of cast removal, without sensory emphasis. A *control* group heard no recorded message. Children's pulse rate was taken at four intervals during the removal procedure. In addition, an observer recorded children's behavioral responses indicative of major or minor distress.

Observation of children's distress behavior during cast removal indicated a significantly lower level of upset among sensory group children than control group subjects. The procedure group ratings fell between those of the other two conditions, but did not differ significantly from either. The rank order of mean differences in pulse rates from the time children were in the waiting room to fifteen to thirty seconds into cast removal was the same as for distress scores, with control group children showing the greatest change. However, group differences on this measure were not significant.

The principle of providing sensory information to children has been applied in two other medical preparation studies, neither of which demonstrates the superiority of sensory explanations over more basic instruction (Abrams, 1982; Eland, 1981). Abrams (1982) incorporated a sensory explanation component in her study of the preparation of children for day surgery. Sixty children, four to eleven years of age, were assigned to one of three conditions. The day before surgery, children in two of the groups viewed the same six-minute slide presentation of hospital scenes, with each group hearing a different taped narration. One tape presented the impending events in "traditional" terms, emphasizing the procedures and activities children would encounter, with the second describing the sensations children would experience while hospitalized. Subjects in the third group were shown no preparation program.

Observations were made of children's "resistance behaviors" (i.e., overt behaviors indicating anxiety, stress, or poor coping) before and during anesthesia induction and following surgery. Only a cursory description of the observation procedures is provided. Two days postoperatively, parents were contacted by telephone to complete the Posthospital Behavior Questionnaire (Vernon, et al., 1966).

Resistance behaviors were found to occur with insufficient frequency to permit statistical analysis of the data. However, according to Abrams, the raw data suggest that subjects viewing either slide-tape presentation were less upset than control group children. The posthospital parent reports indicated that "nearly all" children had recovered from the day surgery in the intervening two-day period with little or no behavioral alteration.

Eland (1981; see Chapter 4) used a 2 × 2 factorial design in her study of the preparation of children for an injection, varying the type of aerosol that was sprayed on the injection site of subjects (a skin coolant or air), as well as the type of message given to children before the procedure. Subjects in one instruction group were merely told that they would have "something sprayed on their leg" before the injection. The others were given a more detailed explanation, including the sensory information that the spray would not hurt, but would feel cool. The latter message was not purely sensory, however, since it also included the suggestion that the spray (either coolant or air, depending on the child's group assignment) would reduce the pain of the shot. Children receiving the skin coolant reported less pain during the injection than those given the air spray. Pain levels did not differ with the type of message provided to children, nor was a significant spray by message interaction found.

Two related dental preparation studies conducted by Siegel and Peterson (1980, 1981) have contrasted the effects of providing sensory information versus the instruction of children in coping skills. In both instances, sensory explanation was found to be superior to a control condition, though it did not differ significantly from the coping skills treatment. Subjects in the 1980 study were 42 children (3 to 6 years of age, with no prior dental experience) who were scheduled for a dental restoration procedure that would include an injection. Each was assigned to one of three experimental treatments. Prior to the restoration procedure, children in the *sensory group* were given a description of the events to occur, emphasizing the physical sensations, sights and sounds likely to be experienced. *Coping skills* subjects were given instruction in general body relaxation, use of pleasant imagery, and comforting self-talk. Those in the *contact control group* were read a chapter from a children's book. Responses of subjects during dental treatment were assessed using the Behavior Profile Rating Scale (Melamed, Hawes, et al., 1975), a summary rating of children's behavior, children's self-reported anxiety, and pulse rates.

Siegel and Peterson (1980) report that both the sensory information and the coping skills subjects exhibited fewer disruptive responses and greater cooperation during treatment than did control group children. No significant differences in the *behavioral* ratings of subjects in the two experimental groups were noted, though coping skills children had lower pulse rates *before* treatment than either sensory or control group children. Following treatment, pulse rates of control group subjects were significantly higher than those of children in both experimental groups. Posttreatment pulse rates of sensory and coping group children were not significantly different.

Twenty-six of these dental patients were observed when they returned for additional treatment one week later (Siegel and Peterson, 1981). No further preparation was provided prior to this session. The authors report that the beneficial effects of the interventions were maintained over a week's time, with children in the sensory information and coping skills groups exhibiting less disruptive behavior, less anxiety, and greater cooperation than control group children during the second dental treatment session. Again, no differences were noted between the experimental groups on these indices.

To summarize these studies, it appears that providing children with sensory information is an effective method of preparing children when compared with control conditions in which children receive no relevant instruction. However, the sensory information approach has not been demonstrated to be significantly better than other preparation techniques such as the providing of procedural information (Johnson, et al., 1975; Abrams, 1982) or instruction in coping skills (Siegel & Peterson, 1980, 1981).

THE USE OF PLAY IN PREPARATION

Basic, informational forms of preparation have been further enhanced through the inclusion of play experiences. Though the rationale for including a play component in preparation interventions is not always explicitly stated, several functions of play have been suggested. For example, the use of play materials is believed to facilitate the acquisition of information. Concrete models, puppets, and medical equipment are used to familiarize children with procedures and to demonstrate their performance, thereby making abstract information more comprehensible. Furthermore, through play sessions in which children repeat the procedures demonstrated, information may be reinforced and children's understanding of the information assessed. In the affective domain, the use of play materials encourages expression of fears and concerns, and may contribute to children's sense of well-being by allowing them to manipulate and master potentially threatening items and situations.

The research design of few of the preparation studies incorporating a play component permit isolation of the unique contribution of play to a reduction of children's upset. Play activities are invariably accompanied by the presentation of information and by contact with a supportive adult. The value of this combination of interventions is typically assessed by comparing the responses of children exposed to this program with those of subjects receiving no intervention at all. Preparation research following this model includes Cassell (1965), Johnson and Stockdale (1975), Schulz, Raschke, Dedrick, and Thompson (1981), Hackett (1976), Crocker (1980), and McCaffery (1971).

Cassell (1965; also reported in Cassell & Paul, 1967) considered the preparation of children for cardiac catheterization through use of puppet play. Forty children, three to eleven years of age, were assigned to either the experimental or control condition. On the day of admission to the hospital, children in the experimental group were instructed by a therapist who used miniature models, puppets, and toy medical instruments to demonstrate the catheterization procedure. Following this demonstration, the child being prepared was allowed to become the "doctor" and play through the procedure. Questions arising during the play were answered honestly. A second, similar play session was conducted following catheterization, on the morning of discharge from the hospital. Control group children received no instruction.

Parents of children in both groups completed a modified Posthospital Behavior Questionnaire one month prior to hospitalization and again twice after discharge. In addition, ratings of children's behavior were made using the Global Mood Scale at specified times on the ward and during catheterization. Experimental group children were rated as less upset during catheterization, although ratings of control and experimental subjects did not differ at discharge. Children in the experimental condition expressed greater willingness than control group children to return to the hospital for further treatment. No differences in the posthospital behavior of the two groups were found.

Johnson and Stockdale (1975) also used puppet play to prepare children for surgical procedures. Forty-three children (5 to 8 years of age, admitted to the hospital for minor elective surgery) were assigned to the experimental or control condition. Soon after admission, experimental group subjects watched a puppet show designed to familiarize them with the procedures and equipment that would be used in their treatment. Children were allowed to interact with and manipulate the puppets during the course of the presentation. To assess patient anxiety, Palmar Sweat Prints were collected from the prepared subjects, and from control group children who received no intervention, at four separate times. The experimental condition was associated with a significant reduction in anxiety from the time of admission to the period after the puppet show. From the posttreatment period to the evening before surgery, a significant *increase* in anxiety was noted among experimental group subjects. However, from the first to the last assessment period (i.e., from admission to the postsurgical period) a significant decline in the anxiety of experimental subjects was found.

In a study similar to that of Johnson and Stockdale (1975), Schulz, et al. (1981) examined the effects of a puppet presentation on children's anxiety, also using the Palmar Sweat Index. In this instance, 28 children (2 to 7 years of age, admitted to the hospital for short-term surgical procedures) were randomly assigned to the experimental or control condition. The experimental condition included use of medical puppets and models of equipment to familiarize children with the hospital environment and procedures. Following the fifteen-minute presentation, children were permitted to play with the equipment and discuss their reactions to the show. Control group children received no intervention. Palmar Sweat Prints were collected from children upon admission to the hospital and again after the puppet presentation (or, in the case of control group subjects, after a comparable interval). As was true of the Johnson and Stockdale study, a significant reduction in the anxiety of experimental, but not control, children was recorded from the pre- to posttreatment periods. No further assessments of anxiety were made.

Not all interventions incorporating play experiences have proven successful in reducing children's upset. Hackett (1976), for example, examined the effects of structured informational play sessions on the responses of children hospitalized for cardiac surgery. Twenty-five children, one to fifteen years of age, were assigned to the experimental or control condition. Experimental group children participated in two play sessions, during which surgical procedures were explained with the use of dolls and medical props. Children were allowed to manipulate the materials in rehearsal of the events they would encounter. Expression of feelings was also encouraged. In addition to the play intervention for children, mothers of experimental group subjects were given two individual counseling sessions intended to reduce their anxiety and minimize their overprotectiveness of their children.

The effects of the interventions were assessed through questionnaires completed by parents addressing their own anxiety and attitudes, as well as the behavior of their children. The experimental treatment was associated with an increase in discipline exercised by mothers. However, no differences were found in the postoperative adjustment of experimental and control group children.

Crocker (1980) also incorporated structured and free-play components in a comprehensive hospital preparation program. The sample for this study consisted of 130 children between four and ten years of age, hospitalized for minor elective surgery. Children admitted on Sunday, Monday, or Tuesday participated in the group preparation program, which included presentation of a film and a discussion of the hospital setting, as well as the play experiences. The control group consisted of children admitted on Wednesday or Thursday, when no program was presented. Comparisons of experimental and control group subjects were made using inhospital physiological indices (temperature, pulse, respiration, blood pressure, and the incidence and frequency of postoperative vomiting) and posthospital parent report on children's recovery after discharge and their behavioral adjustment. Few significant group differences were recorded.

McCaffery (1971) prepared children for rectal temperatures by briefly demonstrating the procedure on a doll and allowing children an opportunity to handle the doll and thermometer. Experimental group children more frequently exhibited relaxed sphincter muscles during the subsequent procedure than did control children. However, this indicator was not significantly associated with behavioral measures, none of which consistently distinguished experimental and control group subjects.

Of the studies considered thus far, none has systematically varied the amount or type of play to which children are exposed. As noted above, this condition precludes attribution of the results obtained through research to the play component. Three studies, which have attempted to disentangle the contribution of play from other elements of the preparation process, provide limited and conflicting evidence of the value of play interventions. Lende (1971) found a play information condition to be no more effective than other experimental methods of instruction or than an attention control condition. Williams (1980) detected no additional benefits when play experiences were added to a basic preparation program. Schwartz, Albino, and Tedesco (1983), on the other hand, found that the opportunity to play, even when unaccompanied by medical information, may be nearly as effective in reducing children's upset as the combination of medical information and play.

Lende (1971) assigned 72 children (4 to 6 years of age, hospitalized for tonsillectomy and adenoidectomy surgery) to one of four conditions, matching subjects on age, sex, and the physician performing the surgery. Among the treatment conditions was a *puppet play group*, in which children were familiarized with the upcoming surgical procedure through play. Children in two other conditions (a *book group* and a *discussion group*) received essentially the same information as the puppet group children, with the method of presentation altered. Children in a *control group* spent a comparable amount of time with the investigator as did those in the other conditions, while receiving no preparatory information. Significant group differences were not evident in children's behavioral responses during a blood test, nor in parent reports of children's posthospital behavior. Lende notes, however, that the majority of children in each group had received appropriate preparation from parents prior to admission to the hospital—a situation possibly accounting for the lack of group differences.

Williams (1980) considered the effects of providing an opportunity for play in addition to basic preparation for surgery. The sample for this study consisted of 36 children, seven to thirteen years of age, hospitalized in the Philippines for wide range of surgical procedures. One group of subjects received preoperative instruction by being read a brief story. Children in a second group heard the identical story, following which they were allowed to play with a set of toys, containing medical and nonmedical items. Play sessions followed the interview format used by Erickson (1958), with each lasting from 20 to 45 minutes. Children in a *control* group received neither the story nor play intervention. Postoperative measures of children's responses included ratings of their behavior using the Global Mood Scale and a record of the number of analgesics received by each. Reports of children's posthospital behavior were obtained from parents on a return visit to the clinic.

One hour after surgery, children who had heard the preparation story, without subsequent play, were rated as less upset than control group children ($p < .10$). Subjects participating in the play sessions did not differ significantly from either of the other groups at that time. However, two hours postoperatively, both experimental groups were significantly less upset than the control group, but did not differ from each other. No group differences were reported in children's analgesic use in the hospital or in their behavior after discharge.

The final study examining variations in the play component of the preparation process is that of Schwartz, Albino, and Tedesco (1983). In this research, 45 three- or four-year-old children (hospitalized for dental surgery) were assigned to one of three conditions: 1) a *related play condition,* in which instruction was presented through medical play, 2) an *unrelated play condition,* consisting of play with nonmedical toys and no information relevant to the hospital, or 3) a *control condition* of no preoperative intervention. Observations were made of children's behavioral responses at each of a series of stress points. When responses at all stress points are considered together, children prepared through medical play experiences were found to be more cooperative and less upset than subjects in the other two groups. However, when each individual stress point was examined, responses of the prepared group consistently differed from those of the control group, but not from the responses of children receiving unrelated play experiences. This suggests that the activity of play itself, even when separated from specific medical content, may be somewhat beneficial to children, possibly by allowing them to express their feelings about their situation and exercise control in a limited sphere.

THE USE OF MODELING IN PREPARATION

In recent years a new technique for reducing children's upset behavior in health care settings has received considerable research attention—the use of filmed modeling. The theoretical basis of this preparation method is fundamentally different than that of techniques previously reviewed. Other forms of preparation attempt to lower children's level of anxiety by providing information and encouraging emotional expression. Filmed modeling purports to lessen children's emotional distress by allowing them to observe the behavior of a model who encounters a threatening stimulus without suffering adverse consequences (Melamed & Siegel, 1975). Research examining the efficacy of this technique in dental, as well as medical settings is reviewed in the following sections. Two additional studies are considered, which use modeling presentations to alter the medical perceptions of nonhospitalized schoolage children (Penticuff, 1976; Roberts, Wurtele, Boone, Ginther, & Elkins, 1981).

Modeling in Medical Settings

The earliest reported research use of modeling techniques in a pediatric setting was to prepare children for specific medical procedures including anesthesia induction (Vernon, 1973; also reported in Vernon & Bailey, 1974) or injections (Vernon, 1974). In the first of this research, Vernon (1973) assigned 38 children (4 to 9 years of age, hospitalized for minor elective surgery) to either an experimental or control condition. Approximately thirty to sixty minutes prior to surgery, experimental group subjects viewed a film depicting four children (ages 5 to 9 years) responding calmly to anesthesia induction. Equipment and techniques commonly used in the procedure were shown in the movie. Control group children remained in their bedrooms during the presurgical period, viewing no film.

Observations made using the Global Mood Scale indicate that experimental group children were significantly less anxious than subjects in the control group when in the surgical waiting area and upon entering the anesthesia room. However, group differences were not apparent during the induction procedure itself. Nor were there significant differences in the behavior of children following discharge from the hospital.

Vernon (1974) further used filmed modeling to prepare minor, elective surgical patients for injections, varying the content of the modeling films presented to children. Thirty subjects (4 to 9 years of age) were randomly assigned to see: 1) a *no pain movie,* depicting a series of children receiving injections without apparent discomfort or fear, 2) a *pain movie,* which was similar to the first, except that the models exhibited some negative reaction to the injection, or 3) *no movie* at all. Observations of children during preoperative injections (again, using Global Mood Scale) revealed greatest upset among the "no-pain" movie group, with least upset manifested by subjects in the "pain" movie group. Control group children displayed intermediate levels of anxiety. Vernon suggests that modeling which presents inaccurate or distorted information, as did the no-pain movie, may actually contribute to children's discomfort, rather than ameliorating it.

Use of filmed modeling techniques has been expanded to include the preparation of children for general experiences associated with hospitalization and surgery, as well as individual procedures (Melamed & Siegel, 1975; Melamed, Meyer, Gee, & Soule, 1976; Ferguson, 1979; Peterson, 1978; Melamed, Dearborn, & Hermecz, 1983). Melamed and Siegel (1975; also reported in Siegel, 1975) assigned sixty elective surgical patients (4 to 12 years of age) to either an experimental or control condition, matching subjects on age, sex, race, and type of operation. Upon admission to the hospital, children in the experimental group were shown a film depicting a seven-year-old male who, though initially apprehensive, successfully encounters a variety of normal hospital experiences.

To control for the possible beneficial effects of merely viewing a film, regardless of the content (a factor not considered by Vernon), Melamed and Siegel showed control group subjects a nature film of comparable length and interest value. After viewing their respective films, children in both groups were given standard preoperative instruction. Responses were assessed during the period of hospitalization, and on a postoperative return visit to a clinic, using the Palmar Sweat Index (PSI), behavioral observation, parent-report, and self-report measures.

Results of the PSI demonstrate that an *increase* in physiological arousal occurred among children in the modeling group immediately after the film was shown. However, when measured again the evening before surgery, the PSI levels of experimental group subjects were significantly reduced, with this lower level of anxiety also evident during the posthospital assessment. Control group children, on the other hand, exhibited lower anxiety immediately after viewing their film. However, their anxiety was elevated in the preoperative period and during the posthospital clinic visit. A significant increase in the behavior problems of control group children was recorded following hospitalization. Self-report ratings and behavioral observations document a decline in the upset of children in the experimental group during the preoperative and posthospital periods.

Melamed, Meyer, Gee, and Soule (1976) also used filmed modeling to prepare children for hospitalization, varying the timing of presentation of the film and the type of additional inhospital preparation children were provided. The sample consisted of 48 children, four to twelve years of age, who were to be hospitalized for minor, elective surgery. Subjects were shown the same modeling film as that used by Melamed and Siegel (1975), either six to nine days prior to admission, or upon arrival at the hospital. In addition, half of the children in each group received minimal inhospital preparation, while the remainder received "standard" preparation, which included use of picture books and surgical masks. Assessment of anxiety was made through a selection of instruments comparable to that used by Melamed and Siegel (1975).

No significant main effect for *type* of preparation (minimal or standard) was found. However, considering the factor of *timing*, responses to the Children's Manifest Anxiety Scale indicate that subjects who had not seen the film prior to admission were significantly more anxious upon arrival at the hospital than those who had already viewed it. Age of children was also found to influence the optimal time for presentation of a modeling film. When analysis was confined to the older children in the sample, it was found that those who had seen the film prior to hospitalization exhibited a greater reduction in posthospital behavior problems than subjects viewing the film upon admission. Among children who were shown the modeling film upon arrival at the hospital, younger subjects displayed less physiological arousal than did older children. The authors suggest that although older children may benefit from viewing of a modeling film prior to admission, younger subjects may need more immediate preparation for hospitalization.

Information provided by Melamed, Dearborn, and Hermecz (1983) also demonstrates the importance of considering children's age, as well as their prior medical experience, when using filmed modeling or other forms of preparation for health care events. In this research project, 58 elective surgical patients, who ranged in age from four to seventeen years, were assigned to the experimental or control condition, with subjects matched on age, sex, race, type of surgery, and previous surgical experience. After arrival at the hospital, and completion of a blood test and physical examination, experimental group subjects were shown a slide-tape presentation depicting the hospital experiences of a thirteen-year-old male. Control group children were shown an unrelated filmed presentation.

Children who had viewed the hospital-relevant film were found to use significantly less pain medication, to be more cooperative in the operating room, and to have fewer postsurgical problems than control group subjects. However, the data also indicate that presentation of the hospital film may have had a sensitizing effect on subjects younger than eight years of age and those with prior surgical experience. Younger subjects assigned to the experimental condition were rated as more anxious before and after viewing the hospital film than were young children in the control condition. Furthermore, young children with prior surgical experience who saw the experimental film were significantly more anxious than children of the same age and experience who viewed the unrelated presentation. Viewing of the experimental film was also found to negatively affect the medical fears of young or experienced patients, while reducing the medical fears of children who had no previous surgical experience. Melamed, et al. suggest that alternate forms of preparation may be necessary to achieve maximum benefits for young and experienced patients.

Ferguson (1979) examined the effectiveness of two interventions—a filmed modeling presentation upon arrival at the hospital and a pre-hospital home visit. Subjects for this study (82 children, 3 to 7 years of age, scheduled for tonsillectomy and adenoidectomy surgery) viewed either a hospital-related peer modeling film or a film unrelated to the hospital upon admission. Half of the subjects in each film group followed regular inhospital admission procedures; the others were visited prior to admission by a nurse who helped mothers complete the necessary admission documents and provided mothers and children with information about the hospital. Self-report, observational and physiological measures were used to assess children's anxiety.

Though not as dramatic as the Melamed and Siegel (1975) data, Ferguson's results support the positive effects of viewing a modeling film. Subjects in the modeling condition had lower preoperative electromyogram scores than control group children. Moreover, significant reductions are reported in the Posthospital Behavior Questionnaire scores of modeling group subjects. Group differences in behavioral observations or in children's self-reported fears were not apparent.

The home visitation intervention was associated with a reduction in the posthospital behavioral disturbance of children six and seven years of age. Mothers in the home visitation group expressed greater satisfaction with the care and information they were given than did mothers who received no home visit. However, both types of experimental interventions (filmed modeling and the preadmission visit) resulted in reductions of mothers' self-reported anxiety.

The preceding studies are significant in two respects. First, they indicate that filmed modeling is effective when contrasted with conditions of no systematic intervention (Vernon, 1973, 1974). Furthermore, it appears that filmed modeling provides additional benefits beyond that which might be expected from the providing of basic information alone (Melamed & Siegel, 1975). However, none of the studies considered thus far has directly compared filmed modeling techniques with other means of preparing children for hospitalization. Peterson (1978; also reported in Peterson, Hartmann, & Gelfand, 1979, and Peterson & Shigetomi, 1981) conducted such a study, comparing the effects of filmed modeling with instruction in coping skills and a condition of minimal preparation.

Subjects for this study included 66 children between two and eleven years of age, scheduled for tonsillectomy surgery. Children were assigned to one of four groups: 1) *coping*, 2) *filmed modeling*, 3) *coping plus filmed modeling*, or 4) *information only*. All participating children were invited to a preadmission program approximately four days prior to surgery, during which they were provided with basic information about the hospital and were given a tour. Depending on the designated treatment condition, additional interventions were provided at this time. Coping groups received instruction in muscle relaxation, distracting mental imagery, and comforting self-talk. Modeling groups were shown the same film as had been earlier used by Melamed and Siegel (1975), while information group children received no additional treatment. Assessments were made using observational, physiological, and self-report instruments.

Though group differences were typically small and often only marginally significant ($p < .10$), the results suggest that coping skills alone or in combination with modeling were more effective in reducing children's anxiety than modeling alone. Anxiety measures of children receiving *information only* seldom differed from those of subjects in the coping groups, and for certain measures were actually lower than those of children in the modeling only condition.

The latter finding is surprising in view of the results obtained by Melamed and Siegel (1975). Peterson notes, however, that these differences may be attributable to variations in procedures used in the two studies. For example, Melamed and Siegel presented the modeling film upon admission, rather than in the preadmission period, to individual children, rather than to groups, and used an older sample of children than did Peterson. Moreover, the film used in both studies depicted the setting in which children in the Melamed and Siegel study were hospitalized, a setting different than that used by Peterson and colleagues. This fact, Peterson suggests, might have resulted in the conveying of contradictory information by the film and the oral presentation, consequently upsetting children and their parents.

Modeling in Nonhospital Settings

Two studies have examined the effectiveness of modeling procedures in altering the health care attitudes and concerns of nonhospitalized children (Penticuff, 1976; Roberts, et al., 1981). Penticuff (1976) had 57 third-graders view a peer modeling film of a child undergoing hospitalization and surgery. Taped introductions to the film were varied, depending on the child's treatment condition. Subjects in the *sensitization group* heard a message encouraging identification with the model, also drawing their attention to the threatening situations that would be depicted in the film. The introductory message heard by children in the *denial group* emphasized dissimilarities between the subjects and the model, discounting the threatening aspects of the film. A *control group* heard no special introduction to the film. The attitudes of subjects were assessed through a semantic differential task. In addition, the Palmar Sweat Index and self-report measures were gathered to assess children's anxiety.

Penticuff found that children's attitudes toward medical personnel and events improved after viewing the film ($p < .10$), with the extent of attitudinal change directly related to children's degree of physiological arousal, as measured by the PSI. Their levels of self-reported medical fears were also found to decline after viewing the film. However, changes in subjects' attitudes and fears were unrelated to the type of introductory message heard.

Roberts, et al. (1981) also examined the effectiveness of a modeling presentation in altering the medical fears of schoolaged children, in this instance using a sample of 36 children, seven to twelve years of age. The experimental presentation consisted of a *slide-*

tape program depicting two children entering the hospital for tonsillectomies. The children shown in the slides (who also provided the taped narration for the presentation) were said to exemplify a *coping* modeling style, with their words, as well as their behaviors, suggesting an initial anxiety that is overcome. Half of the school children viewed this show, while the remainder saw a slide-tape presentation unrelated to hospitals. Three self-report measures were used to assess children's anxiety one week before, immediately after, and two weeks after viewing the program. In addition, all children answered a set of multiple choice questions after the slide-tape presentation, assessing their knowledge of medical terms and procedures.

Results demonstrate the effectiveness of the hospital slide-tape package in reducing children's medical anxiety. Although no group differences in children's trait anxiety (as measured by the Children's Manifest Anxiety Scale) were detected during any assessment period, children's responses to two self-report measures of medical fears were as expected. In the period immediately following the presentation, and again two weeks later, children viewing the hospital show reported significantly lower levels of anxiety, as compared to both their own initial ratings and to ratings of the control group at each corresponding period. As reported earlier, children given the hospital presentation had a significantly better knowledge of medical items than did those viewing the unrelated slide-tape package.

Modeling in Dental Settings

The use of modeling techniques has been repeatedly examined in dental settings. More than sixty percent of the identified experimental dental preparation studies have included a modeling condition. In contrast, only five of the 31 experimental studies concerning preparation for hospitalization have incorporated this technique. The dental modeling studies to be considered are of three basic types. First to be examined is research comparing modeling techniques with conditions of nonintervention (Melamed, Hawes, Heiby, & Glick, 1975; Melamed, Weinstein, Hawes, & Katin-Borland, 1975). Next, studies investigating the relative effectiveness of modeling and other interventions, such as systematic desensitization, are reviewed (White, Akers, Green, & Yates, 1974; Johnson & Machen, 1973; Machen & Johnson, 1974; Sawtell, Simon, & Simeonsson, 1974). The final group of studies in this section examines variations in the effectiveness of modeling techniques as a product of individual differences in patients' prior dental experience and modifications in the format of the film (Melamed, Yurcheson, Fleece, Hutcherson, & Hawes, 1978; Klorman, Hilpert, Michael, LaGana, & Sveen, 1980).

Filmed Modeling Versus Nonintervention. The efficacy of preparation versus nonpreparation has been considered in two studies conducted by Melamed and colleagues, both of which confirm the benefits of modeling presentations. Melamed, Weinstein, Hawes, and Katin-Borland (1975) assigned fourteen children (5 to 9 years of age) to either an experimental or control condition, matching subjects on race, sex, age, and initial self-reported fear levels. Subjects visited the dental clinic for three separate sessions, the first of which consisted of contact with the hygienist and the second, a screening examination by the dentist.

Upon arrival at the clinic for the third visit, which included an injection of a local anesthetic and at least one dental restoration, children in the experimental group were shown a modeling film. Control group children were taken to the same area where the modeling film was shown, but were asked instead to draw pictures during the corresponding interval. Observation of children during the restoration procedure revealed significantly less disruptive behavior among the experimental than control group children, though groups did not differ in their self-reported levels of fear.

In a similar study, Melamed, Hawes, Heiby, and Glick (1975) showed sixteen children (5 to 11 years of age) either a modeling film or a movie unrelated to the dental setting prior to an appointment for dental restorations. In addition to self-report and observational measures, The Palmar Sweat Index was used to assess children's anxiety. Results indicate that children who viewed the modeling film displayed significantly lower levels of disruptive behavior during dental treatment than did control group children. Self-report and PSI measures did not significantly differentiate children during the restoration procedure.

Modeling Versus Other Techniques. Among the studies comparing the effectiveness of modeling procedures with other types of interventions is that of White, Akers, Green, and Yates (1974). This research represents the only use of a live, instead of filmed, model identified in the pediatric medical or dental preparation literature. The sample consisted of fifteen children, between four and eight years of age, who on at least two previous occasions had exhibited disruptive behavior in the dental clinic. Prior to their dental treatment, subjects in the modeling group, accompanied by an experimenter, watched from behind a one-way mirror as an eight-year-old child (a confederate of the investigators) received dental treatment. Six separate modeling sessions were conducted per child, with a different dental technique presented at each session.

Children in *Control Condition I* also watched a series of demonstrations through a one-way mirror. During these sessions a dental staff member named and manipulated the same instruments that were introduced in the modeling condition, but without the presence of a model. Subjects in *Control Condition II* received no intervention. Ratings of children's behavior were made during the dental treatment that immediately followed the intervention period and again at a follow-up visit six months later. Children in the modeling condition were rated as more cooperative and less disruptive than children receiving no intervention (Control Condition II). However, ratings of children exposed to filmed modeling did not differ significantly from those of children who viewed the demonstration of instruments.

Three studies have contrasted modeling procedures with a program of systematic desensitization to dental instruments and procedures (Johnson & Machen, 1973; Machen & Johnson, 1974; Sawtell, et al., 1974). The desensitization procedure consists of gradually exposing subjects to feared stimuli, ranked in order of anxiety production from least to most threatening, while the subject is in a comfortable environment. Johnson and Machen (1973) randomly assigned 58 children, three to five years of age and having no prior dental experience, to a *modeling*, *desensitization*, or *control* condition. Prior to a dental examination, children in the modeling and desensitization treatment groups received their respective interventions, with control group children receiving no advance preparation.

Children's behavior during the examination was rated using the four-point scale developed by Frankl, et al. (1962). Mothers' anxiety in the clinic was also assessed and was found to be significantly higher in the two experimental groups than in the control condition. Since mother's anxiety was believed to influence that of their children, maternal anxiety scores were used as a covariate in an analysis of covariance of children's behavioral ratings. Comparisons of children's adjusted mean behavioral scores indicate that the model learning condition resulted in significantly less upset than did the control condition. The desensitization group upset scores did not differ significantly from those of either the modeling or control groups.

Thirty-one of the subjects in the Johnson and Machen (1973) sample were found to have at least two carious lesions in need of restoration. The reactions of these children were therefore observed during their second and third visits to the dental clinic for treatment, with the results of these observation reported by Machen and Johnson (1974). Children who had participated in either the desensitization or modeling conditions displayed significantly less negative behavior during treatment procedures than did control group children. The behavioral ratings of children in the two experimental groups did not significantly differ from each other.

In their study of children's reactions to an initial dental examination, Sawtell, et al. (1974) contrasted desensitization and filmed modeling conditions with a third intervention, a "behavior modification" treatment. The behavior modification condition consisted of social reinforcement of children's positive behaviors (defined as those necessary for the completion of dental procedures) and the ignoring of noncooperative behaviors. A so-called placebo condition (contact with a dental assistant prior to treatment) and a control condition (no intervention) were also included. Each treatment was conducted immediately prior to the examination. Assessments of children's responses were made by recording the frequency of occurrence of specific noncooperative behaviors. Also recorded were ratings of children's overall behavior using the Frankl, et al. (1962) scale and the amount of time required to perform the dental procedures (an indirect measure of cooperation). No significant group differences in behavior or timing of events were found, though for each of the measures collected the *placebo* group demonstrated the most favorable results, with *control* group children recording the most disturbance.

Variations Due to Subjects' Previous Experience and the Modeling Film Format. With the exception of the research conducted by White, et al. (1974), subjects in each of the preceding dental modeling studies had no prior dental experience. The final two modeling studies considered in this section have included experienced, as well as inexperienced, dental patients in their samples to determine whether the frequently documented benefits of modeling are generalizable to children who have received previous dental care. In addition, these studies have examined the effects of modifications in the length and format of the modeling films presented to subjects. Melamed, Yurcheson, Fleece, Hutcherson, and Hawes (1978) varied the length of the film, while Klorman, Hilpert, Michael, LaGana, and Sveen (1980) compared "coping model" with "mastery model" film formats.

Melamed, et. al (1978) assigned eighty children (4 to 11 years of age, with differing levels of dental experience) to view one of five video tapes prior to dental treatment. A *long model* tape (ten minutes in length) depicted a seven-year-old male undergoing all major steps in the restoration procedure, while a *short model* tape (four minutes in length) focused only on the anesthetic injection and oral examination. These same procedures were explained, without the presence of a model in corresponding *long demonstration* and a *short demonstration* tapes. A control tape, unrelated to dentistry, was also used.

Self-reported fears of the restoration process were significantly lower among children viewing a modeling rather than a demonstration film. Differences in behavioral indices of anxiety also favored modeling group subjects, though the results were of marginal significance ($p < .10$). Examination of subgroups based on age and prior dental experience revealed other differences. Children four to six years of age reported less fear after viewing the long version of either the demonstration or modeling tape. Subjects with no prior dental experience were less disruptive after viewing a short model or a long demonstration tape, whereas those with previous experience benefited most from the long model tape.

Klorman, et al. (1980) compared the effectiveness of two types of modeling films, coping and mastery formats, in three separate experiments. In *Experiment 1* sixty dental patients who had previously experienced dental treatment were assigned to view either a *mastery modeling* film (i.e., no apparent anxiety exhibited by the model), a *coping modeling* film (initial anxiety evident in the behavior of the model, who then overcomes this anxiety and "copes" with events), or an unrelated *control* film. After viewing the filmed presentation, dental restoration procedures were performed on each subject. Behavioral observations were recorded during the procedure.

To assess children's perceptions of the type of film they had seen, subjects in the modeling conditions were also asked to describe the feelings of the depicted model at the beginning and end of the film. Children's responses indicated that the content of modeling films (coping or mastery) had been successfully manipulated. Nevertheless, observational measures of anxiety did not differentiate the modeling conditions from each other or from the control condition.

Experiment 2 was conducted to determine whether further enhancement of the modeling films might produce effects that were lacking in the first experiment. To accomplish this, a simulated posttreatment interview was inserted at the end of each modeling film. The mastery model confirmed that he felt no fear during the procedure, while the coping model admitted initial reluctance and discussed a technique used to lessen his anxiety during procedures. Follow-up interviews with subjects concerning the model's reactions again indicated that coping and mastery films were perceived differently. However, group differences in behavioral ratings again failed to emerge.

For *Experiment 3,* Klorman, et al. replicated the second experiment, with the exception of the sample composition, which in this case was limited to children who had experienced no prior dental extractions or restorations. Observational data indicate that coping and mastery modeling groups each displayed similar levels of disruptive behavior, with both groups significantly lower in disruptiveness than control group subjects. Moreover, when the behavior of subjects from the second and third experiments were compared, it was determined that inexperienced dental patients were significantly more disruptive. Thus, the Klorman, et al. data suggest that the effects of modeling techniques may be more readily demonstrable among that group of patients more vulnerable to upset—children experiencing dental treatment for the first time.

Summary of Modeling Research

As was true of the studies on filmed modeling in medical settings, dental research documents the value of modeling techniques when compared with conditions of nonintervention (Melamed, Hawes, et al., 1975; Melamed, Weinstein, et al., 1975; White, et al., 1974; Johnson & Machen, 1973; Machen & Johnson, 1974). However, with one possible exception (Melamed, Yurcheson, et al., 1978) modeling in dental settings has not demonstrated clear superiority over other techniques such as desensitization (Machen & Johnson, 1974) or even noninformational attention from dental personnel (Sawtell, et al., 1974).

Moreover, Klorman, et al. (1980) found that modeling procedures, though effective with inexperienced patients (the subjects of most dental studies), were ineffective with subjects who had received previous dental care. This finding is consistent with the medical modeling literature. Three of the five studies concerning preparation for hospitalization and surgery through modeling techniques used samples of children who had not been previously hospitalized (Melamed & Siegel, 1975; Melamed, Meyer, Gee, & Soule, 1976; Ferguson, 1979). Each of these studies, to differing extents, has documented the benefits of modeling techniques.

On the other hand, Peterson (1978) included children with hospital experience in her sample, if their hospitalization had not occurred in the previous year and if they had never undergone surgery. Modeling techniques were found to be beneficial when used in combination with instruction in coping skills, but not when applied alone. Melamed, Dearborn, and Hermecz (1983) found a hospital slide-tape presentation to have detrimental effects on the manifested anxiety and self-reported medical fears of patients who had undergone previous surgery. This pattern of results indicates that alternatives to filmed modeling should be explored for use with children having prior experience in the health care setting.

Additional research is necessary to determine the ways in which individual differences, other than children's previous experience, might alter the value of modeling interventions. For example, research conducted by Melamed and colleagues suggests that the age of children may be used to determine the timing a filmed presentation (Melamed, Meyer, et al., 1976), the length of the presentation (Melamed, Yurcheson, et al., 1978), or indeed whether such a presentation should be made at all (Melamed, Dearborn, & Hermecz, 1983).

The impact of the type of modeling format presented to children, coping or mastery, is also unclear. Though a coping format has been used more frequently in the research reviewed, data pertaining to the two formats in dental settings has failed to demonstrate the clear advantage of either. Both mastery models (Johnson & Machen, 1973; Machen & Johnson, 1974) and coping models (Melamed, Hawes, et al., 1975; Melamed, Weinstein, et al., 1975) have produced favorable results in dental settings. However, the only direct comparison of these formats in the pediatric dental literature found both to be equally effective (Klorman, et al., 1980).

Evidence from the medical modeling literature appears to favor the use of a coping format for filmed presentations. Melamed and Siegel (1975) and Ferguson (1979) each observed positive effects when children were prepared for hospitalization through use of a coping model film. Peterson (1978), who also used a coping format, found the modeling procedure to be effective only when used in in conjunction with instruction in coping skills. Vernon (1973), on the other hand, found use of a mastery modeling film to reduce children's anxiety during events immediately prior to the induction of anesthesia, though the difference between prepared and nonprepared children diminished during the actual induction phase. In his study of the preparation of children for injections through filmed modeling, Vernon (1974) found a coping format to reduce children's upset, while the mastery modeling film (children receiving injections with no apparent discomfort) was associated with significantly higher levels of upset.

INSTRUCTION IN COPING SKILLS

A limited number of studies in medical and dental settings have investigated the potential benefits of instructing children in the use of coping skills prior to health care procedures. Although many of the stressful elements of health care encounters cannot be eliminated, their capacity for producing distress may be reduced if patients exercise specific cognitive techniques to control their emotional responses. In each of the studies considered in this section, subjects were instructed in the use of several types of coping skills, that could be used as desired by the children when facing stressful circumstances. Among the skills typically taught are *relaxation techniques* (e.g., deep and regular breathing), the use of *distracting imagery* (concentration on an imagined pleasant setting or event), and *comforting self-talk* (reassuring oneself that all is well and that the aversive condition will be over soon).

Use of these techniques in medical settings has been considered by Peterson and colleagues (Peterson, 1978; Peterson, Hartmann, & Gelfand, 1979; Peterson & Shigetomi, 1981, 1982), and by Meng and Zastowny (1982). In the previously discussed research of Peterson (1978), comparisons were made of children receiving: 1) instruction in coping skills, 2) a filmed modeling intervention, 3) coping plus filmed modeling, or 4) merely basic information about the hospital, which was given to all subjects during a preadmission hospital visit. Group differences in behavioral, physiological and self-report measures of anxiety were small, though consistently in favor of children receiving coping skills training (with or without a modeling intervention). The largest group differences reported were between the coping only and modeling only conditions, with children instructed in coping skills exhibiting lower anxiety levels.

Forty of the mothers participating in the original research project were contacted one year after the hospitalization to investigate children's reactions upon return home and to determine whether mothers had helped their children apply the coping skills during subsequent threatening situations (Peterson & Shigetomi, 1982). Comparisons of treatment group reactions were not made in this follow-up study.

A majority of the mothers reported that their children continued to speak of the hospitalization one year after discharge, with more references being made to positive rather than negative experiences. Children of thirteen of the mothers contacted, had been trained in coping skills during their hospitalization. Mothers of this group (who had received the training in conjunction with their children) reported a preference for use of distracting imagery over the other techniques of relaxation or comforting self-talk. However, only four of the parents receiving coping instruction had applied the technique in other stressful settings, and none had attempted use of the coping skills with a child other than the one receiving the initial training.

Meng and Zastowny (1982) describe a preadmission "stress inoculation" program designed to provide children and parents with information concerning the nature of stress, as well as instruction and rehearsal in the application of specific coping techniques. Information on stress and coping skills was presented to subjects in a filmed format. After introduction of the basic skills, the film depicted a mother and child applying the technique during simulated hospital stress points. To reinforce the information presented in the film, parents and children were given a booklet for use at home, which reviewed the coping techniques.

Parents were asked to maintain a diary of their children's behavior before and after hospitalization. In addition, inhospital observations were made of children's reactions at stress points. Though presentation of methodology used for this assessment is incomplete, the investigators report that subjects trained in coping skills displayed a smaller increase in anxiety on the day of admission than did children in other, unspecified treatment conditions and were also more cooperative at stress points than subjects in a control group.

The use of coping skills in dental settings has been investigated by Nocella & Kaplan (1982) and by Siegel and Peterson (1980, 1981). Nocella and Kaplan randomly assigned thirty children (5 to 13 years of age, each with prior dental experience) to one of three conditions. Children in a *cognitive-behavioral* group received instruction in relaxation techniques and positive self-talk. Those in an *attention-control* group spent fifteen minutes conversing with the experimenter about topics unrelated to stress management or dental procedures, while subjects in a *no-treatment* control group remained in the waiting area, having no contact with the experimenter. Behavioral observation of children during restoration or extraction procedures indicated that the coping skills group was significantly less upset than either of the two control groups, which did not differ significantly from each other.

Siegel and Peterson (1980) compared the responses of inexperienced dental patients receiving *coping skills* training (relaxation, pleasant imagery, and calming self-talk), *sensory explanations* of events, or mere contact with an experimenter. As reported earlier, both coping skills and sensory information treatments were found to be more effective than the control condition in reducing behavioral and physiological indices of upset. No significant differences in the effectiveness of the two treatment conditions were found. The beneficial effects of both the coping and sensory conditions were still apparent during a second dental treatment session occurring one week later (Siegel & Peterson, 1981).

Though few studies have examined the use of coping skills in the preparation of children for health care procedures, the results reported to date appear promising. Instruction in coping skills was found to be as effective as the providing of sensory information to pediatric dental patients (Siegel & Peterson, 1980, 1981). The evidence further indicates that coping techniques may provide a useful complement to, or perhaps alternative to, modeling techniques, at least for certain populations. For example, the data of Nocella and Kaplan (1982) demonstrate the effectiveness of coping skills among experienced dental patients, a group of children Klorman, et al. (1980) found to be unaffected by modeling interventions. Moreover, Peterson (1978) found the use of coping techniques, either alone or in combination with a modeling intervention, to be more effective in reducing children's anxiety than modeling alone.

PARENT PREPARATION

Unlike the preparation studies reviewed in the preceding sections of this chapter, interventions considered in the present section are primarily directed toward parents rather than children. The goal of this form of preparation is to provide information and support to parents, typically mothers, to reduce their feelings of anxiety and discomfort. Since parental anxiety has been repeatedly associated with the emotional distress of children in health care settings, interventions capable of reducing parents' upset may also be beneficial to children.

The hypothesized benefits of information on parent and child anxiety has received support from several studies, considered more fully in Chapter 6. For example, Mahaffy (1965) found that children's inhospital and posthospital responses were more favorable when mothers were given information and allowed to ask questions of a staff member at admission and other times throughout hospitalization. Skipper and colleagues similarly found that the anxiety of mothers (Skipper, Leonard, & Rhymes, 1968) and children (Skipper & Leonard, 1968) could be reduced by providing mothers with information and emotional support, even when this intervention occurred only at admission.

In addition to reducing parent and child anxiety levels, preparation efforts have also been successful in altering parental behaviors, thereby enabling children to receive greater support. Roskies, Mongeon, and Gagnon-Lefebvre (1978) found that by providing information to mothers on the importance of visiting their hospitalized children, the timing and duration of parent visits, as well as their behavior during those visits, were successfully modified.

Although research in the dental literature demonstrates a concern for the relationship between parent and child anxiety, preparation for dental visits and procedures has seldom been directed toward parents. An exception appears in a study conducted by Wright, Alpern, and Leake (1973), in which 124 children, between three and six years of age, were randomly assigned to either a control or experimental condition. Children in both groups received identical treatment in the dental clinic. However, mothers in the experimental group had been sent a preappointment letter describing the procedures to be performed and offering advice on how children might be prepared for the visit. A significant relationship between mother's self-reported anxiety and children's upset behavior during the dental examination was found for the control group. No such relationship was noted among subjects receiving the preappointment letter. Comparisons of experimental and control subjects on mean levels of mother anxiety or child behavioral ratings are not reported.

The capacity of these interventions to modify parent behavior and reduce or alter the relationship between parent and child anxiety is impressive. However, in each of the cases cited, the parent preparation group was compared with a control group denied any intervention, rather than a group provided with a different type of treatment. Therefore, these studies do not speak to the relative merits of parent preparation versus other forms of intervention, or to the unique contribution parent preparation may make when used in combination with child-oriented interventions. Three studies have attempted to assess the value of a parent component in preparation activities, either contrasting parent-oriented and child-oriented interventions (Landes, 1973; Kuhn, 1980) or investigating whether additional benefits are detectable when a parent component is added to child-oriented preparation (Coleman, 1975). The results of these studies less clearly demonstrate the beneficial effects of parent involvement in the preparation process than those previously considered.

Landes (1973; see Chapter 6) assigned parents and children to one of four conditions: 1) a *parents' group,* in which parents were provided with information and emotional support through a preadmission meeting, 2) a *puppet play* condition, which consisted of a preadmission presentation for children and parents, 3) a *parents' group, plus puppet play* condition, or 4) a *control* condition, consisting of neither experimental intervention. Children's blood pressure during hospitalization (selected for use in data analysis from several outcome measures gathered) was found to be consistently lower among subjects in the *parents' group* condition than among children in other treatment groups. But contrary to the findings of Skipper, Leonard, and Rhymes (1968), parents assigned to this condition were *more* anxious upon admission than were others.

However, attribution of these differences to the individual treatment conditions is suspect, since the results reported by Landes are based on the responses of all subjects *invited* to the preadmission sessions, whether or not they actually attended.

Kuhn (1980) similarly compared *child-oriented* and *parent-oriented* preparation activities with *joint preparation* of parents and children, and with a *control condition*, consisting of neither intervention. A total of sixty children between three and ten years of age, hospitalized for nonemergency surgery, were assigned to the four conditions. Child-oriented preparation consisted of a standardized session in which a videotape on hospitalization was presented, followed by a discussion of the presentation. Children in the parent-oriented condition received no direct preparation. Kuhn reports no significant postsurgical group differences in self-report ratings, behavioral observations, or physiological indices.

The value of providing a parent education component in addition to a child-oriented play therapy preparation session was examined by Coleman (1975). Participants in this study were eighty schoolaged children, eight to eleven years of age. Children in *Experimental Group 1* participated in a play therapy session and orientation upon arrival at the hospital. In addition to these interventions, parents in *Experimental Group 2* participated in a parent education program one week prior to their child's admission. The experimental groups were contrasted with two control conditions, one composed of a children scheduled for hospitalization, yet receiving no preparation, and the other consisting of nonhospitalized school children. All subjects were assessed using the Children's Manifest Anxiety Scale one week prior to hospitalization, the evening of admission, and again one week after discharge (or, in the case of the nonhospitalized children, at comparable intervals). No significant group differences were detected.

A number of other studies have actively involved parents in the preparation process, without attempting to precisely assess the contribution of that involvement to the success of the intervention. For example, the series of stress-point preparation studies conducted by Wolfer and Visintainer (1975, 1979; Visintainer & Wolfer, 1975) have included parents in all phases of the preparation process so that they may obtain information and emotional support along with their children. In each study, the emotional distress of children, as well as their parents, was reduced through the intervention. Similarly, Ferguson (1979) found that a preadmission home visit by a nurse, through which information was provided to children and parents alike, reduced the negative posthospital behavior of six- and seven-year-old subjects and also lowered the anxiety levels of mothers during and after the hospitalization.

Two studies of the preparation of children for cardiac surgery also involved parents in the instructional process. Among the elements included in a comprehensive preparation program described by Gabriel and Danilowicz (1978) was a series of explanations given to parents concerning the treatment of their children. Though the investigators report only one long-term negative reaction among the sixty children (2 to 19 years of age) prepared through this program, the absence of a control condition in the research design prevents clear attribution of these results to the preparation process. In another study discussed above, Hackett (1976) found that a combination of play instruction for children facing cardiac surgery and counseling sessions for their mothers altered parents' attitudes toward discipline, but did not affect children's postoperative adjustment or parents' anxiety.

Involvement of parents in the preparation of their children, in itself, may not be sufficient for benefits to be realized by the child. Gutstein (1980) hypothesized that specific parental behaviors may serve to either encourage or discourage children's participation in preparation activities. To examine this hypothesis, Gutstein videotaped a series of children (N = 34) between the ages of four and nine years while they played with hospital and surgical equipment alone, with an experimenter, and with their parents. Sessions were conducted within three days of children's hospitalization for tonsillectomy surgery.

Videotapes were subsequently reviewed to assess children's *active involvement* in the preparatory activities (i.e., information seeking and behavioral rehearsal) and two categories of parental behaviors: *structuring* (defined as the pointing out of salient aspects of the environment and the focusing of children's attention on specific activities) and *congruence* (in which the focus of parents' behavior is derived from children's immediately preceding behavior).

Gutstein believed that child involvement would be facilitated by parents who apply these behaviors in response to children's behavioral changes, for example structuring the situation when children's interest wanes, and using congruent behaviors with those who are already involved. Ratings of the types and contingency of parent behaviors were correlated with measures of the active involvement demonstrated by children. The results indicate that parent use of congruence and contingent structuring were associated with increased involvement of children in the preparation activities, while noncontingent structuring and incongruence were associated with reductions of child involvement.

THE CONTRIBUTION OF EMOTIONAL SUPPORT

In addition to providing children and parents with the information, skills, or experiences that form the core of an intervention, the preparation process also frequently exposes subjects to periods of extended contact with supportive representatives of the health care setting. Interaction with hospital personnel, may enhance the development of a relationship, foster trust, and facilitate the expression of emotions and concerns. This contact in itself, regardless of the information provided, may contribute to the reduction of anxiety in children and their parents.

Two studies in medical settings have been specifically designed to investigate the role of emotional support in the preparation process (Minde & Maler, 1968; Fassler, 1980). A less direct source of data on the potential value of structured contact with hospital personnel is provided by those studies including an attention control condition (i.e., contact with an experimenter, but no relevant information) in their experimental design. Research of this sort has been conducted in hospitals (Lende, 1971; Schwartz, Albino, & Tedesco, 1983) and in dental clinics (Sawtell, et al., 1974; Siegel & Peterson, 1980, 1981; Nocella & Kaplan, 1982). Much of this data suggests that emotional support is at least somewhat effective in reducing children's upset in health care settings.

As reported above, Minde and Maler (1968) found that the self-reported anxiety and the length of stay of children hospitalized for medical conditions could be reduced by providing them with explanations of their condition. Recognizing that this effect might be the product of nonthreatening contact with a member of the hospital staff, rather than of the information provided, the researchers conducted a second investigation. In this case, 41 children (5 to 11 years of age) received either an explanation of their condition, as was done in the first phase, or a similar amount of contact with an experimenter who talked or played with children, while providing no medical information. Following treatment, both groups reported significantly less anxiety than in a pretreatment assessment. Moreover, the average length of hospitalization of the two groups did not differ significantly, with both being comparable to that of the experimental group in the first investigation.

Fassler (1980) randomly assigned 45 children (6 to 12 years of age) to one of three groups. The *experimental condition* consisted of emotional support and information about hospitalization. Subjects in this group were read a story about the hospital, were asked a series of questions concerning hospitalization, and were then permitted to play with a set of hospital toys. Children in *Control Condition I* received emotional support without information, following a protocol similar to that of the experimental group, but with a story, questions, and toys unrelated to the medical setting. *Control Condition II* received no intervention. Assessments of children's anxiety, using two self-report measures, were made immediately following the intervention period. Although experimental group subjects (emotional support plus information) reported significantly lower levels of anxiety than children in either control condition on both measures, those receiving emotional support without information (Control Condition I) were significantly less upset on one of the two assessments than subjects receiving no treatment.

Two additional hospital-based studies, which incorporate attention-control conditions in their research designs, suggest that emotional support may make some contribution to the reduction of children's anxiety (Lende, 1971; Schwartz, et al., 1983). Lende (1971) found that the inhospital and posthospital behavior of tonsillectomy patients who were given attention, but no information, did not differ significantly from that of children prepared either by the reading of a hospital book, by discussion of the procedure, or by playing through the experience.

Schwartz, et al. (1983) compared the inhospital behavior of three groups of children: a *related-play* group, which received relevant play and information about hospitalization from a child life specialist, an *unrelated-play* group, which also participated in play with the child life specialist, while receiving no information about the hospital, and a *control group,* which received no intervention. Children in the related-play condition were found to be significantly more cooperative and less upset than control group children at each of a series of stress points. However, with the exception of one stress point, reactions of the related-play and unrelated-play groups did not significantly differ. Of course, the question remains unresolved as to whether the factor influencing the behavior of children in the unrelated-play group was the "emotional support" of the adult, the opportunity for play, or the combination of both (see Chapter 9).

Among the dental research including an attention control condition are studies conducted by Sawtell, et al. (1974), Siegel and Peterson (1980, 1981), and Nocella and Kaplan (1982). Data from these studies provide less indication of the value of noninformational contact with an adult than do the medical studies. Sawtell, et al. examined the responses of children assigned to one of five conditions: 1) *filmed modeling,* 2) *desensitization,* 3) *behavior modification,* 4) *placebo* (i.e., attention-control, consisting of interaction with a friendly dental assistant), and 5) *control* (no intervention). No significant group differences were found, though indices of noncooperative behavior and the amount of time required to perform procedures were most favorable for the *placebo group* and least favorable for *control group* children.

Siegel and Peterson (1980, 1981) compared the reactions of children who were either instructed in coping techniques or given sensory information about forthcoming dental care, with those of children who spent comparable time with an adult, but received no relevant instruction. Both experimental conditions were found to be significantly more effective in reducing children's stress than the attention control condition, with this difference still observable during treatment one week after the intervention.

Though Siegel and Peterson did not incorporate a nontreatment control group in their design (a condition that may have permitted detection of possible benefits due to supportive contact with an adult), Nocella and Kaplan (1982) included such a group. Children trained in coping techniques were, therefore, compared with attention-control subjects (who engaged in conversation with an experimenter on nondental topics) and with those receiving no intervention. The behavior of children instructed in coping skills was significantly better during dental a restoration or extraction than that of subjects in either control condition, which, in turn, did not significantly differ from each other.

The latter dental studies offer no evidence of the potential value of children's noninformational contacts with representatives of the health care setting. Nevertheless, the majority of studies providing data pertinent to this topic indicate that such contact may be a beneficial component of the preparation process. Fassler (1980) and Sawtell, et al. (1974) suggest that children receiving the attention of an adult may be less upset than subjects receiving no systematic intervention. Others, such as Minde and Maler (1968), Lende (1971), and Schwartz, et al. (1983), have failed to demonstrate a clear superiority of informational interventions over interaction with a supportive individual.

STRESS POINT PREPARATION

The research reviewed to this point has identified several elements as possibly contributing to the success of preparation interventions. Among these are the presentation of information, both procedural and sensory (Johnson, et al., 1975), provided in a manner appropriate to the individual child's level of cognitive development, using play experiences for preschool and early schoolaged children in particular (Cassell, 1965). Preparation of parents, as well as children (Mahaffy, 1965; Skipper & Leonard, 1968), and the emotional support of both (Skipper, Leonard, & Rhymes, 1968; Minde & Maler, 1968; Fassler, 1980) have also been associated with reductions in psychological upset. A comprehensive form of preparation, combining these elements and adding an opportunity for rehearsal of children's behavior during designated periods of threat, is *stress point preparation.* Research examining this approach has been conducted by Wolfer and Visintainer (1975, 1979; Visintainer & Wolfer, 1975) and by McGrath (1979).

Wolfer and Visintainer (1975) assigned eighty children (3 to 14 years of age, hospitalized for elective surgery) to either a *control condition,* which included no systematic preparation or emotional support for children or parents, or the experimental *stress-point preparation* group. As indicated above, children in the latter condition received procedural and sensory information, rehearsal in behavioral responses, and emotional support prior to and during a series of stress points. Parents were included in the process so that they, too, might benefit from the information and support.

Children in the experimental group were found to be significantly less upset and more cooperative during the stress points, to register lower pulse rates in response to blood tests and injections, to void earlier following surgery, and to have fewer problems in posthospital adjustment than children in the control condition. In addition, parents of children receiving stress-point preparation were lower in self-reported anxiety and expressed greater satisfaction with the care and information they received than control group parents.

Visintainer and Wolfer (1975) further examined the effectiveness of stress point preparation by contrasting this intervention with two others: *single-session preparation,* which included presentation of information similar to that of stress-point preparation, but was given in a single 45-minute session upon admission rather than prior to each period of threat, or *consistent supportive care,* in which a nurse offered parents and children support and reassurance at stress points, but without systematic presentation of information. Eighty-four minor elective surgery patients between three and twelve years of age were assigned to one of these three conditions or to a control group.

Children receiving stress point care had more favorable ratings of cooperation and upset behavior at stress points, lesser need for postoperative medications, greater ease of fluid intake following surgery, and fewer posthospital behavioral disturbances than subjects in each of the remaining three conditions. Similarly, parents participating in stress-point preparation rated themselves as less anxious, more adequately informed, and better satisfied with the care they had received than did parents of other children.

In a subsequent study, Wolfer and Visintainer (1979) compared the effectiveness of stress-point preparation, as applied in the earlier research, with that derived through use of home preparatory materials incorporating similar information and techniques. The sample consisted of 163 children between three and twelve years of age who were scheduled for tonsillectomy surgery. Children were assigned to one of five conditions: 1) *stress-point preparation only,* 2) *home-booklet preparation only,* in which parents were asked to prepare their children for hospitalization by means of a packet containing a story booklet, hospital toys for play and demonstration, and an instruction booklet explaining the preparation protocol, 3) *home preparation, plus stress-point preparation,* 4) *home preparation, plus consistent supportive care,* or 5) a *control condition.*

On most outcome measures (which were comparable to those used in the earlier studies), stress-point preparation alone (condition 1) was not significantly more effective than treatments involving a home preparation component (conditions 2, 3, or 4). When compared with the control group, each of the experimental conditions resulted in lower levels of children's upset, as well as greater parent satisfaction with the information and care received. However, parents' self-reported anxiety was reduced by the stress-point intervention (condition 1), but not by any of the three conditions incorporating home preparation. Perhaps the added responsibility for a portion of the preparation process contributed to the anxiety of these parents, as Landes (1973) suggested when he obtained similar results.

McGrath (1979) examined the effectiveness of stress-point preparation provided to children in groups, rather than individually as had Wolfer and Visintainer. Forty-four children (three to twelve years of age, hospitalized for tonsillectomies) were assigned to either the *group preparation* or *control* condition. Experimental instruction groups were formed soon after children's admission, meeting again before and after a blood test, prior to receiving preoperative medications, and upon return from the recovery room following surgery. During group sessions, the usual components of the stress point preparation procedure were applied.

Responses of children in the group preparation and control conditions were also compared with those of forty children who had received individualized stress-point preparation in another study conducted three months earlier in the same institution (Wolfer & Visintainer, unpublished). The group preparation condition was associated with lower upset and greater cooperation of children at stress points than were either the individual preparation or the control condition. The benefits of the individualized preparation sessions also exceeded those of the control condition.

NONEXPERIMENTAL PREPARATION STUDIES

The experimental studies in the preceding sections have consistently demonstrated the beneficial effects of providing preparation to children and parents, whether the intervention comes in the form of informative explanations, medical play experiences, filmed modeling presentations, or instruction in coping skills. Despite documentation of the advantages, not all children receive adequate preparation for hospitalization or surgical procedures. This situation may be due to the lack of a systematic preparation program in the admitting institution (in which case, any preparation children receive must come from other sources), or to the failure of families to participate in activities provided by the hospital.

Both conditions have been considered by nonexperimental studies, which examine the type of preparation received by children and families, relating this information to varying outcome measures. For example, the adequacy of children's preparation for hospitalization in the absence of formalized programming has been assessed and related to variables such as children's perceptions of stress (Menke, 1972, 1981) and to their inhospital adjustment (Milosavljević, Kondić-Petrović, & Pjanović, 1972). Another group of studies has considered family participation in preadmission orientation sessions, comparing the family characteristics and child responses of attenders and nonattenders (Sauer, 1968; Meng, 1979; Nurse & Deber, 1982; Schmeltz & White, 1982; Schrier & Kaplan, 1983).

The Adequacy of Children's Preparation

Three studies address the relationship between the adequacy of children's preparation for hospitalization and their subsequent inhospital responses (Menke, 1972, 1981; Milosavljević, et al., 1972). Menke (1972) interviewed 104 hospitalized children (4 to 12 years of age) using a projective game developed for the research to identify the stimuli perceived by children as stressful. Comparisons were made between the stress perceptions of "prepared" and "unprepared" children, with subjects considered to be prepared if they were so identified by their parents and if they could tell the investigator why they were in the hospital. It was found that children who were prepared for hospitalization were less likely to perceive situations as stressful than were unprepared children. However, an attempted replication of this study with fifty hospitalized children (6 to 12 years of age) failed to reveal the same relationship (Menke, 1981).

In a study conducted in Yugoslavia, Milosavljević, et al. (1972) interviewed the parents of fifty tonsillectomy patients, three to ten years of age, to assess the quality of information given to children about their hospitalization. In addition, data on prior separations and hospitalizations were obtained. Through interviews with children and examination of their drawings, the investigators assessed their emotional status upon admission.

Three categories of emotional response were identified, though the method of categorizing children is not adequately described. Children in *Group I* (N = 17) were said to display realistic fear of hospitalization and surgery. All children in this group had been adequately prepared. *Group II* (N = 25) consisted of children who manifested some degree of depression before the operation. Preparation of subjects in this group was rated as inadequate. Children in *Group III* (N = 8) were characterized as displaying "unusual euphoria" prior to surgery, as well as depression postoperatively. No mention is made of the preparation of subjects in this group, but the investigators note that all had experienced prior separation. Milosavljević, et al. summarize their findings as indicating that children who are adequately prepared display smaller fluctuations in behavior in response to hospitalization and surgery than those who are not.

Participation In Preparation Activities

Family Characteristics. The sociodemographic or behavioral characteristics of families that choose to attend or avoid preadmission preparation programs have been examined in four studies. Schmeltz and White (1982) considered participation in preoperative sessions for parents of children scheduled for cardiac surgery. The remaining studies concern orientation programs for families prior to children's hospitalization for surgical procedures (Schrier & Kaplan, 1983; Meng, 1979; Nurse & Deber, 1982).

Schmeltz and White (1982) found that the average attendance at preadmission sessions for parents of cardiac patients was only 45 percent of those invited. To determine whether specific family characteristics might be related to parents' decision to participate, a survey was conducted. Fifty parents, who were invited to attend preoperative sessions over a two-month period, responded to a questionnaire upon their child's admission to the hospital. Twenty-six of the fifty parents had participated in scheduled sessions.

Among the characteristics distinguishing participants and nonparticipants were the age of the child, sociodemographic status of the family, distance the family lived from the hospital, and the severity of the child's condition. In particular, greater participation was noted among parents of younger children. Correspondingly, parents attending sessions were younger than nonparticipants. A higher percentage of middle income parents participated than those in either upper or lower income groups. Furthermore, a smaller percentage of parents living more than two hours away attended group sessions than did parents living closer. Finally, participation was related to the child's diagnosis. Although more than eighty percent of the parents of children with "mild" or "moderate" conditions attended the scheduled sessions, only 39 percent of the parents of children with "severe" diagnoses did so.

Schrier and Kaplan (1983) report on participation in weekly preadmission sessions conducted by a hospital in South Africa. The program was publicized through posters displayed in the hospital and leaflets distributed in clinics. Subjects for this study were fifteen mothers and their children (3 to 8 years of age) who were scheduled for tonsillectomy surgery. Three separate groups were compared. *Group A* consisted of mothers and children who came to the program of their own accord, without special invitation from the hospital. *Group B* mothers and children attended the program after receiving an invitation by telephone, while subjects in *Group C* did not participate in the preadmission sessions.

Though statistical comparisons of these small samples of subjects were not made, Schrier and Kaplan describe certain characteristics possibly differentiating the groups. Group A families were of higher socioeconomic status than those in groups B or C. Moreover, the majority of mothers in Group C (nonattenders) held jobs, while only one mother in either of the attending groups (A or B) was employed outside of the home. Differences in family composition were also noted. All children in Group A, but none of those in Group C, were either eldest or only children.

Meng (1979) reports on the relationship between family participation in a preadmission program and parents' self-initiated preparation efforts. In this study, the families of one hundred elective surgical patients (4 to 10 years of age) were randomly assigned to either an experimental group, in which subjects were invited to participate in a preadmission orientation program, or a control condition. The investigators found, however, that 24 of the 59 families assigned to the experimental condition chose not to attend. The present study, therefore, focused on the differences among experimental, control, and "no show" families.

Reasons offered by the "no show" families for not attending sessions appear to be less related to social factors (such as those cited by Schrier and Kaplan, 1983) than to parents' perceived need for additional information. The majority of parents (59%) stated that they chose not to attend because they were already knowledgeable about the hospital setting. In fact, it appears that nonattending parents may have drawn upon past experience to prepare children for hospitalization. The preparation provided to children by no-show families was found to parallel that given by experimental families. Eighty percent of the parents in both groups said that they had talked with their children about hospitalization prior to admission, compared with only 54 percent of those in the control condition.

Moreover, no-show parents reported discussing a broader range of hospital topics with their children than did other parents, while their children posed a greater number of questions than experimental or control group subjects.

Nurse and Deber (1982) examined the association between family participation in a preadmission program and parent behavior once in the hospital. Thirty families who had attended a preadmission tour were compared with a second group of families who had not participated, with children in each group matched on age, sex, surgical procedure, prior hospital experience, and distance from the hospital. Upon admission, parents' anxiety, knowledge of hospital routines, and their preparedness for the admission process were rated by members of the hospital staff. No difference in either anxiety or preparedness for admission was noted between attenders and nonattenders. However, more of the parents who had participated in the preadmission tour had their children bring along personal possessions to the hospital. They were also rated as more knowledgeable than nonattending parents about where they would wait during their child's surgery.

Children's Responses. Differences have also been examined in the levels of psychological upset exhibited by children who have or have not participated in preadmission programs. For example, Sauer (1968) compared the responses of fifty patients who had attended a preadmission tour with those of another group of 59 children who had not. Subjects in both groups were three to thirteen years of age, scheduled for minor surgery. Each child was rated as being either a difficult patient or not by a pediatric nurse (who was not, in all cases, unaware of children's preparation condition). Significantly fewer patients who had participated in the preadmission tour were rated as difficult.

Nurse and Deber (1982) also report on the relationship between children's inhospital and posthospital behavior and their participation in preadmission programming. Children's behavior was assessed upon separation from parents prior to surgery and while in a preoperative playroom. During both periods of assessment, fewer instances of upset were observed among children who had attended a preadmission orientation. No significant group differences in parent reports of children's posthospital behavior were found.

Additional data on the effects of preadmission programming on children are provided by Schrier and Kaplan (1983) and by Meng (1979). Schrier and Kaplan found participation in a preadmission program to be associated with reductions in children's fears and fantasies, though the method of assessing these reductions is not presented. Meng reports that the effects of preadmission orientation varied with the age of the patient. According to parent ratings, participation in the program lowered the anxiety of older children (7 to 10 years of age) prior to admission, but raised that of younger subjects (4 to 6 years of age). Data on inhospital reactions are not provided.

A final nonexperimental study addresses inhospital, rather than preadmission, preparation services. Taylor (1977) compared the responses of children admitted for short-term surgical procedures to one of two hospitals: a pediatric hospital that provided preparation services, or a general hospital offering no organized preparation. Few significant differences were found in the reactions of children in the two settings. However, because of the multitude of factors, in addition to preparation, that likely distinguished the two research settings, attribution of the differences observed to preparation is unwarranted.

THE PREVALENCE AND FUNCTIONING OF PREPARATION PROGRAMS

Two major surveys of the pediatric preparation services of hospitals in the United States have been conducted (Peterson & Ridley-Johnson, 1980; Azarnoff & Woody, 1981). Peterson and Ridley-Johnson (1980) obtained information on the preadmission preparation of children and parents provided by 62 pediatric hospitals. Seventy-four percent of the facilities reported conducting some formal prehospital preparation programming, with 42 percent offering preparation to all children prior to hospitalization, 31 percent to all surgical patients, and 19 percent limiting preparation to children undergoing specific procedures, such as cardiac catheterization. A variety of preparation materials and formats were used by the hospitals surveyed: 61 percent used narrative explanations, 55 percent distributed booklets, 48 percent used play therapy, 37 percent used filmed modeling, 21 percent puppet shows, and 16 percent relaxation techniques.

A majority of the hospitals conducting preparation programs included parents as well as children. The estimated percentage of children receiving preparation varied widely among the institutions surveyed, ranging from 0 to 100 percent, with the average being 42 percent. Attitudes of the hospitals toward preparation were highly positive, with 86 percent of the respondents viewing prehospital preparation as essential.

Azarnoff and Woody (1981) received responses from 1,427 hospitals providing inpatient pediatric care, a figure representing nearly half of all such facilities in the United States. Although Peterson and Ridley-Johnson found that some three-fourths of the pediatric hospitals provided preparation prior to hospitalization, Azarnoff and Woody report that only one-third of hospitals surveyed (which included both general and pediatric facilities) offered any form of preparation on a regular basis.

Characteristics of hospitals providing preparation experiences were contrasted with those that did not. Hospitals offering preparation services had significantly more pediatric beds, greater average length of patient stay, and admitted a wider age range of pediatric patients. Those failing to provide preparation services had significantly larger populations of black, Mexican-American, and Native-American children. The most frequently given reasons for not providing preparation services were that the number of pediatric patients was too small to warrant such a program, that the size of the staff was insufficient to prepare children, and that funding was not available.

Methods of preparing children prior to and during hospitalization were also examined. The hospital tour was the most common means of offering preadmission information, used by 64 percent of the hospitals offering preparation. The most frequently used methods of providing inhospital information were described as "the child learns as events occur" (cited by 89.3% of the hospitals offering preparation) and "conversation" (87.2%), methods that the investigators note were the most informal among items on a list presented to respondents.

The gap between the findings of the research reviewed earlier in this chapter and the practices of hospitals as described by Azarnoff and Woody is evident. For example, medical toys and models, which allow for the active participation of children in the preparation process, have been frequently incorporated in successful interventions (Cassell, 1965; Johnson & Stockdale, 1975). However, use of these materials during preparation was found to be less common than the strictly verbal approaches. Similarly, data on the effects of filmed modeling have been impressive (Melamed & Siegel, 1975), but Azarnoff and Woody found that films and videotapes were among the least used of preparation materials. The unfortunate conclusion that must be drawn from this study is that despite a preponderance of material demonstrating the benefits of systematic preparation and emotional support, children's access to preparation for hospitalization and medical events is still limited. Moreover, when preparation is available, it is likely to be conducted using approaches that are demonstrably less effective than the best available methods.

Chapter 11

SUMMARY AND CONCLUSIONS

A considerable amount of data lies in the more than 300 research articles examined in this text, a greater amount than can be readily summarized in a single chapter. Nonetheless, before concluding this review, it would be helpful to cast a view back over this material, with the goal of highlighting major trends and evaluating the current state of research. The framework for this discussion will build upon that used by Vernon, Foley, Sipowicz, and Schulman (1965) to bring closure to their own review. In particular, they considered the question of whether hospitalization is, in fact, upsetting to children, also identifying several possible determinants of the degree of upset experienced by individuals, with these being age, unfamiliarity, separation, and prehospital personality. Evidence from the research reviewed in the present text pertaining to children's immediate, posthospital, and longer term reactions is considered in this chapter. In addition, the determinants of upset suggested by Vernon, et al. (1965) are reconsidered in light of current research knowledge.

Vernon, et al. further delineated a series of limitations evident in the literature they evaluated—limitations in the design, analysis, and reporting of research that constrain interpretation and frustrate replication. The applicability of each of these criticisms to current research is examined. In addition, other concerns characteristic of research published over the past two decades are raised. Finally, the need for broadening the focus of research on the psychosocial aspects of childhood hospitalization is discussed.

DOES HOSPITALIZATION PRODUCE UPSET?

The evidence reviewed in Chapter 2, some of which was expanded upon in subsequent chapters, indicates that immediate and posthospital fluctuations do occur in behavioral, subjective, and physiological indices of children—fluctuations that are commonly interpreted as evidence of upset. In question, however, are the validity of this interpretation and the frequency with which these changes occur, as well as the severity and duration of the responses.

Immediate Responses

Given the standards by which emotional distress is most often measured, one must conclude that the experience of hospitalization or health care frequently results in children's short-term or immediate upset. Changes in behavior, in subjective reports of fear, and in selected physiological indicators such as heart rate or Palmar Sweat Index have been repeatedly documented among children receiving treatment in hospitals or outpatient settings. Moreover, in absence of experimental interventions, measurements of these indices are commonly found to be more extreme.

Posthospital Responses

Posthospital alterations in children's behavior, indicating difficulty in adjustment, have also been repeatedly (though not universally) reported. In most cases, these behavioral problems have been found to subside within a period ranging from days to a month or more, though individual cases of persistent difficulties are not uncommon. As was true of immediate responses, posthospital reactions (including physiological recovery, as well as behavioral changes) have proven to be modifiable through interventions such as parents' rooming-in and psychological preparation.

Long-term Responses

Several retrospective studies conducted in recent years suggest that children who have experienced hospitalization (especially, *repeated* hospitalizations) or severe illness at an early age may be at an increased risk for socioemotional difficulties at a later age. Much of this research is based on samples of subjects whose periods of hospitalization occurred two or more decades ago, under conditions that were presumably quite different from that existing today. Whether children currently experiencing hospitalization for comparable medical conditions are similarly at risk is unknown.

Researchers examining the posthospital period should, however, be alert to the possibility that some forms of posthospital response may persist, or perhaps reemerge, after physical recovery has been achieved and after the more obvious behavioral symptoms of distress have disappeared.

DETERMINANTS OF UPSET

Though hospitalization and health care experiences appear to have the potential for producing either immediate or deferred reactions indicative of upset, not all children are similarly affected. A considerable range of factors possibly influencing the degree of upset experienced by children has been proposed and investigated (see Chapter 2), but few variables have been examined with sufficient frequency, or have yielded results with sufficient consistency, to permit firm conclusions. Among the exceptions are the four determinants of upset identified by Vernon, et al. (age, unfamiliarity, separation, and prehospital adjustment), which have continued to receive extensive research attention.

Age

After reviewing the available data, Vernon, et al. concluded that a curvilinear relationship exists between children's age and their psychological upset. Children between six months and three to four years of age were found to be considerably more vulnerable to emotional distress than were those older or younger than this age range. Research conducted since 1965 assessing age-related responses has, almost without exception, confirmed this general pattern.

This rare display of research consensus notwithstanding, further consideration of influence of age is necessary for at least two reasons (discussed more fully in Chapter 2). First, virtually no systematic research has been conducted documenting the reactions of subjects beyond the late schoolage years. One of the few studies tracing the relationship between age and upset beyond these years (Gabriel & Danilowicz, 1978) hints that a second period of vulnerability may emerge in adolescence. A more rigorous examination of this possibility is necessary.

A second problem lies in the nature of the instruments (particularly the behavioral measures) used to assess upset, which may contain a bias toward accentuating distress exhibited by preschoolers. Indications of upset among late schoolaged children or adolescents may take more subtle forms than the instruments commonly in use are capable of detecting. Researchers investigating changes in upset across age groups should carefully select their measures for applicability to each of the ages examined.

Unfamiliarity

Vernon, et al. cite data from the limited amount of preparation research available in 1965 as evidence that a lack of familiarity with the hospital environment contributes to children's upset. In that group of studies, subjects provided with additional information about their circumstances were found to be less upset than those receiving no experimental treatment. Subsequent investigations have reaffirmed the association between informationally oriented preparation and reduced distress. However, attribution of this change to an increase in subjects' familiarity with the health care environment or procedures has not been firmly established. There have been few efforts to directly examine the relationship either between preparation and increased knowledge, or between knowledge and diminished upset, though the research addressing this question to date appears to confirm the importance of an accurate understanding of health care (see Chapter 10). Nevertheless, the possibility remains that another element of the preparation process, such as interaction with the person providing instruction, accounts for or contributes to the observed benefits.

Separation

Separation from parents was found by Vernon, et al. to be associated with to children's upset, both during and immediately following the period of hospitalization. Studies in the current review also indicate that the presence of parents, through rooming-in, visiting frequently, or remaining with their children during procedures, is capable of affecting children's immediate and posthospital responses.

There is some debate in the literature as to the meaning of a portion of the behavior manifested by children when in the presence of their parents. On initial consideration, certain responses, such as increased crying during procedures or greater aggression, appear to be indicative of emotional distress. Yet behavior of this type has most frequently been given a positive interpretation, being viewed as evidence of children's greater comfort when with their parents, which permits expression of normal feelings.

More unambiguous has been the research on the posthospital reactions of children whose parents remained with them during hospitalization. Studies in this category indicate that rooming-in is associated with reductions in behavioral disturbances and physical complications following discharge.

Prehospital Personality

Several of the studies reviewed by Vernon, et al. (1965) examined the possibility that children's prehospital adjustment would be predictive of the frequency or severity of their psychological responses to hospitalization. Only limited evidence of such a relationship was found. The few studies published since 1965 examining this possibility indicate that children with poorer emotional adjustment prior to hospitalization may, indeed, manifest greater inhospital and posthospital upset. However, questions concerning the nature of this relationship remain. In particular, does the inhospital or posthospital disturbance displayed by children with poor prior adjustment represent a continuation of preexisting difficulties, occurring with relative independence of the stresses of hospitalization, or does their prior emotional status make them more vulnerable to these stresses? Explication of this relationship has important implications for the type of interventions practitioners may use to minimize children's upset.

Other Factors

Aside from those factors just discussed, few other major candidates have emerged from the research as possible determinants of upset. Perhaps the most promising factors are related to the nature of children's interpersonal relationships with their parents and with members of the health care staff. Though these areas have not been as widely or systematically researched as others, evidence from several sources is strongly suggestive that children's immediate, and possibly deferred, responses are affected by factors such as parents' style of interacting with and disciplining their children and by the manner in which health care personnel approach and interact with patients. Excesses in either permissiveness or harshness of parental discipline have been associated with greater child upset in response to health care, while modeling behaviors and positive reinforcement are associated with declines (see Chapter 2). Concerning staff-child interactions, reductions in children's emotional distress have been documented when health care personnel adopt an empathic, child-oriented approach to these encounters, provide clear instructions, and offer appropriate behavioral reinforcement during examinations and treatment (see Chapter 8).

LIMITATIONS OF THE RESEARCH

Upon concluding their review of the literature on childhood hospitalization, Vernon, et al. (1965) identified a number of weaknesses evident in the research they had examined. Each of these identified limitations is considered in the following sections to determine the extent to which research published since 1965 differs from the earlier work. Many of the criticisms offered by Vernon, et al. are most directly applicable to research using experimental or quasiexperimental methodologies. Therefore, for purposes of assessing the quality of recent research in relation to these characteristics, information will be presented from a select group of studies—the 52 experimental and eleven nonexperimental preparation studies reviewed in Chapter 10. It should be noted that, as a group, the preparation studies are somewhat atypical of the literature reviewed in this text (much of which is correlational or descriptive) and generally represents a more rigorous approach to investigation. Nevertheless, even among this select group of studies, many of the limitations persist.

Adequacy of Descriptions

The concern was raised by Vernon, et al. that numerous studies failed to provide clear and complete descriptions of the procedures followed. Frequently omitted were adequate descriptions of systems used for categorizing subjects' upset responses or for collapsing data obtained from several sources to yield a single measure of upset. In the present review, a description was considered inadequate if it failed to provide information precisely delineating sample characteristics, methods of collecting or combining data, treatment procedures, or other information that would prohibit reasonable replication of the study. Judging by these criteria, the descriptions of recent experimental, if not nonexperimental, preparation studies were found to be quite good. Of the 52 experimental preparation studies, 48 (92.3%) were judged to provide an adequate description of the procedures used. Seven of the eleven nonexperimental studies (63.6%) also provided adequate descriptions.

Though descriptions provided were generally sufficient to allow replication of the research, one additional item of information, important to interpretation of the data, was seldom reported—the percentage of subjects accepting or rejecting participation in the project. Omission of this information may be due to limitation of space in the published reports. Nevertheless, its absence raises questions about the generalizability of the findings. A low acceptance rate may indicate that participants are of a select group, differing in certain, unspecified characteristics from those refusing to cooperate. Thus, for example, the effectiveness of a program of preparation of children by their parents may be demonstrated. However, if acceptance rates are low, one can only conclude that the intervention is of value when applied by parents sufficiently motivated and able to engage in research when most others decline. A high acceptance rate would remove these doubts.

Control of Observer Bias

The studies appearing prior to 1965 were further criticized for their infrequent use of blind observers or multiple, independent raters of subjects' behavior. This problem appears to persist in the more recent research. A study was designated as controlling for observer bias if procedures for achieving blind ratings were specified. Control of bias was not considered to be adequate if the research design included separate experimental and control phases—a practice that increases the difficulty of blinding observers.

Thirty of the experimental preparation studies (57.7%), and only two of the nonexperimental studies (18.2%) were judged to provide for adequate control of observer bias.

Use of Statistical Tests

Vernon, et al. (1965) observed that, "Many of the studies either have not employed statistical tests or have neglected to thoroughly report the results of such tests" (p. 162). This criticism is less applicable to the experimental preparation research conducted since 1965. Forty-nine of the 52 studies in this category (94.2%) used statistical analyses in consideration of their data. Slightly more than half (54.5%) of the nonexperimental studies have also incorporated statistical tests. These figures merely reflect the use and reporting of statistical analyses in the research under examination. No judgment has been made of the appropriateness of the techniques used or the degree to which assumptions underlying the procedures were met.

Confounding of Theoretical Implications

Vernon, et al. expressed the concern that, in an effort to develop effective programs for reducing hospitalized children's upset, researchers would frequently vary several elements of the hospital experience simultaneously in their experimental conditions. This confounding of interventions hinders determination of the individual factors possibly responsible for the effects achieved. Since quantification of the recent research regarding this practice, for purposes of comparison, is less easily accomplished, several subjective comments must suffice.

Examples may be found in the experimental preparation studies published since 1965 of the conscientious use of control groups. Perhaps the best use of control conditions for disentangling causal elements may be found in research examining the value of filmed modeling or instruction in coping techniques. For example, factors such as the effects the viewing of a film, regardless of its content, or of mere contact with an investigator who provides no relevant information, have been isolated through control conditions.

The importance of the latter type of control (commonly referred to as an attention control condition) has been illustrated by recent investigations. The opportunity for children to interact with a representative of the health care setting, without additional treatment, has been found to be at least somewhat effective in reducing children's upset (see Chapter 10). Therefore, researchers investigating an intervention involving interaction with health care personnel, are advised to use an attention control group, if they wish to demonstrate the effects of their experimental treatment beyond that potentially caused by the contact alone.

The desire to investigate comprehensive interventions, combining several therapeutic techniques as is frequently done in practice, need not result in the serious confounding of causal factors. A limited number of investigators have adopted a programmatic approach, examining the effects of several interventions applied in concert, while conducting complementary studies designed to assess the contribution of the individual elements (e.g., see Wolfer & Visintainer, 1975; Visintainer & Wolfer, 1975). Unfortunately, when the research literature is considered as a whole, studies adopting the commendable approaches discussed in this section still appear to be the exception.

Measurement of Direct Effects

Experimental research conducted prior to 1965 (which includes a small number of preparation studies) was criticized by Vernon, et al. for its failure to measure the direct effects of the treatment. For example, no attempt was made to determine whether preparation programs actually resulted in an increase in children's knowledge—data considered necessary to an understanding of the psychological processes operating during preparation.

Only a few of the more recent preparation studies in either the experimental or nonexperimental category have included a posttreatment assessment of the knowledge or understanding of either children (Lende, 1971; Rie, et al., 1968; Roberts, et al., 1981; Melamed, Dearborn, & Hermecz, 1983) or parents (Nurse & Deber, 1982; Wright, et al., 1973). Instead, most research has followed the pattern of earlier investigations, examining only the secondary effects of preparation, such as changes in subjects' behavioral, subjective, and physiological responses.

It may be argued that assessment of knowledge is inappropriate as a means of measuring the direct effects of certain forms of intervention appearing since 1965. For example, in research examining coping techniques, the ability of subjects to apply the procedures demonstrated, or the frequency with which the techniques are actually employed during stressful situations, may constitute a reasonable measure of the direct effects of the experimental treatment. For research on filmed modeling, behavioral indices (measures that for most forms of intervention would be considered secondary) might be used as direct assessment, if the target behaviors observed in children are closely linked to those demonstrated by the model. Though the question of the form of direct measure most appropriate to specific categories of interventions is unresolved, the Vernon, et al. criticism of lack of concern for direct effects remains valid.

Concern for Reliability and Validity

Vernon, et al. found documentation of the reliability and validity of research measures to be almost totally ignored in the literature they reviewed. The research covered in the present text demonstrates an increased concern for interrater reliability, though consideration of other forms of reliability, or of the validity of measures, remains rare. Thirty-eight of the 52 experimental studies (73.1%) report data on some form of reliability for at least one of the measures used in that research, with nearly all of this information pertaining to interrater agreement. Referral to test-retest reliability (Peterson, 1978; Melamed, Dearborn, & Hermecz. 1983) or the internal consistency of instruments (Coleman, 1975) is infrequent. Only three of the nonexperimental studies mention reliability, with each of these making reference to interrater agreement.

Studies were considered to have addressed the topic of validity if, in referring to at least one measure used in a given research project, the authors commented on its face or content validity, its previous demonstrated ability to distinguish experimental conditions, or its relationship to other, independent means of assessing the same construct. Not counted were studies using instruments for which *others* have examined validity (e.g., the Posthospital Behavior Questionnaire, Vernon, et al., 1966), unless the subsequent researcher demonstrated awareness of this prior effort. Despite these liberal criteria, only sixteen of the experimental studies (30.8%) and one of the nonexperimental studies were found to address the validity of any measure.

Consideration of Psychological Benefits

The early research on childhood hospitalization was further criticized for its pathological orientation, which concentrated on identification of the negative responses of children to health care and precluded assessment of positive effects associated with the experience. One group of studies appearing since 1965 (that documenting the coping responses of children) has argued against the pathological orientation, preferring instead to interpret children's immediate reactions to health care as normal, adaptive behavior.

Other research examining the posthospital adaptation of children has provided for assessment of improvements, as well as deterioration, in children's emotional state following discharge (Vernon, et al., 1966; Sides, 1977; Simons, et al., 1980). Nevertheless, only a minority of the recent preparation research (12 experimental studies and 1 nonexperimental study) is designed to permit consideration of positive effects. Of this research, all but the single nonexperimental study (Gabriel & Danilowicz, 1978) accomplish this objective through use of the Posthospital Behavior Questionnaire (Vernon, et al., 1966)—an instrument through which parents make a retrospective comparison of children's pre- and posthospital behavior, thereby allowing for detection of improvement in behavior.

ADDITIONAL CONCERNS

In conducting the present review of the literature, several other limitations in the existing research have become apparent. Unlike those identified by Vernon, et al., which primarily concerned technical aspects of conducting and reporting research, the additional limitations to be discussed below relate to the content examined. Of major concern is the relatively narrow range of children and topics considered by researchers—a condition that signals the need to broaden the focus of investigation. By so doing, it is hoped that we may gain a more comprehensive view of the effects of hospitalization on children of all ages and on other members of their family, and that we may further identify new forms of interventions that are applicable to subjects varying in age and diagnosis, and compatible with recent changes in the nature of health care delivery.

Limited Research on Involvement of Fathers and Siblings

The need for additional research on the reactions and influence of fathers during the hospitalization of their children is discussed in Chapter 6. An appreciable amount of data exists concerning mothers' involvement in children's hospitalization. For example, research attention has been devoted to topics such as the impact of mothers' presence on children's reactions, the magnitude of their anxiety, the effect of this anxiety on their children, the factors influencing their responses when in the medical setting, and the utility of informational and emotional support interventions designed to reduce their distress. In contrast, virtually nothing has been reported concerning fathers' responses to the hospitalization of a child. A similar lack of information concerning the adjustments and reactions of siblings of hospitalized children is apparent, though there have been indications of a change in this situation in recent years.

Restricted Range of Subjects used in Experimental Research

The majority of the experimental research on childhood hospitalization has been restricted to a relatively narrow sample of the hospital population. Specifically, most of these studies have examined subjects of a limited age range, admitted to the hospital for minor, elective surgery. For example, one may consider the data on the 31 experimental studies in this text concerning preparation for hospitalization. Figure 1 (see Chapter 10) depicts the percentages of these 31 studies that include subjects of various ages. As can be seen, this group of experimental studies has concentrated on children in the late preschool through early schoolage years, with nearly 84 percent of the research including subjects six years of age.

It is perhaps understandable that relatively fewer of the preparation studies would include subjects younger than four years of age, given the cognitive orientation of these interventions. More surprising is the failure of experimental preparation studies to consider adolescents. Only three of the 31 hospital preparation studies included subjects older than twelve years of age, with none focusing exclusively on this population.

The data on *diagnoses* of subjects participating in experimental research reveals an even greater homogeneity of sample characteristics. Of the 31 experimental studies concerning preparation for hospitalization, all but three limited their samples to surgical patients. Twenty-six of these, or more than eighty percent of all experimental preparation studies, involved short-term, elective surgical patients. A similar, though not quite so extreme, situation is observed among nonexperimental preparation studies, 64 percent of which examined patients admitted for minor, elective surgery. Even among the thirteen experimental and nonexperimental studies concerning interventions designed to minimize difficulties associated with separation (research in which the need for access to subjects prior to or immediately following admission would seem to be less acute than for preparation research), nearly half (46%) were limited to children in the minor surgical category.

The problem inherent in this concentration of research on children of restricted age and diagnosis is that little is known about the effects of intervention on a substantial portion of the pediatric population. For example, children admitted to the hospital for *medical* conditions have been virtually ignored. Ironically, that population with which most of the experimental research has been conducted (i.e., young patients facing minor surgery) represents a declining proportion of the pediatric inpatient census. Fewer tonsillectomies (the principal diagnosis in much of this research) are being performed than in years past. Moreover, when performed, tonsillectomies and other forms of minor, elective surgery are increasingly conducted on an outpatient basis.

The paradox of this situation is that categories of children for whom experimental interventions have been of demonstrated effectiveness are now less often in a position to receive this additional inpatient care. On the other hand, those who can take advantage of these treatments (e.g., medical patients, or those admitted for nonelective or more involved surgical procedures) have seldom been included in the research. The changing nature of health care, and the state of our current knowledge dictate at least two directions for future study. First, research on inpatient, experimental interventions must be extended to patients not previously considered. Second, as the move toward increased utilization of outpatient surgery continues, reactions of patients to this form of care must be examined, and interventions successful in the inpatient setting must be reevaluated and adapted for use under new conditions.

Restricted Range of Interventions Examined

Of the interventions typically used with hospitalized children, psychological preparation for procedures has been the most frequently researched. Within this category of studies are a number of theoretically distinct approaches, including the use of filmed modeling, training in coping techniques, and the provision of procedural and sensory information. However, aside from preparation, and a smaller group of studies varying parent presence (see Chapter 5), few other forms of intervention have received experimental assessment. For example, play is often incorporated in the hospital experience of children, yet few studies have attempted to assess the value of this activity. Also limited has been research varying the approach adopted by hospital personnel in their interactions with children, though results from outpatient medical and dental clinics have been encouraging (see Chapter 8).

Of perhaps greater concern is the complete absence of research in other areas. As discussed earlier, Vernon, et al. (1965) considered unfamiliarity to be one of several factors responsible for hospitalized children's upset. Most of the data suggesting the importance of this factor, however, has come from the preparation research, through which children are acquainted with unfamiliar aspects of their hospitalization. Unexamined have been changes made in the hospital environment designed to reduce the discrepancy between hospital and home—an approach commonly referred to as normalization. Among the activities that might be included in this category are efforts to limit environmental intrusions (e.g., restricting the number of persons with whom children must interact, or limiting disruptions of periods of rest or play) and to return to the child the autonomy, responsibility, and freedom of choice that he or she might experience at home.

REFERENCES

Abrams, L. Resistance behaviors and teaching media for children in day surgery. *AORN Journal,* 1982, *35,* 244–258.

Abu-Saad, H., & Holzemer, W. L. Measuring children's self-assessment of pain. *Issues in Comprehensive Pediatric Nursing,* 1981, *5,* 337–349.

Aisenberg, R. B., Wolff, P. H., Rosenthal, A., & Nadas, A. S. Psychological impact of cardiac catheterization. *Pediatrics,* 1973, *51,* 1051–1059.

Akins, D. L., Mace, G. S., & Akins, F. R. *The hospitalized child: Psychosocial issues.* New York: Plenum, 1981.

Alcock, D. Hey, what about the kids? *The Canadian Nurse,* 1977, *73,* 38–41.

Ammon, K. J. The effects of music on children in respiratory distress. *ANA clinical sessions, 1968, Dallas.* New York: Appleton-Century-Crofts, 1968, 127–133.

Aply, J., Barbour, R. F., & Westmacott, I. Impact of congenital heart disease on the family: Preliminary report. *British Medical Journal,* 1967, *1,* 103–105.

Astin, E. W. Self reported fears of hospitalized and non-hospitalized children aged ten to twelve. *Maternal-Child Nursing Journal,* 1977, *6,* 17–24.

Azarnoff, P., Bourque, L. B., Green, J. A., & Rakow, S. *The preparation of children for hospitalization.* National Institute of Mental Health Report. Department of Pediatrics, University of California, Los Angeles, 1975.

Azarnoff, P., & Woody, P. D. Preparation of children for hospitalization in acute care hospitals in the United States. *Pediatrics,* 1981, *68,* 361–368.

Barker, R. G., Dembo, L., & Lewin, K. Frustration and regression: An experiment with young children. *University of Iowa Studies in Social Welfare.* 1941, *18,* No. 386.

Barnes, C. M. Levels of consciousness indicated by responses of children to phenomena in the intensive care unit. *Maternal-Child Nursing Journal,* 1975a, *4*(4, Monograph #4), 215–285.

Barnes, C. M. School-age children's recall of the intensive care unit. *ANA clinical sessions, San Francisco, 1974.* New York: Appleton-Century-Crofts, 1975b.

Barnes, C. M., Kenney, F. M., Call, T., & Reinhart, J. B. Measurement in management of anxiety in children for open heart surgery. *Pediatrics,* 1972, *49,* 250–259.

Barton, P. H. The relationship between fantasy and overt stress reactions of children to hospitalization (Doctoral dissertation, University of Florida, 1964). *Dissertation Abstracts,* 1968, *29,* 809-A. (University Microfilms No. 68-12979)

Beardslee, C. I. Factors which influence the sleep-wakefulness pattern of young, hospitalized children at nap time (Doctoral dissertation, University of Pittsburgh.

1974). *Dissertation Abstracts International,* 1974, *35,* 345-B. (University Microfilms No. 74-15, 603)

Beardslee, C. The sleep-wakefulness pattern of young hospitalized children during nap time. *Maternal-Child Nursing Journal,* 1976, *5,* 15–24.

Beavers, B. C. An exploratory study of the psychological sequelae of surgery and hospitalization in male children (Doctoral dissertation, University of Southern California, 1974). *Dissertation Abstracts International,* 1974, *34,* 5160–B. (University Microfilms No. 74-9054)

Beck, M. Attitudes of parents of pediatric heart patients toward patient care units. *Nursing Research,* 1973, *22,* 334–338.

Becker, R. D. Recent developments in child psychiatry: Clinical pediatrics liaison consultation. *Israeli Annals of Psychiatry and Related Disciplines,* 1975, *13,* 239–258.

Bernheimer, L. P. Well children's perceptions of routine health care: Coping behaviors during the physical examination (Doctoral dissertation, University of California, Los Angeles, 1981). *Dissertation Abstracts International,* 1982, *42,* 3426-A. (University Microfilms No. 82-01073)

Bernstein, A., & Cowan, P. Children's concepts of how people get babies. *Child Development,* 1975, *46,* 77–91.

Beverly, B. I. The effect of illness upon emotional development. *Journal of Pediatrics,* 1936, *8,* 533–543.

Bibace, R., & Walsh, M. E. Development of children's concepts of illness. *Pediatrics,* 1980, *66,* 912–917.

Bibace, R., & Walsh, M. E. Developmental stages in children's conceptions of illness. In G. Stone, F. Cohen, & N. Adler (Eds.), *Health psychology: A handbook.* San Francisco: Josey-Bass, 1978.

Blitzer, E. C., Zuckerman, B., Pozen, J. T., & Blitzer, P. H. Another myth: Reduced hospital visiting by inner-city mothers. *Pediatrics,* 1983, *71,* 504–509.

Binger, C. M., Ablin, A. R., Feuerstein, R. C., Kushner, J. H., Zoger, S., & Mikkelsen, C. Childhood leukemia: Emotional impact on patient and family. *New England Journal of Medicine,* 1969, *280,* 414–418.

Bolig, R. The relationship of personality factors to responses to hospitalization in young children admitted for medical procedures (Doctoral dissertation, Ohio State University, 1980). *Dissertation Abstracts International,* 1981, *41,* 3732-B. (University Microfilms No. 81-07304).

Bothe, A., & Galdston, R. The child's loss of consciousness: A psychiatric view of pediatric anesthesia. *Pediatrics,* 1972, *50,* 252–263.

Brain, D. J., & Maclay, I. Controlled study of mothers and children in hospital. *British Medical Journal,* 1968, *1,* 278–280.

Branstetter, E. The young child's response to hospitalization: Separation anxiety or lack of mothering care? *American Journal of Public Health,* 1969a, *59,* 92–97.

Branstetter, E. The young child's response to hospitalization: Separation anxiety or lack of mothering care? *Communicating Nursing Research,* 1969b, *2,* 13–25.

Brewster, A. B. Chronically ill hospitalized children's concepts of their illness. *Pediatrics,* 1982, *69,* 355–362.

Brodie, B. M. An exploratory study of the perceptions of healthy children toward illness (Doctoral dissertation, Michigan State University, 1970). *Dissertation Abstracts International*, 1971, *31*, 5838-A. (University Microfilms No. 71-11795)

Brodie, B. Views of healthy children toward illness. *American Journal of Public Health*, 1974, *64*, 1156–1159.

Brown, B. Beyond separation: Some new evidence on the impact of brief hospitalization on young children. In D. Hall and M. Stacey (Eds.), *Beyond separation: Further studies of children in hospital*. London: Routledge & Kegan Paul, 1979.

Brunswick, A. F. Health needs of adolescents: How the adolescent sees them. *American Journal of Public Health*, 1969, *59*, 1730–1745.

Burling, K. A., & Collipp, P. J. Emotional responses of hospitalized children: Results of a pulse-monitor study. *Clinical Pediatrics*, 1969, *8*, 641–646.

Burstein, S., & Meichenbaum, D. The work of worrying in children undergoing surgery. *Journal of Abnormal Child Psychology*, 1979, *7*, 121–132.

Burton, L. *The family life of sick children*. London: Routledge & Kegan Paul, 1975.

Caldwell, B. S., & Lockhart, L. H. A care-by-parent unit: Its planning, implementation and patient satisfaction. *Children's Health Care*, 1981, *10*, 4–7.

Campbell, E. H. Effects of mothers' anxiety on infants' behavior (Doctoral dissertation, Yale University, 1957).

Campbell, J. D. Illness is a point of view: The development of children's concepts of illness. *Child Development*, 1975, *46*, 92–100.

Campbell, J. D. The child in the sick role: Contributions of age, sex, parental status, and parental values. *Journal of Health and Social Behavior*, 1978, *19*, 33–51.

Cannell, R. T. Effects of physical disorders on the adjustment of hospitalized children (Doctoral dissertation, University of Missouri-Columbia, 1970). *Dissertation Abstracts International*, 1971, *31*, 3987-A. (University Microfilms No. 71-3317)

Carandang, M. L. A., Folkins, C. H., Hines, P. A., & Steward, M. S. The role of cognitive level and sibling illness in children's conceptualizations of illness. *American Journal of Orthopsychiatry*, 1979, *49*, 474–481.

Carty, R. M. Identification of behavioral responses of preschool-age children before, during, and after hospitalization in a pediatric intensive care unit (Doctoral dissertation, Catholic University of America, 1977). *Dissertation Abstracts International*, 1977, *38*, 1380–1381-B. (University Microfilms No. 77-19,967)

Cassell, S. Effect of brief puppet therapy upon the emotional responses of children undergoing cardiac catheterization. *Journal of Consulting Psychology*, 1965, *29*, 1–8.

Cassell, S., & Paul, M. H. The role of puppet therapy on the emotional response of children hospitalized for cardiac catheterization. *Journal of Pediatrics*, 1967, *71*, 233–239.

Cassell, S. E. The effects of brief puppet therapy upon the emotional responses of children undergoing cardiac catheterization (Doctoral dissertation, Northwestern University, 1963). *Dissertation Abstracts*, 1964, *25*, 2042. (University Microfilms No. 64-05859)

Castaneda, A., McCandless, B. R., & Palermo, D. S. The children's form of the Manifest Anxiety Scale. *Child Development*, 1956, *27*, 317–326.

Cataldo, M. F., Bessman, C. A., Parker, L. H., Pearson, J. E. R., & Rogers, M. C. Behavioral assessment for pediatric intensive care units. *Journal of Applied Behavior Analysis*, 1979, *12*, 83–97.

Clatworthy, S. M. The effect of therapeutic play on the anxiety behaviors of hospitalized children (Doctoral dissertation, Boston University, 1978). *Dissertation Abstracts International*, 1978, *38*, 6142-B. (University Microfilms No. 78-08055)

Clatworthy, S. Therapeutic play: Effects on hospitalized children. *Children's Health Care*, 1981, *9*, 108–113.

Cleary, J. Demands and responses: The effects of the style of work allocation on the distribution of nursing attention, in D. Hall and M. Stacey (Eds.), *Beyond separation: Further studies of children in hospital.* London: Routledge & Kegan Paul, 1979.

Cleary, J. The distribution of nursing attention in a children's ward. *Nursing Times*, occasional papers, 1977, *73*, 93–96.

Clegg, R. L. Effects of a child life program upon the anxiety levels of children hospitalized for major elective surgery (Doctoral dissertation, University of Maryland, 1972). *Dissertation Abstracts International*, 1973, *33*, 4882-B. (University Microfilms No. 73-9688)

Clough, F. Staff ratings of children's behaviour in hospital: Comparability of factor structures. *British Journal of Psychology*, 1978, *69*, 59–68.

Clough, F. The validation of meaning in illness-treatment situations. In D. Hall and M. Stacey (Eds.), *Beyond separation: Further studies of children in hospital.* London: Routledge & Kegan Paul, 1979.

Coleman, K. P. Preventing and reducing anxiety in pediatric surgical patients: An educational and direct treatment approach (Doctoral dissertation, Kent State University, 1975). *Dissertation Abstracts International*, 1976, *36*, 5819-A. (University Microfilms No. 76-4920)

Conway, B. The effect of hospitalization on adolescence. *Adolescence*, 1971, *6*, 77–92.

Cook, S. D. The development of causal thinking with regard to physical illness among french children (Doctoral dissertation, University of Kansas, 1975). *Dissertation Abstracts International*, 1976, *37*, 454–455-B. (University Microfilms No. 76-16,710)

Cormier, P. Identification of typologies derived from child behaviors in the hospital as predictors of psychological upset (Doctoral dissertation, University of Virginia, 1975). *Dissertation Abstracts International*, 1976, *36*, 4376-B. (University Microfilms No. 76-612)

Cormier, P. P. Identification of typologies derived from child behaviors in the hospital as predictors of psychological upset. *Journal of Psychiatric Nursing and Mental Health Services*, 1979, *17*, 28–35.

Couture, C. J. The psychological response of young children to brief hospitalization and surgery: The role of parent-child contact and age (Doctoral dissertation,

Boston University, 1976). *Dissertation Abstracts International,* 1976, *37,* 1427-B. (University Microfilms No. 76-21,275)

Craft, M. Preferences of hospitalized adolescents for information providers. *Nursing Research,* 1981, *30,* 205–211.

Crocker, E. Preparation for elective surgery: Does it make a difference? *Journal of the Association for the Care of Children's Health,* 1980, *9,* 3–11.

Crocker, E. A review of the literature concerning the effects of hospitalization and illness on children, or we know less than we think we do! *Journal of the Association for the Care of Children in Hospitals,* 1974, *3,* 3–9.

Dabbs, J. M., Johnson, J. E., & Leventhal, H. Palmar sweating: A quick and simple measure. *Journal of Experimental Psychology,* 1968, *78,* 347–350.

Danilowicz, D. A., & Gabriel, H. P. Postoperative reactions in children: "Normal" and abnormal responses after cardiac surgery. *American Journal of Psychiatry,* 1971, *128,* 185–188.

Dart, R. J. Reducing stress in young children: Effects of mother's picture and voice recordings on response to hospitalization (Doctoral dissertation, University of Waterloo, 1980). *Dissertation Abstracts International,* 1980, *41,* 1104–1105-B.

Davenport, H. T., & Werry, J. S. The effect of general anesthesia, surgery and hospitalization upon the behavior of children. *American Journal of Orthopsychiatry,* 1970, *40,* 806–824.

Dearden, R. The psychiatric aspects of the case study sample. In M. Stacey (Ed.), *Hospitals, children and their families: The report of a pilot study.* London: Routledge & Kegan Paul, 1970.

Dew, T. A., Bushong, M. E., & Crumrine, R. S. Parents in pediatric RR. *AORN Journal,* 1977, *26,* 266–272.

Dombro, R. H. Child life programs in ninety-two pediatric departments of general hospitals in the United States and Canada. In J. A. Haller, J. L. Talbert, & R. H. Dombro (Eds.), *The hospitalized child and his family.* Baltimore: Johns Hopkins Press, 1967a.

Dombro, R. H. Child life programs in ninety-one children's hospitals in the United States and Canada. In J. A. Haller, J. L. Talbert, & R. H. Dombro (Eds.), *The hospitalized child and his family.* Baltimore: Johns Hopkins Press, 1967b.

Douglas, J. W. B. Early hospital admissions and later disturbances of behaviour and learning. *Developmental Medicine and Child Neurology,* 1975, *17,* 456–480.

Dowd, E. L., Novak, J. C., & Ray, E. J. Releasing the hospitalized child from restraints. *MCN: American Journal of Maternal Child Nursing,* 1977, *2,* 370–373.

Earthrowl, B., & Stacey, M. Social class and children in hospital. *Social Science and Medicine,* 1977, *11,* 83–88.

Eland, J. M. Minimizing pain associated with prekindergarten intramuscular injections. *Issues in Comprehensive Pediatric Nursing,* 1981, *5,* 361–372.

Elkind, D. The child's conception of prayer. *Journal for the Scientific Study of Religion,* 1967, *6,* 101–109.

Erickson, F. Play interviews for four-year-old hospitalized children. *Monographs of the Society for Research in Child Development*, 1958, *23* (3, Serial No. 69).

Erikson, E. H. *Childhood and society.* New York: Norton, 1963.

Evans, R. G., & Robinson, G. C. An economic study of cost savings on a care-by-parent ward. *Medical Care*, 1983, *21*, 768–782.

Fagin, C. M. *The effects of maternal attendance during hospitalization on the posthospital behavior of young children.* Philadelphia: F. A. Davis, 1966.

Fagin, C. M. Mothers and children in hospital. *British Medical Journal*, 1969, *2*, 311.

Fagin, C. M. Rooming in and its effects on the behavior of young children: A comparative survey on the effects of maternal attendance during hospitalization on the posthospital behavior of young children (Doctoral dissertation, New York University, 1964). *Dissertation Abstracts*, 1965, *25*, 4657–4658. (University Microfilms No. 65–968)

Fagin, C. M., & Nusbaum, J. G. Parental visiting privileges in pediatric units: A survey. *Journal of Nursing Administration*, 1978, *8*, 24–27.

Fassler, D. Reducing preoperative anxiety in children: Information versus emotional support. *Patient Counselling and Health Education*, 1980, *2*, 130–134.

Ferguson, B. F. Preparing young children for hospitalization: A comparison of two methods. *Pediatrics*, 1979, *64*, 656–664.

Fernald, C. D., & Corry, J. J. Empathic versus directive preparation of children for needles. *Children's Health Care*, 1981, *10*, 44–47.

Finkelstein, J. W., Medina, M., & Vegehla, M. Hospital-based employees' opinions about adolescents of four racial-ethnic groups. *Journal of Adolescent Health Care*, 1981, *2*, 1–7.

Fiser, D. H., Stanford, G., & Dorman, D. J. Services for parental stress reduction in a pediatric intensive care unit, *Critical Care Medicine*, 1984, *12*, 504–507.

Fleece, E. L. Contingency management as a method of reducing children's disruptive behaviors during dental treatment. (Doctoral dissertation, Case Western Reserve University, 1979). *Dissertation Abstracts International*, 1979, *39*, 5549-B. (University Microfilms No. 79-09351)

Fletcher, B. Psychological upset in posthospitalized children: A review of the literature. *Maternal-Child Nursing Journal*, 1981, *10*, 185–195.

Fletcher, B. Rooming-in: A reassessment. *Maternal-Child Nursing Journal*, 1981, *10*, 85–98.

Foley, J. M. Children's responses to frustration: Relationship with child rearing practices and infant reaction patterns (Doctoral dissertation, Northwestern University, 1962). *Dissertation Abstracts*, 1963, *23*, 3990. (University Microfilms No. 63-01288)

Francis, V., Korsch, B. M., & Morris, M. J. Gaps in doctor-patient communication: Patients' response to medical advice. *The New England Journal of Medicine*, 1969, *280*, 535–540.

Frankl, S. N., Shiere, F. R., & Fogels, H. R. Should the parent remain with the child in the dental operatory? *Journal of Dentistry for Children*, 1962, *29*, 150–163.

Freemon, B., Negrete, V. F., Davis, M., & Korsch, B. M. Gaps in doctor-patient communication: Doctor-patient interaction analysis. *Pediatric Research*, 1971, *5*, 298–311.

Freud, A. The role of bodily illness in the mental life of children. In R. S. Eissler, A. Freud, M. Kris, & A. J. Solnit (Eds.), *The psychoanalytic study of the child.* New York: International Universities Press, 1952.

Frieberg, K. H. How parents react when their child is hospitalized. *American Journal of Nursing*, 1972, *72*, 1270–1272.

Furth, G. M. Impromptu paintings by terminally ill, hospitalized and healthy children: What can we learn from them? (Doctoral dissertation, Ohio State University, 1973). *Dissertation Abstracts International*, 1974, *34*, 4739–4740-A. (University Microfilms No. 74-3170)

Gabriel, H. P., & Danilowicz, D. Postoperative responses in 'prepared' child after cardiac surgery. *British Heart Journal*, 1978, *40*, 1046–1051.

Gardner, B. A. The guilt reactions of parents of children with severe physical diseases. *American Journal of Psychiatry*, 1969, *126*, 636–644.

Gardner, G. G., & Simkins, R. A. Does it really matter what nurses wear in the intensive care unit? *MCN: American Journal of Maternal Child Nursing*, 1976, *1* 239–242.

Gath, A. The mental health of siblings of congenitally abnormal children. *Journal of Child Psychology and Psychiatry*, 1972, *13*, 211–218.

Gellert, E. *Children's concepts about bodily illness.* Paper presented at the meeting of the American Psychological Association, New York, 1961.

Gellert, E. Children's conceptions of the content and functions of the body. *Genetic Psychology Monographs*, 1962, *65*, 293–411.

Gilmore, J. B. The role of anxiety and cognitive factors in children's play behavior. *Child Development*, 1966, *37*, 397–416.

Gips, C. How illness experiences are interpreted by hospitalized children (Doctoral dissertation, Columbia University, 1956).

Gofman, H., Buckman, W., & Schade, G. H. Parents' emotional responses to hospitalization. *American Journal of Diseases of Children*, 1957, *93*, 629–637.

Gohsman, B. Differences in attitude toward hospitalization between pediatric staff and parents of hospitalized children. *Communicating Nursing Research*, 1977, *9*, 51–58.

Goslin, E. R. The effects of crisis intervention therapy in reducing anxiety in emergency hospitalization of preschool children (Doctoral dissertation, Florida State University, 1979). *Dissertation Abstracts International*, 1979, *40*, 3394-B. (University Microfilms No. 80-01099)

Goslin, E. R. Hospitalization as a life crisis for the preschool child: A critical review. *Journal of Community Health*, 1978, *3*, 321–346.

Gozzi, E. K., Morris, M. J., & Korsch, B. M. Gaps in doctor-patient communication: Implications for nursing practice. *American Journal of Nursing*, 1969, *69*, 529–533.

Grant, V. J. Pedestrian traffic in a paediatric ward. *New Zealand Medical Journal*, 1983, *96*, 91–93.

Gratz, R. R. Children's responses to emergency room care: An exploratory study of personal, situational, and parental variables (Doctoral dissertation, University of Wisconsin, 1977). *Dissertation Abstracts International,* 1978, *38,* 5834–5835-B. (University Microfilms No. 78-04419)

Green, M. M. Adolescent boys' expressions about their body experiences following surgery (Doctoral dissertation, University of Pittsburgh, 1976). *Dissertation Abstracts International,* 1977, *37,* 3349–3350-B. (University Microfilms No. 76-30431)

Gutstein, S. E. Parental facilitation of children's involvement in preparation for elective surgery (Doctoral dissertation, Case Western Reserve University, 1980). *Dissertation Abstracts International,* 1981, *41,* 2761-B. (University Microfilms No. 81-00533)

Guttentag, D. N. W., Albritton, W. L., & Kettner, R. B. Daytime television viewing by hospitalized children. *Pediatrics,* 1981, *68,* 672–676.

Guttentag, D. N. W., Albritton, W. L., & Kettner, R. B. Daytime television viewing by hospitalized children: The effect of alternative programming. *Pediatrics,* 1983, *71,* 620–625.

Hackett, J. M. Preoperative psychological preparation for children undergoing cardiac surgery (Doctoral dissertation, California School of Professional Psychology, 1976). *Dissertation Abstracts International,* 1978, *38,* 4457-B. (University Microfilms No. 77-32477)

Hagemann, V. P. Night sleep of children in a hospital (Doctoral dissertation, University of Pittsburgh, 1978). *Dissertation Abstracts International,* 1979, *39,* 3762-B. (University Microfilms No. 79-02794)

Hagemann, V. Night sleep of children in a hospital, part I: Sleep duration. *Maternal-Child Nursing Journal,* 1981a, *10,* 1–13.

Hagemann, V. Night sleep of children in a hospital, part II: Sleep disruption. *Maternal-Child Nursing Journal,* 1981b, *10,* 127–142.

Hall, D. J. Bedside blues: The impact of social research on the hospital treatment of sick children. *Journal of Advanced Nursing,* 1978, *3,* 25–37.

Hall, D. J. *Social relations and innovation: Changing the state of play in hospitals.* London: Routledge & Kegan Paul, 1977.

Hanna, W. J., & Sherlock, H. Recall and fears of anaesthesia and surgery in 50 Jamaican paediatric patients. *West Indian Medical Journal,* 1983, *32,* 75–82.

Harder, L., & Bowditch, B. Siblings of children with cystic fibrosis: Perceptions of the impact of the disease. *Children's Health Care,* 1982, *10,* 116–120.

Hardgrove, C. B. Living-in accommodations and practices for parents in hospital pediatric units: An update. *Journal of the Association for the Care of Children in Hospitals,* 1975, *4,* 24–26.

Hardgrove, C. B., & Dawson, R. B. *Parents and children in the hospital: The family's role in pediatrics.* Boston: Little, Brown and Company, 1975.

Hardgrove, C. B., & Kermoian, R. Parent-inclusive pediatric units: A survey of policies and practices. *American Journal of Public Health,* 1978, *68,* 847–850.

Harper, J. R., & Varakis, G. Children in adult intensive care therapy units. *British Medical Journal,* 1970, *1,* 810–813.

Heffernan, M., & Azarnoff, P. Factors in reducing children's anxiety about clinic visits. *HSMHA Health Reports,* 1971, *86,* 1131–1135.

Heisel, J. S., Ream, S., Raitz, R., Rappaport, M., & Coddington, R. D. The significance of life events as contributing factors in the diseases of children, III: A study of pediatric patients. *Journal of Pediatrics*, 1973, *83*, 119–123.

Hennessey, J. A. Hospitalized toddlers' responses to mothers' tape recordings during brief separations (Doctoral dissertation, University of Pittsburgh, 1974). *Dissertation Abstracts International*, 1974, *35*, 1766–1767-B. (University Microfilms No. 74-20823)

Hennessey, J. A. Hospitalized toddlers' responses to mothers' tape recordings during brief separations. *Maternal-Child Nursing Journal*, 1976, *5*, 69–91.

Herbertt, R. M., & Innes, J. M. Familiarization and preparatory information in the reduction of anxiety in child dental patients. *Journal of Dentistry for Children*, 1979, *46*, 319–323.

Hester, N. K. O. The preoperational child's reaction to immunization. *Nursing Research*, 1979, *28*, 250–255.

Hetherington, M., Cox, M., & Cox, R. Play and social interaction in children following divorce. *Journal of Social Issues*, 1979, *35*, 26–49.

Hill, C. J. S. The mother on the pediatric ward: Insider or outlawed? *Pediatric Nursing*, 1978, *4*, 26–29.

Hofmann, A. D., Becker, R. D., & Gabriel, H. P. *The hospitalized adolescent: A guide to managing the ill and injured youth*. New York: Free Press, 1976.

Hollenbeck, A. R., Susman, E. J., Nannis, E. D., Strope, B. E., Hersh, S. P., Levine, A. S., & Pizzo, P. A. Children with serious illness: Behavioral correlates of separation and isolation. *Child Psychiatry and Human Development*, 1980, *11*, 3–11.

Holt, J. L. Children's recall of a pre-school age hospital experience after an interval of five years (Doctoral dissertation, University of Pittsburgh, 1967). *Dissertation Abstracts*, 1968, *28*, 3352-B. (University Microfilms No. 68-1979)

Holt, J. L. Discussion of the method and the clinical implications from the study "Children's recall of a preschool age hospital experience after an interval of five years." *Communicating Nursing Research*, 1968, *1*, 56–72.

Howe, J. Children's ideas about injury. *ANA Clinical Regional Conferences, 1967, Philadelphia/Kansas City*. New York: Appleton-Century-Crofts, 1968, 189–195.

Hunt, G. M. Implications of the treatment of myelomeningocele for the child and his family. *Lancet*, 1973, *2*, 1308–1310.

Hymovich, D. P. The pediatric nursing role as perceived by nursing personnel and four- to eight-year-old hospitalized children (Doctoral dissertation, University of Maryland, 1973). *Dissertation Abstracts International*, 1974, *34*, 5534–5535-B. (University Microfilms No. 74-9800)

Hyson, M. C. Going to the doctor: A developmental study of stress and coping. *Journal of Child Psychology and Psychiatry*, 1983, *24*, 247–259.

Hyson, M. C., Snyder, S. S., & Andujar, E. M. Helping children cope with checkups: How good is the "good patient"? *Children's Health Care*, 1982, *10*, 139–144.

Irwin, E. C., & Kovacs, A. Analysis of children's drawings and stories. *Journal of the Association for the Care of Children in Hospitals*, 1979, *8*, 39–48.

Jackson, D. W. The adolescent and the hospital. *Pediatric Clinics of North America* 1973, *20*, 901–910.

Jackson, K. Psychologic preparation as a method of reducing the emotional trauma of anesthesia in children. *Anesthesiology*, 1951, *12*, 293–300.

Jackson, K., Winkley, R., Faust, O. A., Cermak, E. G., & Burtt, M. M. Behavior changes indicating emotional trauma in tonsillectomized children. *Pediatrics*. 1953, *12*, 23–27.

Jackson, P. B., Bradham, R. F., & Burwell, H. K. Child care in the hospital: A parent/staff partnership. *MCN: American Journal of Maternal Child Nursing*, 1978, *3*, 104–107.

James, V. L., & Wheeler, W. E. The care-by-parent unit. *Pediatrics*, 1969, *43*, 488–494.

Janis, I. L. *Psychological stress*. New York: Wiley, 1958.

Jessner, L., Blom, G. E., & Waldfogel, S. Emotional implications of tonsillectomy and adenoidectomy in children. In R. S. Eissler, A. Freud, M. Kris, & A. Solnit (Eds.), *The psychoanalytic study of the child*. New York: International Universities Press, 1952.

Johnson, J. E., & Dabbs, J. M. Enumeration of active sweat glands: A simple physiological indicator of psychological changes. *Nursing Research*, 1967, *16*, 273–275.

Johnson, J. E., Kirchhoff, K. T., & Endress, M. P. Altering children's distress behavior during orthopedic cast removal. *Nursing Research*, 1975, *24*, 404–410.

Johnson, P. A., & Stockdale, D. F. Effects of puppet therapy on palmar sweating of hospitalized children. *Johns Hopkins Medical Journal*, 1975, *137*, 1–5.

Johnson, R., & Baldwin, D. C. Relationship of maternal anxiety to the behavior of young children undergoing dental extraction. *Journal of Dental Research*, 1968, *47*, 801–805.

Johnson, R., & Baldwin, D. C. Maternal anxiety and child behavior. *Journal of Dentistry for Children*, 1969, *36*, 13–18.

Johnson, R., & Machen, J. B. Behavior modification techniques and maternal anxiety. *Journal of Dentistry for Children*, 1973, *40*, 272–276.

Kaplan, S., Achtel, R. H., & Callison, C. B. Psychiatric complications following open-heart surgery. *Heart and Lung*, 1974, *3*, 423–428.

Kaplan, S. L., Rosenstein, J., Skomorowsky, P., Shenker, I. R., & Ramsey, P. The hospitalized adolescent interaction scale: An instrument to measure patient behavior on an adolescent medicine ward. *Journal of Adolescent Health Care*, 1981, *2*, 101–105.

Kashani, J. H., Hodges, K. K., Simonds, J. F., & Hilderbrand, E. Life events and hospitalization in children: A comparison with a general population. *British Journal of Psychiatry*, 1981, *139*, 221–225.

Kay, B. Outpatient anaesthesia, especially for children. *Acta Anaesthesiologica Scandinavica*, 1966, *25* (Supp.), 421–425.

Kessler, E. R. A comparative analysis of distress among mothers of hospitalized two through four year old children and its relation to social class membership

(Doctoral dissertation, New York University, 1969). *Dissertation Abstracts International*, 1969, *30*, 2771–2772-B. (University Microfilms No. 69-21215)

Kister, M. C., & Patterson, C. J. Children's conceptions of the causes of illness: Understanding of contagion and use of immanent justice. *Child Development*, 1980, *51*, 839–846.

Klinzing, D. R., Klinzing, D. G., & Schindler, P. D. A preliminary report of a methodology to assess the communicative interaction between hospital personnel and hospitalized children. *American Journal of Public Health*, 1977, *67*, 670–672.

Klorman, R., Hilpert, P. L., Michael, R., LaGana, C., & Sveen, O. B. Effects of coping and mastery modeling on experienced and inexperienced pedodontic patients' disruptiveness. *Behavior Therapy*, 1980, *11*, 156–168.

Klorman, R., Michael, R., Hilpert, P. L., & Sveen, O. B. A further assessment of predictors of the child's behavior in dental treatment. *Journal of Dental Research*, 1979, *58*, 2338–2343.

Knafl, K. A. Parents' views of the response of siblings to a pediatric hospitalization. *Research in Nursing and Health*, 1982, *5*, 13–20.

Knafl, K. A., & Dixon, D. M. The role of siblings during pediatric hospitalization. *Issues in Comprehensive Pediatric Nursing*, 1983, *6*, 13–22.

Knight, R. B. Coping mechanisms used by children hospitalized for elective surgery (Doctoral dissertation, Yeshiva University, 1977). *Dissertation Abstracts International*, 1978, *38*, 4465-B. (University Microfilms No. 77-32520)

Knight, R. B., Atkins, A., Eagle, C. J., Evans, N., Finkelstein, J. W., Fukushima, D., Katz, J., & Weiner, H. Psychological stress, ego defenses, and cortisol production in children hospitalized for elective surgery. *Psychosomatic Medicine*, 1979, *41*, 40–49.

Knight, R. B., Atkins, A., Eagle, C., Evans, N., Finkelstein, J. W., Fukushima, D., & Weiner, H. A study of the coping mechanisms used by children undergoing elective surgery in the hospital. *Psychosomatic Medicine*, 1977, *39*, 56.

Koenigsberg, S. R., & Johnson, R. Child behavior during sequential dental visits. *Journal of the American Dental Association*, 1972, *85*, 128–132.

Kornfeld, D., Zimberg, S., & Malm, J. Psychiatric complications of open-heart surgery. *New England Journal of Medicine*, 1965, *273*, 287–292.

Korsch, B. M., Gozzi, E. K., & Francis, V. Gaps in doctor-patient communication: I. Doctor-patient interaction and patient satisfaction. *Pediatrics*, 1968, *42*, 855–871.

Kramer, M., Chamorro, I., Green, D., & Knudtson, F. Extra tactile stimulation of the premature infant. *Nursing Research*, 1975, *24*, 324–334.

Kueffner, M. Passage through hospitalization of severely burned isolated school-age children. *Communicating Nursing Research*, 1975, *7*, 181–197.

Kueffner, M. C. A qualitative study of the passage through hospitalization of severely burned, isolated school-age children (Doctoral dissertation, University of California, San Francisco, 1973). *Dissertation Abstracts International*, 1975, *35*, 4520-B. (University Microfilms No. 75-2498)

Kuhn, I. F. Children's psychological preparation for surgery: A comparison of child-oriented, parent-oriented, and joint-preparation techniques (Doctoral dissertation, Auburn University, 1980). *Dissertation Abstracts International,* 1981, *41,* 3895-B. (University Microfilms No. 81-07123)

Lampe, J, Trause, M. A., & Kennell, J. Parental visiting of sick infants: The effect of living at home prior to hospitalization. *Pediatrics,* 1977, *59,* 294–296.

Landes, H. R. Treatment of anxiety in the families of children undergoing tonsillectomy (Doctoral dissertation, Northwestern University, 1973). *Dissertation Abstracts International,* 1973, *34,* 2938-B. (University Microfilms No. 73-30640)

Larsen, C. A. The child life professions: Today and tomorrow. In *Child life activities: An overview.* Washington, D.C.: Association for the Care of Children's Health, 1980.

Lasater, K. L., & Grisanti, D. J. Postcardiotomy psychosis: Indications and interventions. *Heart and Lung,* 1975, *4,* 724–729.

Laurendeau, M., & Pinard, A. *Causal thinking in the child.* New York: International Universities Press, 1962.

Lavigne, J. V. The pediatric hospital staff's knowledge of normal adolescent development. *Journal of Pediatric Psychology,* 1977, *2,* 98–100.

Lavigne, J. V., & Ryan, M. Psychologic adjustment of siblings of children with chronic illness. *Pediatrics,* 1979, *63,* 616–627.

Lee, J. S., & Greene, N. M. Parental presence and emotional state of children prior to surgery. *Clinical Pediatrics,* 1969, *8,* 126–130.

Lehman, E. J. The effects of rooming-in and anxiety on the behavior of preschool children during hospitalization and followup (Doctoral dissertation, Cornell University, 1975). *Dissertation Abstracts International,* 1975, *36,* 3052-B. (University Microfilms No. 75-27037)

Lende, E. W. The effect of preparation on children's response to tonsillectomy and adenoidectomy surgery. (Doctoral dissertation, University of Cincinnati, 1971). *Dissertation Abstracts International,* 1971, *32,* 3642-B. (University Microfilms No. 72-1440)

Lerner, M. J., Haley, J. V., Hall, D. S., & McVarish, D. Hospital care-by-parent: An evaluative look. *Medical Care,* 1972, *10,* 430–436.

Levenson, P. M., Pfefferbaum, B. J., Copeland, D. R., & Silberberg, Y. Information preferences of cancer patients ages 11–20 years. *Journal of Adolescent Health Care,* 1982, *3,* 9–13.

Levenson, P. M., Pfefferbaum, B., & Overall, J. E. A factor analysis of the informational concerns of adolescent cancer patients. *Children's Health Care,* 1983, *11,* 148–153.

Levenson, P. M., Pfefferbaum, B., Silberberg, Y., & Copeland, D. R. Sources of information about cancer as perceived by adolescent patients, parents, and physicians. *Patient Counselling and Health Education,* 1981, *3,* 71–76.

Levy, D. M. The infant's earliest memory of inoculation: A contribution to public health procedures. *Journal of Genetic Psychology,* 1960, *96;* 3–46.

Lewandowski, L. A. Stresses and coping styles of parents of children undergoing open-heart surgery. *Critical Care Quarterly,* 1980, *3,* 75–84.

Lincoln, L. Effects of illness and hospital procedures on body image in adolescents: A review of the literature. *Maternal-Child Nursing Journal,* 1978, *7,* 55–60.

Lindheim, R., Glaser, H. H., & Coffin, C. *Changing hospital environments for children.* Cambridge, Mass.: Harvard University Press, 1972.

Lockwood, N. L. The effects of situational doll play upon the preoperative stress reactions of hospitalized children. *ANA Clinical Sessions, Miami.* New York: Appleton-Century-Crofts, 1970, 133–120.

Lord, R., & Schowalter, J. Visiting on an adolescent ward. *Journal of the Association for the Care of Children in Hospitals,* 1979, *8,* 5–9.

Lord, R., & Schowalter, J. E. A ten-year comparison of fathers' and mothers' reactions toward their hospitalized adolescents. *Children's Health Care,* 1982, *10,* 87–89.

Louis, M., & Lovejoy, F. H. Adolescent attitudes in a general pediatric hospital: A survey of 87 inpatient admissions. *American Journal of Diseases of Children,* 1975, *129,* 1046–1049.

MacDonald. E. M. Parents participate in care of the hospitalized child. *Canadian Nurse,* 1969, *65,* 37–39.

Machen, J. B., & Johnson, R. Desensitization, model learning, and the dental behavior of children. *Journal of Dental Research,* 1974, *53,* 83–87.

Mahaffy, P. R. The effects of hospitalization on children admitted for tonsillectomy and adenoidectomy. *Nursing Research,* 1965, *14,* 12–19.

Mahon, B. F. Adaptive personality traits as predictors of physical recovery rate and psychological state following surgery for adolescent idiopathic scoliosis (Doctoral dissertation, New York University, 1980). *Dissertation Abstracts International,* 1981, *41,* 3186-B. (University Microfilms No. 80-27463)

Mason, W. A. Determinants of social behavior in young chimpanzees. In A. M. Schier, H. F. Harlow, & F. Stollnitz (Eds.), *Behavior of nonhuman primates* (*Vol. 2*). New York: Academic Press, 1965.

Mather, P. L., & Glasrud, P. H. Child life workers: Who are they and what are they doing? *Children's Health Care,* 1981, *10,* 11–15.

Mattsson, A., & Weisberg, I. Behavioral reactions to minor illness in preschool children. *Pediatrics,* 1970, *46,* 604–610.

May, J. G. A psychiatric study of a pediatric intensive therapy unit. *Clinical Pediatrics,* 1972, *11,* 76–82.

McCaffery, M. Children's responses to rectal temperatures: An exploratory study. *Nursing Research,* 1971, *20,* 32–45.

McCain, G. C. Parent created recordings for hospitalized children. *Children's Health Care,* 1982, *10,* 104–105.

McCollum, A. T., & Schwartz, A. H. Pediatric research hospitalization: Its meaning to parents. *Pediatric Research,* 1969, *3,* 199–204.

McCue, K., Wagner, M., Hansen, H., & Rigler, D. A survey of a developing health care profession: Hospital "play" programs. *Journal of the Association for the Care of Children in Hospitals,* 1978, *7,* 15–22.

:uddy, M. C. A study of the relationship between mothers' rooming-in ...ng their children's hospitalization and changes in selected areas of children's behavior (Doctoral dissertation, New York University, 1976). *Dissertation Abstracts International,* 1976, *37,* 700-B. (University Microfilms No. 76-19034)

McGrath, M. M. Group preparation of pediatric surgical patients. *Image,* 1979, *11,* 52–63.

McKeever, D. A., III. Religious ideation in selected hospitalized children (Doctoral dissertation, Southern Baptist Theological Seminary, 1974). *Dissertation Abstracts International,* 1974, *35,* 2385–2386-A. (University Microfilms No. 74-22661)

McTigue, D. J., & Pinkham, J. Association between children's dental behavior and play behavior. *Journal of Dentistry for Children,* 1978, *45,* 218–222.

Melamed, B. G., Bennett, C. G., Jerrell, G., Ross, S. L., Bush, J. P., Hill, C., Courts, F., & Ronk, S. Dentists' behavior management as it affects compliance and fear in pediatric patients. *Journal of the American Dental Association,* 1983, *106,* 324–330.

Melamed, B. G., Dearborn, M., & Hermecz, D. A. Necessary considerations for surgery preparation: Age and previous experience. *Psychosomatic Medicine,* 1983, *45,* 517–525.

Melamed, B. G., Hawes, R. R., Heiby, E., & Glick, J. Use of filmed modeling to reduce uncooperative behavior of children during dental treatment. *Journal of Dental Research,* 1975, *54,* 797–801.

Melamed, B. G., Meyer, R., Gee, C., & Soule, L. The influence of time and type of preparation on children's adjustment to hospitalization. *Journal of Pediatric Psychology,* 1976, *1,* 31–37.

Melamed, B. G., & Siegel, L. J. Reduction of anxiety in children facing hospitalization and surgery by use of filmed modeling. *Journal of Consulting and Clinical Psychology,* 1975, *43,* 511–521.

Melamed, B. G., Weinstein, D., Hawes, R., & Katin-Borland, M. Reduction of fear-related dental management problems with use of filmed modeling. *Journal of the American Dental Association,* 1975, *90,* 822–826.

Melamed, B. G., Yurcheson, R., Fleece, E. L., Hutcherson, S., & Hawes, R. Effects of film modeling on the reduction of anxiety-related behaviors in individuals varying in level of previous experience in the stress situation. *Journal of Consulting and Clinical Psychology,* 1978, *46,* 1357–1367.

Meng, A. L. Parents' and children's reactions toward impending hospitalization for surgery. *Maternal-Child Nursing Journal,* 1980, *9,* 83–98.

Meng, A., & Zastowny, T. Preparation for hospitalization: A stress inoculation training program for parents and children. *Maternal-Child Nursing Journal,* 1982, *11,* 87–94.

Menke, E. M. Factors related to children's perception of stress in the hospital (Doctoral dissertation, Ohio State University, 1972). *Dissertation Abstracts International,* 1973, *33,* 4093-A. (University Microfilms No. 73-2070)

Menke, E. M. School-aged children's perceptions of stress in the hospital. *Children's Health Care,* 1981, *9,* 80–86.

Merrow, D. L., & Johnson, B. S. Perceptions of the mother's role with her hospitalized child. *Nursing Research*, 1968, *17*, 155–156.

Meyers, E. F., & Muravchick, S. Anesthesia induction technics in pediatric patients: A controlled study of behavioral consequences. *Anesthesia and Analgesia*, 1977, *56*, 538–542.

Miles, M. S., & Carter, M. C. Sources of parental stress in pediatric intensive care units. *Children's Health Care*, 1982, *11*, 65–69.

Millstein, S. G., Adler, N. E., & Irwin, C. E. Conceptions of illness in young adolescents. *Pediatrics*, 1981, *68*, 834–839.

Milosavljević, L., Kondić-Petrović, K., & Pjanović, Z. Pre- and post-operative anxiety in children. In A. L. Annell (Ed.), *Depressive states in childhood and adolescence*. New York: Halsted Press, 1972.

Minde, K., & Maler, L. Psychiatric counseling on a pediatric medical ward: A controlled evaluation. *Journal of Pediatrics*, 1968, *72*, 452-460.

Myers-Vando, R., Steward, M. S., Folkins, C. H., & Hines, P. The effects of congenital heart disease on cognitive development, illness causality concepts, and vulnerability. *American Journal of Orthopsychiatry*, 1979, *49*, 617–625.

Natapoff, J. N. Children's views of health: A developmental study. *American Journal of Public Health*, 1978, *68*, 995–1000.

Neuhauser, C., Amsterdam, B., Hines, P., & Steward, M. Children's concepts of healing: Cognitive development and locus of control factors. *American Journal of Orthopsychiatry*, 1978, *48*, 335–341.

Nocella, J., & Kaplan, R. M. Training children to cope with dental treatment. *Journal of Pediatric Psychology*, 1982, *7*, 175–178.

Nurse, R., & Deber, R. Conquering fear of surgery. *Dimensions in Health Service*, 1982, *59*, 34–36.

O'Donnell, R. L. The psychological effects of childhood hospitalization: Implications for pediatric health care delivery (Doctoral dissertation, University of Iowa, 1976). *Dissertation Abstracts International*, 1978, *38*, 3121–3122-B. (University Microfilms No. 77-28498)

Oelberg, D. G., & Finkelstein, J. W. Hospitalization of adolescents: Collecting the data base. *Journal of Adolescent Health Care*, 1981, *1*, 283–288.

Pantell, R. H., Stewart, T. J., Dias, J. K., Wells, P., & Ross, A. W. Physician communication with children and parents. *Pediatrics*, 1982, *70*, 396–402.

Parcel, G. S., Nader, P. R., & Meyer, M. P. Adolescent health concerns, problems, and patterns of utilization in a triethnic urban population. *Pediatrics*, 1977, *60*, 157–164.

Parker, G., & Gibson, C. Development of the hospitalized adolescent anxiety tool. *Journal of Psychiatric Nursing and Mental Health Services*, 1977, *15*, 21–24.

Pearson, J. E. R., Cataldo, M., Tureman, A., Bessman, C., & Rogers, M. C. Pediatric intensive care unit patients: Effects of play intervention on behavior. *Critical Care Medicine*, 1980, *8*, 64–67.

Penticuff, J. H. The effect of filmed peer modeling, cognitive appraisal, and autonomic reactivity in changing children's attitudes about health care procedures and personal (Doctoral dissertation, Case Western Reserve University, 1976). *Dissertation Abstracts International*, 1976, *37*, 3089-B. (University Microfilms No. 76-28404)

Perrin, E. C., & Gerrity, P. S. There's a demon in your belly: Children's understanding of illness. *Pediatrics*, 1981, *67*, 841–849.

Perrin, E. C., & Perrin, J. M. Clinicians' assessments of children's understanding of illness. *American Journal of Diseases of Children*, 1983, *137*, 874–878.

Peters, B. M. Concepts of hospitalized children about causality of illness and intent of treatment (Doctoral dissertation, University of Pittsburgh, 1975). *Dissertation Abstracts International*, 1976, *36*, 6074-B. (University Microfilms No. 76-14158)

Peters, B. M. School-aged children's beliefs about causality of illness: A review of the literature. *Maternal-Child Nursing Journal*, 1978, *7*, 143–154.

Peterson, E. T. The impact of adolescent illness on parental relationships. *Journal of Health and Social Behavior*, 1972, *13*, 429–437.

Peterson, L. The use of a self-control procedure to minimize pain and anxiety in hospitalized children (Doctoral dissertation, University of Utah, 1978). *Dissertation Abstracts International*, 1978, *39*, 3000-B. (University Microfilms No. 78-22817)

Peterson, L., Hartmann, D. P., & Gelfand, D. M. Prevention of child behavior disorders: A lifestyle change for child psychologists. In P. Davidson & S. Davidson (Eds.), *Behavior medicine: Changing health lifestyles*. New York: Brunner/Mazel, 1979.

Peterson, L., & Ridley-Johnson, R. Pediatric hospital responses to survey on prehospital preparation for children. *Journal of Pediatric Psychology*, 1980, *5*, 1–7.

Peterson, L., & Shigetomi, C. One-year follow-up of elective surgery child patients receiving preoperative preparation. *Journal of Pediatric Psychology*, 1982, *7*, 43–48.

Peterson, L., & Shigetomi, C. The use of coping techniques to minimize anxiety in hospitalized children. *Behavior Therapy*, 1981, *12*, 1–14.

Pfefferbaum, B., & Levenson, P. M. Adolescent cancer patient and physician responses to a questionnaire on patient concerns. *American Journal of Psychiatry*, 1982, *139*, 348–351.

Piaget, J. *The moral judgment of the child*. New York: Free Press, 1964.

Piaget, J. *Play, dreams, and imitation in childhood*. New York: Norton, 1962.

Pidgeon, V. A. Children's concepts of the rationale of isolation technic. *ANA clinical sessions, 1966, San Francisco*. New York: Appleton-Century-Crofts, 1967, 21–27.

Pidgeon, V. A. Functions and content of verbal contacts initiated by disadvantaged and advantaged preschool children with adults in a hospital (Doctoral dissertation, University of Pittsburgh, 1974a). *Dissertation Abstracts International*, 1974, *34*, 5041-B. (University Microfilms No. 74-8696)

Pidgeon, V. A. Functions and content of verbal contacts initiated by disadvantaged and advantaged preschool children with adults in a hospital.

Maternal-Child Nursing Journal, 1974b, *3*(4, Monograph #3).

Pinkham, J. R., & Kerber, P. E. Association between school-age children's dental behavior and play behavior. *Pediatric Dentistry*, 1979, *1*, 221–225.

Porter, C. S. Grade school children's perceptions of their internal body parts. *Nursing Research*, 1974, *23*, 384–391.

Porter, L. S. Health care workers' role conceptions and orientation to family-centered child care. *Nursing Research*, 1979, *28*, 330–337.

Porter, L. S. The impact of physical-physiological activity on infants' growth and development. *Nursing Research*, 1972, *21*, 210–219.

Post, S. Trends in peadiatric hospitals (sic). *Dimensions in Health Service*, 1979, *56*, 51–53.

Powazek, M., Goff, J. R., Schyving, J., & Paulson, M. A. Emotional reactions of children to isolation in a cancer hospital. *Journal of Pediatrics*, 1978, *92*, 834–837.

Prugh, D. G., Staub, E., Sands, H. H., Kirschbaum, R. M., & Lenihan, E. A. A study of the emotional reactions of children and families to hospitalization and illness. *American Journal of Orthopsychiatry*, 1953, *23*, 70–106.

Quiggin, V. Children's knowledge of their internal body parts. *Nursing Times*, 1977, *73*, 1146–1151.

Quinton, D., & Rutter, M. Early hospital admissions and later disturbances of behaviour: An attempted replication of Douglas' findings. *Developmental Medicine and Child Neurology*, 1976, *18*, 447–459.

Rausch, P. B. Effects of tactile and kinesthetic stimulation on premature infants. *Journal of Obstetric, Gynecologic, and Neonatal Nursing*, 1981, *10*, 34–37.

Resnick, M., Blum, R. W., & Hedin, D. The appropriateness of health services for adolescents. *Journal of Adolescent Health Care*, 1980, *1*, 137–141.

Resnick, R., & Hergenroeder, E. Children and the emergency room. *Children Today*, 1975, *4*, 5–8.

Richter, H. G. Emotional disturbance of constant pattern following nonspecific respiratory infections. *Journal of Pediatrics*, 1943, *23*, 315–325.

Ricks, F., & Faubert, T. Canadian child life/non-medical programs in hospitals. *Children's Health Care*, 1981, *10*, 16–19.

Riddle, I. I. Communicative behaviors of hospitalized school age children with binocular bandages. *Maternal-Child Nursing Journal*, 1972, *1*, 291–354.

Rie, H. E., Boverman, H., Grossman, B. J., & Ozoa, N. Immediate and long-term effects of interventions early in prolonged hospitalization. *Pediatrics*, 1968, *41*, 755–764.

Rieveschl, J. L. Regression in spatial and affective role-taking skill and its implications for young tonsillectomy patients (Doctoral dissertation, University of Michigan, 1979). *Dissertation Abstracts International*, 1979, *40*, 2385-B. (University Microfilms No. 79-25216)

Riffee, D. M. Self-esteem changes in hospitalized school-age children. *Nursing Research*, 1981, *30*, 94–97.

Rigg, C. A., & Fisher, R. C. Is a separate adolescent ward worthwhile? *American Journal of Diseases of Children*, 1971, *122*, 489–493.

Rigg, C. A., & Fisher, R. C. Some comments on current hospital medical services for adolescents. *American Journal of Diseases of Children*, 1970, *120*, 193–196.

Roberts, M. C., Wurtele, S. K., Boone, R. R., Ginther, L. J., & Elkins, P. D. Reduction of medical fears by use of modeling: A preventive application in a general population of children. *Journal of Pediatric Psychology*, 1981, *6*, 293–300.

Robinson, D. Illness behaviour and children's hospitalization: A schema of parents' attitudes toward authority. *Social Science and Medicine*, 1972, *6*, 447–468.

Robinson, D. Mothers' fear, their children's well-being in hospital, and the study of illness behaviour. *British Journal of Preventive and Social Medicine*, 1968, *22*, 228–233.

Robinson, D. The social milieu. In M. Stacey (Ed.), *Hospitals, children and their families: The report of a pilot study*. London: Routledge & Kegan Paul, 1970.

Rose, M. H. The effects of hospitalization on the coping behaviors of children. In M. V. Batey (Ed.), *Communicating nursing research*. Boulder, Colorado: Western Interstate Commission for Higher Education, 1972.

Roskies, E., Bedard, P., Gauvreau-Guilbault, H., & LaFortune, D. Emergency hospitalization of young children: Some neglected psychological considerations. *Medical Care*, 1975, *13*, 570–581.

Roskies, E., Mongeon, M., & Gagnon-Lefebvre, B. Increasing maternal participation in the hospitalization of young children. *Medical Care*, 1978, *16*, 765–777.

Rothbaum, F., Wolfer, J., & Visintainer, M. Coping behavior and locus of control in children. *Journal of Personality*, 1979, *47*, 118–135.

Rothstein, P. Family reaction to acute overwhelming illness in children. *Critical Care Medicine*, 1979, *7*, 130.

Rothstein, P. Psychological stress in families of children in a pediatric intensive care unit. *Pediatric Clinics of North America*, 1980, *27*, 613–620.

Roy, M. C. Role cues and mothers of hospitalized children. *Nursing Research*, 1967, *16*, 178–182.

Roy, C. Role cues for the mother of the hospitalized child. *ANA clinical sessions, 1968, Dallas*. New York: Appleton-Century-Crofts, 1968, 199–206.

Rumfelt, J. J. M. How five year old children perceive the role of the nurse. *Maternal-Child Nursing Journal*, 1980, *9*, 13–24.

Rutkowski, J. A survey of child life programs. *Journal of the Association for the Care of Children in Hospitals*, 1978, *6*, 11–16.

Rutter, B. A. Children's beliefs about the locus of control in illness situations. (Doctoral dissertation, University of Minnesota, 1970). *Dissertation Abstracts International*, 1970, *31*, 3006-B. (University Microfilms No. 70-20233)

Sackett, G. P. Measurement in observational research. In G. P. Sackett (Ed.), *Observing behavior, Vol. II*. Baltimore: University Park Press, 1978.

Sauer, J. E. Preadmission orientation: Effect on patient manageability. *Hospital Topics*, 1968, *46*, 79–83.

Savedra, M. Parental responses to a painful procedure performed on their child. In P. Azarnoff & C. Hardgrove (Eds.), *The family in child health care*. New York: John Wiley & Sons, 1981.

Savedra, M., & Tesler, M. Coping strategies of hospitalized school-age children. *Western Journal of Nursing Research,* 1981, *3,* 371–384.

Savedra, M., Tesler, M., Ward, J., Wegner, C., & Gibbons, P. Description of the pain experience: A study of school-age children. *Issues in Comprehensive Pediatric Nursing,* 1981, *5,* 373–380.

Sawtell, R. O., Simon, J. F., & Simeonsson, R. J. The effects of five preparatory methods upon child behavior during the first dental visit. *Journal of Dentistry for Children,* 1974, *41,* 367–375.

Scarr-Salapatek, S., & Williams, M. L. The effects of early stimulation on low-birth-weight infants. *Child Development,* 1973, *44,* 94–101.

Schachter, S. *The psychology of affiliation.* Stanford: Stanford University Press, 1959.

Schaffer, H. R. Activity level as a constitutional determinant of infantile reaction to deprivation. *Child Development,* 1966, *37,* 595–602.

Schmeltz, K., & White, G. A survey of parent groups: Prehospital admission. *Maternal-Child Nursing Journal,* 1982, *11,* 75–86.

Schowalter, J. E. Psychological reactions to physical illness and hospitalization in adolescence. *Journal of the American Academy of Child Psychiatry,* 1977, *16,* 500–516.

Schowalter, J. E., & Anyan, W. R. Experience on an adolescent inpatient division. *American Journal of Diseases of Children,* 1973, *125,* 212–215.

Schowalter, J. E., & Lord, R. D. Admission to an adolescent ward. *Pediatrics,* 1969, *44,* 1009–1011.

Schrier, A., & Kaplan, D. The effectiveness of a preoperation preparation program in reducing anxiety in children. *Children's Health Care,* 1983, *11,* 142–147.

Schulman, J. L., Foley, J. M., Vernon, D. T. A., & Allen, D. A study of the effect of the mother's presence during anesthesia induction. *Pediatrics,* 1967, *39,* 111–114.

Schulman, J. L., Kaspar, J. C., & Child, D. Videotape sampling of the child's day in the hospital. *The Journal of Pediatrics,* 1970, *76,* 728–731.

Schultz, T. R. Play as arousal modification. In B. Sutton-Smith (Ed.), *Play and learning.* New York: Gardner Press, 1979.

Schulz, J. B., Raschke, D., Dedrick, C., & Thompson, M. The effects of a preoperational puppet show on the anxiety levels of hospitalized children. *Children's Health Care,* 1981, *9,* 118–121.

Schwab, F., Tolbert, B., Bagnato, S., & Maisels, M. J. Sibling visiting in a neonatal intensive care unit. *Pediatrics,* 1983, *71,* 835–838.

Schwartz, A. H. Children's concepts of research hospitalization. *New England Journal of Medicine,* 1972, *287,* 589–592.

Schwartz, B. H., Albino, J. E., & Tedesco, L. A. Effects of psychological preparation on children hospitalized for dental operations. *Journal of Pediatrics,* 1983, *102,* 634–638.

Seidl, F. W. Pediatric nursing personnel and parent participation. *Nursing Research,* 1969, *18,* 40–44.

Seidl, F. W., & Pillitteri, A. Development of an attitude scale on parent participation. *Nursing Research,* 1967, *16,* 71–73.

Sermet, O. Emotional and medical factors in child dental anxiety. *Journal of*

Child Psychology and Psychiatry, 1974, *15*, 313–321.

Shade-Zeldow, Y. Attachment and separation: The effects of hospitalization on pediatric patients (Doctoral dissertation, Purdue University, 1976). *Dissertation Abstracts International*, 1977, *37*, 5376-B. (University Microfilms No. 77-7526)

Shanley, P. J. The effects of maternal attendance in the care of young hospitalized children with a diagnosis of cancer (Doctoral dissertation, Columbia University Teachers College, 1981). *Dissertation Abstracts International*, 1981, *42*, 1823-B. (University Microfilms No. 81-23291)

Shapiro, R. Psychological sequalae of childhood cancer and heart surgery (Doctoral dissertation, Ohio State University, 1977). *Dissertation Abstracts International, 1978, 38, 5549-B. (University Microfilms No. 78-06200*

Shaw, E. G., & Routh, D. K. Effect of mother presence on children's reactions to aversive procedures. *Journal of Pediatric Psychology*, 1982, *7*, 33–42.

Shrand, H. Behavior changes in sick children nursed at home. *Pediatrics*, 1965, *36*, 604–607.

Shuler, S. N., & Reich, C. A. Sibling visitation in pediatric hospitals: Policies, opinions, and issues. *Children's Health Care*, 1982, *11*, 54–60.

Sibinga, M. S., & Friedman, C. J. Restraint and speech. *Pediatrics*, 1971, *48*, 116–122.

Sibinga, M. S., Friedman, C. J., Steisel, I. M., & Sinnamon, H. M. The effect of immobilization and sensory restriction on children with phenylketonuria. *Pediatric Research*, 1968, *2* 371–377.

Sides, J. P. Emotional responses of children to physical illness and hospitalization (Doctoral dissertation, Auburn University, 1977). *Dissertation Abstracts International*, 1978, *38*, 917-B. (University Microfilms No. 77-16832)

Siegel, L. J. Preparation of children for hospitalization: A selected review of the research literature. *Journal of Pediatric Psychology*, 1976, *1*, 26–30.

Siegel, L. J. Reduction of anxiety in children facing hospitalization and surgery by use of filmed modeling (Doctoral dissertation, Case Western Reserve University, 1975). *Dissertation Abstracts International*, 1975, *36*, 3071–3072-B. (University Microfilms No. 75-27964)

Siegel, L. J., & Peterson, L. Maintenance effects of coping skills and sensory information on young children's responses to repeated dental procedures. *Behavior Therapy*, 1981, *12*, 530–535.

Siegel, L. J., & Peterson, L. Stress reduction in young dental patients through coping skills and sensory information. *Journal of Consulting and Clinical Psychology*, 1980, *48*, 785–787.

Simeonsson, R. J., Buckley, L., & Monson, L. Conceptions of illness causality in hospitalized children. *Journal of Pediatric Psychology*, 1979, *4*, 77–83.

Simeonsson, R. J., & McHale, S. M. Research on handicapped children: Sibling relationships. *Child: Care, Health, and Development*, 1981, *7*, 153–171.

Simons, B., Bradshaw, J., & Silva, P. A. Hospital admissions during the first five years of life: A report from the Dunedin multidisciplinary child development study. *New Zealand Medical Journal*, 1980, *91*, 144–147.

Sines, J. O., Pauker, J. D., & Sines, L. K. *The Missouri children's picture series manual.*

Iowa City: Psychological Assessment & Services, 1974.

Singer, J. L. Television, imaginative play and cognitive development: Some problems and possibilities. Paper presented at the meeting of the American Psychological Association, San Francisco, 1977.

Sipowicz, R. R., & Vernon, D. T. A. Psychological responses of children to hospitalization. *American Journal of Diseases of Children,* 1965, *109,* 228–231.

Skipper, J. K. Mothers' distress over their children's hospitalization for tonsillectomy. *Journal of Marriage and the Family,* 1966, *28,* 145–151.

Skipper, J. K., & Leonard, R. C. Children, stress, and hospitalization: A field experiment. *Journal of Health and Social Behavior,* 1968, *9,* 275–287.

Skipper, J. K., Leonard, R. C., & Rhymes, J. Child hospitalization and social interaction: An experimental study of mothers' feelings of stress, adaptation and satisfaction. *Medical Care,* 1968, *6,* 496–506.

Smith, E. C. School-age children's concepts of body organs and illness. (Doctoral dissertation, University of Pittsburgh, 1973). *Dissertation Abstracts International,* 1973, *34,* 1167-B. (University Microfilms No. 73-21340)

Smith, J. C. Spending time with the hospitalized child. *MCN: American Journal of Maternal Child Nursing,* 1976, *1,* 164.

Spicher, C. M. Children's perceptions of their covered operative sites. *Maternal-Child Nursing Journal,* 1982, *11,* 181–192.

Spielberger, C. D., Gorsuch, R. L., & Luchene, R. E. *Test manual for the state-trait anxiety inventory.* Palo Alto: Consulting Psychologists Press, 1970.

Stacey, M. Dearden, R., Pill, R., & Robinson, D. (Eds). *Hospitals, children and their families.* London: Routledge & Kegan Paul, 1970.

Sternlieb, J. J., & Munan, L. A survey of health problems, practices, and needs of youth. *Pediatrics,* 1972, *49,* 177–186.

Steward, M., & Regalbuto, G. Do doctors know what children know? *American Journal of Orthopsychiatry,* 1975, *45,* 146–149.

Stocking, M., Rothney, W., Grosser, G., & Goodwin, R. Psychopathology in the pediatric hospital: Implications for community health. *American Journal of Public Health,* 1972, *62,* 551–556.

Stocking, M., Rothney, W., Grosser, G., & Goodwin, R. Psychopathology in the pediatric hospital: Implications for the pediatrician. *Psychiatry in Medicine,* 1970, *1,* 329–338.

Suran, B. G., & Lavigne, J. V. Rights of children in pediatric settings: A survey of attitudes. *Pediatrics,* 1977, *60,* 715–720.

Sutarman & Thomson, M. L. A new technique for enumerating active sweat glands in man. *Journal of Physiology,* 1952, *117,* 51–52.

Tarnow, J. D., & Gutstein, S. E. Children's preparatory behavior for elective surgery. *Journal of the American Academy of Child Psychiatry,* 1983, *22,* 365–369.

Taylor, F. L. Educational preparation for surgery: An examination of physical and behavioral parameters post-operatively (Doctoral dissertation, Case Western Reserve University, 1977). *Dissertation Abstracts International,* 1978, *38,* 6416-A. (University Microfilms No. 78-00555)

Taylor, P. L. Post-operative pain in toddler and pre-school age children. *Maternal Child Nursing Journal*, 1983, *12*, 35–50.

Taylor, S. C. The effects of chronic childhood illnesses upon well siblings. *Maternal Child Nursing Journal*, 1980, *9*, 109–116.

Tesler, M. D., Wegner, C., Savedra, M., Gibbons, P. T., & Ward, J. A. Coping strategies of children in pain. *Issues in Comprehensive Pediatric Nursing*, 1981, *5*, 351–359.

Tew, B., & Laurence, K. M. Mothers, brothers and sisters of patients with spina bifida. *Developmental Medicine and Child Neurology*, 1973, *15*, (Supp. 29) 69–76.

Thompson, R. H. An investigation of factors related to five-year-old children's psychological upset during an outpatient physical examination (Doctoral dissertation, University of Wisconsin-Madison, 1983). *Dissertation Abstracts International*, 1983, *44*, 2376B. (University Microfilms No. 83-16237)

Thompson, R. H., & Stanford, G. *Child life in hospitals: Theory and practice*. Springfield, Ill.: Charles C Thomas, 1981.

Thomson, E. Preop visits—for the nurse—for the patient? *AORN Journal*, 1972, *16*, 75–81.

Thomson, M. L., & Sutarman. The identification and enumeration of active sweat glands in man from plastic impressions of the skin. *Transactions of the Royal Society of Tropical Medicine and Hygiene*, 1953, *47*, 412–417.

Thornes, R. Parental access and family facilities in children's wards in England. *British Medical Journal*, 1983, *287*, 190–192.

Tisza, V. B., Hurwitz, I., & Angoff, K. The use of a play program by hospitalized children. *Journal of the American Academy of Child Psychiatry*, 1970, *9*, 515–531.

Tonkin, R. S., Ng, S. S. H., & Sheps, S. B. Hospitalization of adolescents in a new children's hospital. *Journal of Adolescent Health Care*, 1981, *1*, 202–207.

Torrance, J. T. *Children's reactions to intramuscular injections: A comparative study of needle and jet injections*. Cleveland: Case Western Reserve University (Francis Payne Bolton School of Nursing), 1968.

Trause, M. A., Voos, D., Rudd, C., Klaus, M., Kennell, J., & Boslett, M. Separation for childbirth: The effect on the sibling. *Child Psychiatry and Human Development*, 1981, *12*, 32–39.

Tsigounis, S. A. The relationship between parent-child perceptions of hospitalization and the child's subsequent psychological response (Doctoral dissertation, California School of Professional Psychology, 1977). *Dissertation Abstracts International*, 1978, *38*, 3915-B. (University Microfilms No. 77-32253)

Turiel, E. Developmental processes in the child's moral thinking. In P. Mussen, J. Langer, & M. Covington, (Eds.), *New directions in developmental psychology*. New York: Holt, Rinehart, & Winston, 1969.

Umphenour, J. H. Bacterial colonization in neonates with sibling visitation. *Journal of Obstetric, Gynecologic, and Neonatal Nursing*, 1980, *9*, 74–75.

Vardaro, J. A. Preadmission anxiety and mother-child relationships. *Journal of the Association for the Care of Children in Hospitals*, 1978, *7*, 8–15.

Vaughan, G. F. Children in hospital. *Lancet*, 1957, *272*, 1117–1120.

Venham, L. L., Murray, P., & Gaulin-Kremer, E. Child-rearing variables affecting the preschool child's response to dental stress. *Journal of Dental Research*, 1979a, *58*, 2042–2045.

Venham, L. L., Murray, P., & Gaulin-Kremer, E. Personality factors affecting the preschool child's response to dental stress. *Journal of Dental Research*, 1979b, *58*, 2046–2051.

Vermilion, B. D., Ballantine, T. V., & Grosfeld, J. L. The effective use of the parent care unit for infants on the surgical service. *Journal of Pediatric Surgery*, 1979, *14*, 321–324.

Vernon, D. T. A. Modeling and birth order in responses to painful stimuli. *Journal of Personality and Social Psychology*, 1974, *29*, 794–799.

Vernon, D. T. A. Use of modeling to modify children's responses to a natural, potentially stressful situation. *Journal of Applied Psychology*, 1973, *58*, 351–356.

Vernon, D. T. A., & Bailey, W. C. The use of motion pictures in the psychological preparation of children for induction of anesthesia. *Anesthesiology*, 1974, *40*, 68–72.

Vernon, D. T. A., Foley, J. M., & Schulman, J. L. Effects of mother-child separation and birth order on young children's responses to two potentially stressful experiences. *Journal of Personality and Social Psychology*, 1967, *5*, 162–174.

Vernon, D. T. A., Foley, J. M., Sipowicz, R. R., & Schulman, J. L. *The psychological responses of children to hospitalization and illness*. Springfield, Ill.: Charles C Thomas, 1965.

Vernon, D. T. A., Schulman, J. L., & Foley, J. M. Changes in children's behavior after hospitalization. *American Journal of Diseases of Children*, 1966, *111*, 581–593.

Visintainer, M. A., & Wolfer, J. A. Psychological preparation for surgical pediatric patients: The effect on children's and parents' stress responses and adjustment. *Pediatrics*, 1975, *56*, 187–202.

Vredevoe, D. L., Kim, A. C., Dambacher, B. M., & Call, J. D. Aggressive post-operative play responses of hospitalized preschool children. *Nursing Research Report*, 1969, *4*, 1,4–5.

Wälder, R. The psychoanalytic theory of play. *Psychoanalytic Quarterly*, 1933, *2*, 208–224.

Wallach, M. A., & Kogan, N. *Modes of thinking in young children*. New York: Holt, Rinehart, & Winston, 1965.

Weinick, H. M. Psychological study of emotional reactions of children to tonsillectomy (Doctoral dissertation, New York University, 1958). *Dissertation Abstracts*, 1959, *19*, 2140. (University Microfilms No. 58-07625)

Weinstein, P., Getz, T., Ratener, P., & Domoto, P. The effect of dentists' behaviors on fear-related behaviors in children. *Journal of the American Dental Association*, 1982a, *104*, 32–38.

Weinstein, P., Getz, T., Ratener, P., & Domoto, P. Dentists' responses to fear- and nonfear-related behaviors in children. 1982b, *104*, 38–40.

White, J. L., & Labarba, R. C. The effects of tactile and kinesthetic stimulation on neonatal development in the premature infant. *Developmental Psychobiology,* 1976, *9,* 569–577.

White, W. C., Akers, J., Green, J., & Yates, D. Use of imitation in the treatment of dental phobia in early childhood: A preliminary report. *Journal of Dentistry for Children,* 1974, *41,* 106–110.

Williams, P. D. Children's concepts of illness and internal body parts. *Maternal-Child Nursing Journal,* 1979, *8,* 115–123.

Williams, P. D. Preparation of school-age children for surgery: A program in preventive pediatrics—Philippines. *International Journal of Nursing Studies,* 1980, *17,* 107–119.

Williams, T. K. Infants' reactions to restraint of motility: A review of the literature. *Maternal-Child Nursing Journal,* 1973, *2,* 229–235.

Williams, Y. B., & Powell, M. Documenting the value of supervised play in a pediatric ambulatory care clinic. *Journal of the Association for the Care of Children's Health,* 1980, *9,* 15–20.

Winer, G. A. A review and analysis of children's fearful behavior in dental settings. *Child Development,* 1982, *53,* 1111–1133.

Wolfer, J., & Visintainer, M. *Preparation and hospitalized children's adjustment.* Unpublished manuscript, Yale University School of Nursing, 1974.

Wolfer, J. A., & Visintainer, M. A. Pediatric surgical patients' and parents' stress responses and adjustment. *Nursing Research,* 1975, *24,* 244–255.

Wolfer, J. A., & Visintainer, M. A. Prehospital psychological preparation for tonsillectomy patients: Effects on children's and parents' adjustment. *Pediatrics,* 1979, *64,* 646–655.

Woodward, J. Emotional disturbances of burned children. *British Medical Journal,* 1959, *1,* 1009–1013.

Woodward, J., & Jackson, D. Emotional reactions in burned children and their mothers. *British Journal of Plastic Surgery,* 1961, *13,* 316–324.

Wright, G. Z., & Alpern, G. D. Variables influencing children's cooperative behavior at the first dental visit. *Journal of Dentistry for Children,* 1971, *38,* 60–64.

Wright, G. Z., Alpern, G. D., & Leake, J. L. The modifiability of maternal anxiety as it relates to children's cooperative dental behavior. *Journal of Dentistry for Children,* 1973, *40,* 265–271.

Youssef, M. M. S. Self control behaviors of school-age children who are hospitalized for cardiac diagnostic procedures. *Maternal-Child Nursing Journal,* 1981, *10,* 219–284.

Zabin, M. A., & Melamed, B. G. Relationship between parental discipline and children's ability to cope with stress. *Journal of Behavioral Assessment,* 1980, *2,* 17–38.

Ziegler, S., & King, J. Evaluating the observable effects of foster grandparents on hospitalized children. *Public Health Reports,* 1982, *97,* 550–557.

AUTHOR INDEX

SUBJECT INDEX

R